T0316725

Sickness in the Workhouse

Rochester Studies in Medical History

Series Editor: Christopher Crenner
Robert Hudson and Ralph Major Professor and Chair
Department of History and Philosophy of Medicine
University of Kansas School of Medicine

Additional Titles of Interest

Of Life and Limb: Surgical Repair of the Arteries in War and Peace, 1880–1960
Justin Barr

The Hidden Affliction: Sexually Transmitted Infections and Infertility in History
Edited by Simon Szreter

China and the Globalization of Biomedicine
Edited by David Luesink, William H. Schneider, and Zhang Daqing

Explorations in Baltic Medical History, 1850–2015
Edited by Nils Hansson and Jonatan Wistrand

Health Education Films in the Twentieth Century
Edited by Christian Bonah, David Cantor, and Anja Laukötter

The History of the Brain and Mind Sciences: Technique, Technology, Therapy
Edited by Stephen T. Casper and Delia Gavrus

Technological Change in Modern Surgery:Historical Perspectives on Innovation
Edited by Thomas Schlich and Christopher Crenner

Setting Nutritional Standards: Theory, Policies, Practices
Edited by Elizabeth Neswald, David F. Smith, and Ulrike Thoms

Fit to Practice: Empire, Race, Gender, and the Making of British Medicine, 1850–1980
Douglas M. Haynes

Reasoning against Madness: Psychiatry and the State in Rio de Janeiro, 1830–1944
Manuella Meyer

A complete list of titles in the Rochester Studies in Medical History series
may be found on our website, www.urpress.com.

Sickness in the Workhouse

Poor Law Medical Care in Provincial England, 1834–1914

Alistair Ritch

UNIVERSITY OF ROCHESTER PRESS

First published 2019

University of Rochester Press
668 Mt. Hope Avenue, Rochester, NY 14620, USA
www.urpress.com
and Boydell & Brewer Limited
PO Box 9, Woodbridge, Suffolk IP12 3DF, UK
www.boydellandbrewer.com

ISBN-13: 978-1-58046-975-3
ISSN: 1526-2715

Cataloging-in-Publication data available from the Library of Congress

For Christina, Mark, David, Gavin, Olivia, Mia, and Noah

Contents

Tables

Acknowledgments

For just over twenty-seven years, I looked after patients in the former Birmingham workhouse and infirmary. Working in an environment surrounded by poor law history stimulated my interest in poor law medicine. The workhouse was still vivid in the minds of many of my patients and their families and some still expressed fear at being admitted to a former poor law institution. This whetted my appetite to determine the kind of medicine that was practiced within poor law infirmaries. *Sickness in the Workhouse* is the result of my endeavors.

I wish to express my gratitude to Jonathan Reinarz, director, The History of Medicine Unit, and Malcolm Dick, director, Centre for West Midlands History, at the University of Birmingham, for their guidance and constructive criticism concerning the progress of the research, the preparation of the manuscript on which this book is based, and for their assistance in gathering the additional material requested by the manuscript reviewers. The majority of the research was undertaken at the Archives and Heritage Service at Birmingham Central Library and Wolverhampton Archives and Local Studies, with additional material from The National Archives in London, Cadbury Research Library, University of Birmingham, and the Royal College of Physicians of London. I am grateful to the staff at these centers for their assistance in identifying relevant documents and for the retrieval of the volumes from the archives. Several individuals assisted in a variety of ways. I am grateful to Dr. Stuart Wildman for his comments and suggestions relating to the chapter on nursing, to Dr. Leonard Smith for drawing my attention to the volume concerning "insane" inmates in Birmingham workhouse and for his advice on mental health issues, and to Alison Smith for drawing my attention to the letters of Martha Beatrice Webb. I am grateful to Sonia Kane and her staff at the University of Rochester Press for guiding me painlessly through the publication process. I would particularly like to thank my wife, Christina, for her support and encouragement throughout the long years of study and preparation of the book and for undertaking the typing of the manuscript from my, at times, illegible handwriting.

Introduction

Pauperism and Sickness

In July 1841, Charles Hodgkins reported to the Board of Guardians of Wolverhampton Union that Anne, the wife of John Walford, was suffering from a disorder of her liver and bowels that was likely to last for six or seven weeks and resulted in her being "unable to follow any employ." He added that both her sons required constant attention: John, aged two years, was "labouring under water on the brain," and George, seven weeks old, also had a bowel disorder. Hodgkins, who had been appointed by the guardians as medical officer for Wolverhampton Union, arranged for them to receive four pounds of mutton and four loaves of bread per week for two weeks and planned to admit Anne after that time to the union workhouse, which had opened only two years previous. However, at the end of the two weeks, her condition had deteriorated to such an extent that Hodgkins regarded her recovery as very doubtful and removal to the workhouse as not prudent. The rations were continued for a further four weeks.[1] Whether she recovered or not, we shall never know, but Hodgkins clearly saw the workhouse as a suitable place for treating a sick pauper.

Yet many poor law historians have claimed that workhouses did not develop a significant medical role until the late nineteenth century and emerged as the most important institutions for medical care only in the early twentieth century. Some have been highly critical of the standard of medical care provided in the early years after the New Poor Law, claiming a significant deterioration in the provision of medical services. As evidence, they point to the restriction of funding, the understaffing of infirmaries, and the undermining of medical officers' decisions by guardians, who sought to treat patients as cheaply as possible.[2] The conventional viewpoint denigrates medical care after the act as of such poor quality as to bring little benefit to sick paupers. However, the traditional history of the Poor Law Amendment Act (1834), usually referred to as the New Poor Law, as a watershed in the provision of medical services is now being challenged in favor of one of continuity of care across the eighteenth and nineteenth centuries. This book will offer a fresh perspective of institutional poor law medicine by examining the character, scope, and scale of medical care in Birmingham and Wolverhampton workhouses in the West Midlands of England after the enactment of the New Poor Law in 1834. By delineating the range and intensity of diseases suffered by workhouse inmates, it will bring to the fore this disadvantaged group of sick paupers, previously neglected by medical historians.

It will cover the period from 1834 to the start of World War I, at which time the Birmingham workhouse infirmary was evacuated for use as a military hospital. The Victorian era was a time of huge change, both in social terms and in medical theory and practice. Rapid industrialization caused a massive shift of people from the countryside to the towns in search of work. This was compounded by the increasing size of the population enhanced by a declining mortality rate, particularly among children and younger adults. The mid-nineteenth century was the era of the ideology of laissez-faire and economic liberalism, of not interfering in the natural state of the country and the market. However, as historian Felix Driver has pointed out, it was accompanied by increased state regulation as central government augmented its infrastructural capacities in significant ways.[3] By the 1880s these ideological certainties had been rudely shaken and the issues of poverty and overcrowding appeared on the social agenda as requiring attention, raising the possibility of state action. In the following decade, Charles Booth in London and Seebolm Rowntree in York revealed the extent of poverty to be greater than expected and concluded that it was mostly due to low wages and irregular employment, absolving the poor of blame for their condition. Medicine saw radical developments with the rise of the germ theory of disease and laboratory practice. By the end of the century, science was embedded in medical teaching and hospitals had become sanctuaries of medical knowledge.[4] Nursing evolved from being little more than a housekeeping role with little in the way of personal attention to a profession after the introduction of nurse education. According to medical historian John Pickstone, the increased technicality of late nineteenth-century medicine sharpened the distinction between medical care and general relief, between assistance to cure specific lesions and a more general nursing support.[5]

Poverty and Sickness

Within the literature on poor law history, sick paupers have been relatively neglected. Yet, as poor law historian Steven King has pointed out, sickness was *the* pivotal experience for people on the margins.[6] Furthermore, by the mid-nineteenth century, nearly three-quarters of the cases of pauperism in England and Wales involved sickness.[7] Ill health was a major cause of destitution, giving rise to the need for relief under the poor law system, traditionally viewed as the result of restricted earning power, but more recent insights into the relationship between poverty and sickness have shown that the poor were more likely to suffer ill health.[8] Research has been hampered by the scarcity of sources relating to poor law medical relief and the fleeting references to medical care within poor law archives. However, of more importance has been the lack of definition of ill health as a cause for poor law relief, leading some historians to suggest that distinguishing medical relief from other forms of help is not important and that the sick poor are not worthy of study as a specific subgroup. For instance, in her study of the poor in eighteenth-century Bristol, the historian Mary Fissell found that medical care for many paupers was such an integral part of their welfare support that it was not possible to make a clear distinction between health care and poor relief. The support provided to families often defied separation into medical and welfare components. This is hardly surprising given the inextricable link between illness, disability, and poverty. However, she did accept that illness could be a clearly defined point of entry to relief for some paupers.[9] Indeed, even when sickness or physical disability was not a key reason for an application for relief, it was often a necessary accompaniment for success. Furthermore, relief granted on the basis of unemployment often unmasked underlying sickness.[10] The view of welfare historian Alannah Tomkins is that there is much to be learned from trying to distinguish "the sick from the total pool of 'the poor'" and from examining the provision of identifiable medical relief.[11] As a result of the limited dedicated research on sick paupers, we have a limited understanding of the type of medical care that was offered in workhouses and how important it was in the life course of paupers.[12]

Sickness was very often the major reason for admission to a workhouse and yet the poor law institutional medical service has been less intensively researched than outdoor medical relief. Kevin Siena argues that medical historians have been slow to explore workhouses prior to the New Poor Law and, as a result, these important medical spaces have not been integrated into the history of eighteenth-century institutional medicine.[13] Jeremy Boulton and Leonard Schwarz affirm that medical services provided by the parish workhouse under the Old Poor Law have been neglected within the history of institutional provision, despite delivering increasing amounts of medical care in the latter part of the eighteenth century.[14] From his analysis of the medical responses to sickness and disease in Newcastle-upon-Tyne between

1750 and 1850, Graham Butler concluded that workhouse medicine was an important element in the care of the sick and was more complex than has been described in other provincial workhouses.[15] With the exception of the study discussed in this book, there is a paucity of literature exploring poor law medicine in the late nineteenth century. King has highlighted a number of issues that have remained unresolved as a result of sick paupers escaping historical attention. What was the intended medical function of the workhouse? What illnesses did workhouse inmates suffer? What medical treatment did they receive and how meaningful was it for their lives? What was the relationship between workhouse care and background medical standards? He sums up the situation by stating that "an understanding of the exact medical role of the workhouse remains elusive."[16] However, he does concede that sick inmates may have been in a better position than their immediate counterparts outside the workhouse.[17] Outdoor medical relief has received more attention than workhouse medicine since it played a larger part in the relief of the sick poor, partially due to sick paupers' attempts to obtain alternative sources of support in order to avoid care in the workhouse. The complexity of arrangements that grew up after the New Poor Law and the considerable interregional and intraregional variation make it difficult to gain a full understanding of the operation and impact of poor law policy, creating the need for research in different geographical localities.[18] Yet, published whole union studies remain rare to this day and comparisons of unions within close proximity to one another are rarer still.[19] Thus, this research into these two workhouses will help promote the importance of poor law infirmaries in the history of medical institutions, an underresearched area within medical history more generally.

The poor adopted a range of strategies to ensure material survival by accessing disparate sources of income, a concept that has been termed "the economy of makeshifts."[20] Similar strategies were employed in times of sickness to access the local mixed economy of health care comprising private, voluntary-funded (that is, funded by charitable donations) and public provision. For those who could not afford to pay for medical treatment, the main avenues for free care were provided by voluntary hospitals (also funded by charitable donations from the public and free to patients) and the poor law as outpatient attendance at dispensaries or institutional care. Voluntary hospitals began to be established in the early eighteenth century and gradually increased in numbers to cover the main centers of population. By 1861, there were 153 voluntary teaching and general hospitals in England and Wales, though the number of beds in them was small, seventy-seven per hospital on average.[21] They were set up as charities and depended on voluntary subscriptions and fund-raising activities for their financial support. Subscribers were given the right to nominate a defined number of patients annually for admission to the hospital. The hospitals were intended for use by members of the working population who had no other means of accessing medical help, "the deserving poor." As the destitute were excluded, patients entering voluntary hospitals in England were a carefully selected group. Jonathan Reinarz has described how in Birmingham steps were taken to identify and eject them from the hospital.[22] The mid-nineteenth century saw the advent of schemes, such as the Hospital Saturday Fund, in which workmen could contribute to the financial support of their local hospital. It was not until late in the century before these schemes also provided contributors with the ability to access free hospital care. An alternative means by which workmen could contribute financially to secure medical treatment was through membership of a Friendly Society. These societies were cooperative associations and sprang up in the late eighteenth century offering mutual sickness insurance. Their main initial focus was income replacement when a worker was sick. However, benefits were gradually reduced for periods of sickness lasting longer than six months and members were required to leave the scheme if unable to continue contributions.[23] Friendly Societies appealed mostly to skilled workers and many nonskilled workingmen and those in irregular employment did not become members; for instance, only 12.5 percent of the British population were members in 1872.[24] By the end of the nineteenth century, they also offered free curative medical care by means of contractual arrangements with doctors.

Poor Law Amendment Act (1834)

Prior to 1834, poor relief in England and Wales was governed by the Acts for the Relief of the Poor of 1595 and 1601 (usually referred to collectively as the Old Poor Law). The system of relief was based on the parish as the unit from which the poor law levy was raised and through which relief was distributed. The main types of help were in the form of money, food, clothing, and bedding provided to paupers living at home, so-called outdoor relief, but it could also include the payment of medical expenses. Institutional care, known as indoor relief, was unusual as the buildings used were usually small in size, often a large adapted house or cottages. By the end of the eighteenth century, the emphasis had moved toward the greater provision of workhouses, stimulated by amalgamation of parishes, enabled by Gilbert's Act of 1782. The major social and economic changes that took place throughout the eighteenth and early nineteenth centuries—with increasing unemployment in rural areas resulting in a mass movement of people into urban areas, rapid industrialization, and a huge increase in the population—resulted in increasing difficulty in financing relief and in an ever-increasing poor rate levy. The resulting dissatisfaction with the system resulted in the establishment of the Royal Commission on the Poor Laws in 1832. At that time, the mood toward the poor in the country was changing from one of "benevolence" rooted in a "moral economy" to one of an austere "political economy."[25] Amid concerns over the rapidly increasing population, especially among the poor, the availability of relief was felt to have a demoralizing effect, causing the recipients to become lazy and improvident. Pauperism became seen as a social sickness and a moral failing on the part of paupers. Thus, reform meant lowering the costs by disciplining the poor. The aim was to inspire self-discipline and promote the moral authority of government against a background of a crisis of social authority throughout rural England.[26]

The report of the Royal Commission on the Poor Laws in 1834 was principally concerned with "the increase in the number of the able-bodied paupers," which the commissioners considered to be "the principal evil of the system" of poor law relief. Thus, the report's first recommendation stated that all relief to able-bodied people and their families, other than in well-regulated workhouses, should cease.[27] The main architect of the report of the Royal Commission on the Poor Laws was Edwin Chadwick, a barrister and a disciple of the philosopher, Jeremy Bentham, the founder of Unitarianism. Although Bentham's ideas were based on self–interest as the root motive for human action, they assumed that individual interest would coincide with the general interest and this led him to promote regulative solutions for social problems.[28] Chadwick's major interest had been in keeping the poor rate down and he had suggested to the commission that the pain of pauperism should be made greater than the pain of poverty. In other words, an automatic deterrent mechanism was required.[29] The subsequent act, commonly referred to as the New Poor Law, was aimed at the management of pauperism in order to control the "unacceptably burdensome poor rates."[30] It recommended restricting outdoor relief other than for medical attention. It required parishes to join together to form unions in order to provide larger workhouses for indoor relief, and the erection of general mixed workhouses gradually spread across the country. These institutions became the central component of poor law policy, their layout and appearance designed to make a powerful impact on the poor.[31] The act also established the principles of "less eligibility" for relief, namely a lower standard of living for a pauper compared to a wage-earning laborer. It promoted the "workhouse test," whereby a pauper would receive relief only if he or she was prepared to enter a workhouse, where conditions would theoretically have been worse than for the poorest in the community. The workhouse test was intended as a means of distinguishing those who were destitute from those who were seen as merely poor and thereby limiting relief to the former and reducing expenditure from the poor law rates. Because it was difficult to make physical conditions inside the workhouse worse than the homes of the poor, the enforcement of less eligibility could be achieved only by psychological means, such as the deprivation of identity and dignity.[32] According to historical geographer Felix Driver, the workhouse was "designed to be a disciplinary institution, its inmates subject to the rule of official regulations," although public health historian Christopher Hamlin maintains that the public wanted workhouses to be humane as well as deterrent.[33] In one of the earliest comprehensive analyses of the working of the workhouse, Anne Crowther describes it as invariably a place of irresolvable tension since it had the dual role of deterring able-bodied paupers while at the same time providing a refuge for the old and the sick.[34] She has called the rapid development of heavily regulated workhouses the "first national experiment in institutional care," but emphasized the variability and diversity within parishes, where conditions within the workhouse were influenced by the size of the union, the wealth of local ratepayers and the caliber of the local guardians.[35]

The effectiveness of the workhouse system as a deterrent depended upon the classification of paupers, ensuring strict physical segregation of the different classes of pauper within the building.[36] The emphasis was on strict discipline and a monotonous daily routine in which the same activities took place at the same times each day.[37] Paupers were supplied with a workhouse uniform, and their own clothes were returned to them on discharge. The dietaries were repetitive, the food was often adulterated, and dietary restriction played a major role in the disciplinary system. On the other hand, they were nutritionally sound and sufficient to sustain life. One of the most important aspects was the reliance on the surveillance of individual conduct, as was common in projects of moral regulation in the nineteenth century.[38] Discipline was instilled into the inmates by regimentation and regulation of every minute of the day. The forbidding appearance of the buildings and the disciplinary regime were intended to impress on the poor the virtues of independent labor.[39] Together they enhanced the sense of depersonalization by diminishing the more personal contact between paupers and poor law officers that had been usual in the parishes under the Old Poor Law. Whether the disciplinary regime did instill total obedience on the part of inmates is a moot point. Although poor law authorities represented the workhouse as a place where discipline reigned, from the early years of the New Poor Law and across the rest of the century, there was a steady stream of committals of inmates to the courts for misbehavior within workhouses, indicating that paupers did not always passively conform to workhouse routine.[40] In his investigation of the misbehavior of inmates in London workhouses in the first few decades of the New Poor Law, David Green found that all types of paupers questioned authority and challenged workhouse discipline. Most were low-level offenses, but all forms of individual and collective action occurred with regularity, so that maintaining discipline appeared to be an endemic problem. He concluded that the indoor poor were by no means powerless to challenge authority and the workhouse was far from being a total institution that fostered docile bodies.[41] However, there was no mention of sick inmates within the sample population and it is possible that illness may have hampered their ability to rebel. King is of the opinion that inmates did protest when they or their friends experienced inadequate medical care or were subject to unjust discipline.[42]

The New Poor Law created a new system of local management of poor law relief in the form of boards of guardians under the aegis of a central authority, initially the Poor Law Commission, with Chadwick as secretary. It meant that for the first time, poor relief would be organized within a centralized administrative system and determined by fixed rules rather than on a personal basis. The commission exerted its influence over guardians by issuing advice, regulations, and statutory orders supplemented by routine inspections of local arrangements. Indeed, Driver maintains that central inspection was the linchpin of the post-1834 system and that there was something revolutionary in the establishment of a centrally based inspectorate at that time.[43] However, the act proved to be a controversial piece of legislation and spawned an anti-New Poor Law movement that hindered the implementation of the new system throughout the country, but especially in the north of England. The commission was also beset by a number of scandals involving maltreatment of inmates and was left to expire when its term of authority ended in 1847. It was replaced by the Poor Law Board under the charge of a president who was answerable to Parliament. The poor law assistants within the old commission were renamed inspectors in recognition of their key role in ensuring coordination of local practice with central policy.[44] The Poor Law Board never met as a board, being run by permanent officials, and gained a reputation for inactivity. Amid increasing concern at the failure to restrain outdoor relief, it was replaced in 1871 as the major department within the newly formed Local Government Board. Under the Old Poor Law, relief had been in the hands of parish vestries, with the exception of localities where administrative systems, some of which were called unions, had been set up under Gilbert's Act or local acts, as in Birmingham. The New Poor Law unions were administered by the newly established boards of guardians, as occurred in Wolverhampton. The new property and financial qualifications for board members that were set under the New Poor Law favored owners and occupiers of large properties in place of the vestries, which included all householders.[45] This placed boards in the hands of a middle-class elite.[46] Although the nature of guardians has been underexplored by historians, it is clear that the personalities, skills, and experiences of board members could determine how efficiently poor relief was managed and how it influenced the nature of the experiences of paupers.[47]

Workhouse Provision for Sick Inmates

The New Poor Law made no recommendations for a medical service and the Poor Law Commissioners never envisaged that medical relief would be a reason for admission to the workhouse. Unfortunately, the Poor Law Amendment Act (1834) attempted to deal only with the problem of able-bodied pauperism and neglected to consider provision for sick paupers. Pickstone has suggested that this concentration on able-bodied paupers helped to disguise the extent to which workhouses catered for the sick.[48] Additionally, the central authority never produced a definitive medical policy in the early years after the act, and the development of medical relief was influenced solely by the administrative orders of the Poor Law Commissioners. Medical historian Michael Flinn has argued that though the New Poor Law medical service was unintended and unplanned, its expansion in the late 1830s was "really very remarkable" and arose as a spontaneous development, as "an accident of history which only the most pressing social need could have engineered."[49] However, an extensive system of outdoor medical relief had existed prior to the 1834 Act, following which it became more and more restricted as the century progressed. It was workhouse medical care that increased dramatically under the New Poor Law and can rightly lay claim to be the accident of history.

Prior to 1834, sick inmates frequently remained in their beds within the main workhouse dormitories as only larger institutions provided sickrooms or wards for inmates who became unwell. The only reference in the report of the Royal Commission on the Poor Laws to sick paupers was the recognition that appropriate rooms would be required for them within workhouses. Sick wards were included in the plans of the model workhouses in the first annual report of the Poor Law Commissioners in 1835, one type involving an infirmary building separated from the main workhouse. This type of dedicated infirmary, usually consisting of a number of small rooms, became more popular by the 1860s. In some unions, especially in London, they were located in sites some distance from the workhouse. In the late nineteenth century, many were built in the pavilion style, praised by Florence Nightingale, which allowed a high degree of segregation and through-ward ventilation. As workhouses catered for paupers with chronic illnesses on a long-term basis, this necessitated the provision of large infirmaries and the recommended size of 500 to 600 beds was often exceeded. By 1900, some had expanded to over 1,000 beds.[50] The number of sick inmates they could accommodate dwarfed that of the local voluntary hospitals; for instance, there were only 80 beds in Wolverhampton's and 420 in Birmingham's hospitals in the middle of the century. Nationally, poor law institutions provided 81 percent of the country's hospital beds by 1861, so it is not surprising that, ten years later, some workhouses could be described as the "first public hospitals" and those in the larger towns as "infirmaries for the sick."[51]

Poor Law Medical Service

The New Poor Law was instrumental in the development of a new branch of the medical profession, the poor law medical officers, who became the linchpin of the poor law medical service. The orders issued by the Poor Law Commission authorized guardians to appoint medical officers for districts within their union. They were required to attend the sick punctually and provide directions on the diet, classification, and treatment of sick paupers.[52] Thus, they performed an important gatekeeper role within the poor law administration, allocating resources by virtue of their ability to differentiate the truly sick from the malingering poor. However, in Victorian England the social status of poor law medical officers was low, both within the medical profession, where they were regarded as third-rate practitioners who had failed to succeed in private practice, and the poor law administration, where guardians treated them as servants. The main reasons for the former were that they were poorly paid, worked for a state service, were subservient to public officials in the form of the boards of guardians, and treated patients who were destitute.[53] The patients they treated suffered from uninteresting diseases and from the stigma of pauperism, plus their places of work, the workhouse infirmaries, were less prestigious than the voluntary hospitals. Their authority could be challenged by guardians and by lay poor law officers if it clashed with the policy of less eligibility and they were not infrequently held responsible for systemic failures in a poor law medical service that has been described as "not fit for purpose."[54] However, their status within the profession gradually rose and by 1871 poor law doctors were seen as an important branch of the medical profession. They benefited also from the greater respect in the eyes of the public that the profession had gained toward the end of the century with the rise of scientific medicine. Within the workhouse, their position gradually changed from a subordinate role to one of great influence by 1914.[55] Nevertheless, historian Anne Crowther considers that they remained at the bottom of the medical hierarchy.[56]

Medical officers' posts were frequently accepted out of necessity in a highly competitive medical marketplace that was oversubscribed in terms of the number of medical men, even though the positions were despised.[57] Given their status within the profession in the early years after the New Poor Law and the conditions under which they worked, what type of doctor would apply to work for the poor law medical service? The generally accepted opinion is that they were either at the start of their career and hoping to become well enough known in the locality to establish a private practice, or an already established local practitioner wishing to keep out competition.[58] The vast majority of medical officers were employed on a part-time contract to provide services within a district of the union and could continue with private practice. They were able to appoint nonmedical assistants, who were more likely to be allocated the poor law duties. Only a small proportion attended a workhouse, either as part of their district or exclusively. The small minority who were required to reside in the workhouse were more likely to be young doctors at the start of their careers. This held true for the most part for resident medical officers for the Birmingham workhouse and more especially for assistant medical officers. It was not the case for surgeons to the workhouse in the first half of the nineteenth century. For instance, one was Edward Cox, whose son, Sands Cox, assisted him in the workhouse and later became honorary surgeon at the Queen's Hospital, of which he was a founder.[59] Nor was it the case for the visiting physicians and the surgeon appointed in the latter part of the century, of whom five also had honorary appointments with local voluntary hospitals and professorial appointments at Birmingham University. One of the resident medical officers later held an honorary appointment with the Children's Hospital and another became professor of mental diseases at the university.[60] Appointments such as these were not unusual in larger towns. The medical officers to Leicester workhouse also had connections with local medical institutions and were men of standing in the town.[61] Dr. L. M. Guilding at Battle workhouse was also assistant surgeon at the Royal Berkshire Hospital.[62] Alfred Sheen was both medical officer at Cardiff workhouse and senior surgeon at Glamorgan and Monmouthshire Infirmary and published a workbook for medical officers.[63] The medical culture in Birmingham was very different from a town like Wolverhampton because of the presence of formal medical teaching after Thomas Tomlinson, surgeon at Birmingham workhouse, commenced a course of anatomical lectures in the late 1760s.[64] Informal lectures by Birmingham physicians led to the founding of two medical colleges: Queen's College in 1828, attached to Queen's Hospital, and Sydenham's College in 1854, attached to the General Hospital. The workhouse medical officers at Wolverhampton Union were typical of the majority of part-time officers practicing outside the centers of learning and very little is known about them.

Poor law medical officers were at the forefront of the movement for reform of the medical service that grew from the 1840s onward, but there is controversy among historians as to their motivations and achievements. Their early complaints regarding the Poor Law Commission's policy of appointment by lowest tender and encouragement of large medical districts, both intended to reduce poor law expenditure, were rebuffed by the commission's secretary, Edwin Chadwick. He accused medical officers of abusing their powers and turning many simply poor laborers into paupers as a result of being liberal with medical relief. However, behind his attacks lay a strong contempt for curative medicine, but also a narrow interest in keeping the poor rates down.[65] Following the establishment of the Convention of Poor Law Medical Officers in 1846, the reformers' main objectives covered improvements to the conditions of service to provide security of tenure, higher salaries, superannuation, and a limit to the size of medical officers districts; the provision of medicines by the guardians rather than by the doctor; the establishment of a national chain of dispensaries; and a means for channeling to the central authority any perceived defects in the medical service. An early degree of success was achieved in 1845 when a parliamentary committee recommended that they should be employed on a permanent contract, though many unions failed to change the existing annual tendering process. A change in public opinion in favor of reform took place over the 1850s following the scandal in Andover workhouse, where inmates were reputed to have had to resort to eating rotten meat from bones waiting to be crushed in order to stay alive. The impetus for reform was strengthened in the following decade by the untimely deaths of two inmates in London workhouses. This prompted *The Lancet* to set up a Commission to Inquire into the State of Workhouse Hospitals. Following the publication of its reports, the leader of the medical reform movement, Joseph Rogers, a workhouse medical officer in London, met with the president of the Poor Law Board. He succeeded in getting many of his suggestions incorporated into the Metropolitan Poor Act of 1867. These included institutions for sick paupers separated geographically and financially from workhouses, and the employment of resident surgeons with senior supervision. He also stimulated the Poor Law Board to issue a circular recommending that guardians pay for expensive drugs, though once again, uptake was limited. Subsequently, Rogers founded the Poor Law Medical Officers' Association by the amalgamation of the existing metropolitan and provincial bodies. The new association focused its vision on achieving compulsory superannuation, the adoption of the dispensary system, and the promotion of medical officers' interests, principally defending members against oppression on the part of the authorities.[66]

The last measure became necessary after the crusade against outdoor relief, which began in the early 1870s. The Longley Report of 1874 encouraged complete withdrawal of relief outside the workhouse, plus much tighter controls over medical relief. The crusade arose out of the belief that welfare dependency created pauperism and reducing support could eradicate poverty. The sick were thought to be abusing the poor law system by simultaneously claiming charitable support and by feigning illness in order to claim relief on medical rather than unemployment grounds in order to avoid entering a workhouse.[67] Longley's strategy was enforced by the Local Government Board inspectors. This increased encroachment into the medical service by nonmedical officers resulted in an increasing number of charges for medical negligence being brought against medical officers and was seen to impinge on medical independence. Historian Kim Price maintains that poor law historians have underestimated both the impact of the crusade on medical practice and its role in the failure of the medical reform movement after 1870.[68] As a result, only compulsory superannuation was accomplished after the early minor improvements in conditions of service and that had to wait until 1894. Overall, pressure at the national level achieved little as the central authority remained reluctant to become involved in medical matters, and most of the problems remained unresolved throughout the existence of the poor laws.[69] Many of the reformers demands had centered on issues that could be seen as furthering only the doctors' interests, although Ruth Hodgkinson asserts that the improvements they achieved furthered the interests of their patients.[70] She considers that poor law medical officers stand out as "particularly good public servants," striving for "positive health measures," and Jeanne Brand concurs that they repeatedly urged for improvements in medical care to the poor.[71] Poor law historian Anne Crowther considers that medical officers were not in a position to make more than minor changes, but she concedes that little was known about the situation of local doctors.[72] Indeed, Flinn contends that individual medical officers could bring about piecemeal improvements locally by means of "perpetual guerrilla warfare."[73] Price describes poor law medical officers as a "fractious heterogeneous group" with only a few as "prescient reformers." He considers the historiography of these medical men to be contradictory and incomplete, especially with regard to the nature of their day-to-day practice; what he refers to as the "reality of poor law doctoring" and it is this area that will be explored in the book.[74] Notwithstanding the controversy, there is general agreement among historians that poor law doctors were the key figures in the poor law medical welfare system, and poor law historian Lynn Hollen Lees asserts that they "turned paupers into patients."[75] However, they also exerted considerable influence on the way medical services were shaped at the national level. According to medical historian Ruth Hodgkinson, if it had not been for their efforts, "it is doubtful whether many present developments would have come about in the English medical system."[76]

Doctors and State Medicine

Medical relief was first officially acknowledged as a state responsibility toward the poor in the General Medical Order relating to medical administration issued by the Poor Law Commission in 1842.[77] It was reiterated in the system brought about in London by the Metropolitan Poor Act of 1867, a significant step in the development of distinct infirmaries. The act established in London infirmaries for the sick geographically separated from workhouses, plus separate asylums for lunatics and imbeciles and institutions for the isolation of those with infectious diseases. This system of medical care was funded by a centrally controlled Common Poor Fund, into which each metropolitan union contributed on a proportional basis, thus pooling the capital's poor law levies. It also recommended the appointment of a resident medical officer for every 150 patients. The act represented an explicit acknowledgment by the state of its responsibilities for the destitute sick by inaugurating a state hospital service for the poor in London, and in Gwendoline Ayer's view, it was "a significant step towards socialization of medical care in this country."[78]

One year after the act there was hardly a union in the capital without a separate infirmary.[79] In the same year, provincial unions were empowered, rather than legally obliged, to establish separate institutions for the sick, but no centralized funding was organized. Nevertheless, a process of taking hospitals out of workhouses was begun, albeit slowly, firmly establishing the hospital branch of the poor law. These separate infirmaries began to be selective in admitting only those with acute illnesses, leaving the workhouses to accept the remainder, who were predominantly the chronic sick. Medical historian Ruth Hodgkinson claims this differentiation between the two types of admission was in place by 1871.[80] Simon Fowler has described this development of poor law medical care as the "greatest success of the workhouse."[81] However, as Alysa Levene has pointed out, the state of affairs by the time of the Local Government Act in 1929 abolishing boards of guardians was a "patchwork of local provision and uneven services in medical care for the poor."[82]

Although ideas put forward by the medical authorities featured in both the order and the act, resentment built up among the medical profession because of lay resistance to greater reform. Thus, the seeds of the profession's later opposition to a state medical service lay in the poor law system. It was fostered in the steps taken to implement sanitary reform after the Public Health Act of 1848. Chadwick was appointed to the General Board of Health set up by the act, having produced a report six years previously on the sanitary conditions of the laboring population. The report contained a sustained attack on curative medicine and took a strong anticontagionist stance at a time when there was controversy among the medical profession over the mode of transmission of diseases. Later reports from Chadwick's Board of Health on the value of quarantine during a cholera epidemic also drew fire from *The Lancet* medical journal and the Royal College of Physicians in London. The latter, in particular, took exception to lay advice on an issue that lay within their province.[83] In general, the Board of Health operated not merely independently of the medical profession, but in direct opposition to it. Chadwick's views were shared by one of the prominent sanitarians, Thomas Southwood, who also served on the board, but were opposed by another, William Farr, whose views on contagion were closer to the medical profession as a whole. He also placed more emphasis on the effectiveness of medicines. Nevertheless, he supported Chadwick over the issue of quarantine.[84] Another medical man whose opinions were diametrically opposite to Chadwick's was William Pulteney Alison, who held the chair in the Theory and Practice of Medicine in Edinburgh and led the campaign for the reform of the Scottish poor law. Alison had empathy for the poor, was convinced of the centrality of destitution as a cause of disease, and saw public health as a social policy. He also clashed with Chadwick by advocating a more generous policy for relief. Chadwick rejected Alison's view that poverty caused disease and promoted the cause of sanitation as a means to virtually end the social problems of industrialization.[85]

A series of Public Health Acts, masterminded by John Simon, the first medical officer of health, brought further sanitary measures that were accepted as a public responsibility and a legitimate social intervention by government. As a result, he has been credited with bringing in state medicine as a new concept.[86] However, demands had begun to arise for the state to intervene directly in health care after the Metropolitan Poor Act, with the result that appropriate government measures steadily increased.[87] The issue of a free state-controlled medical service surfaced during the Royal Commission on the Poor Laws and Relief of Distress, set up in 1905. Although the majority and minority reports of the commission four years later differed in the degree in which they recommended that the poor laws should be reformed, both were in agreement in rejecting a medical service free to all comers. However, *The Minority Report* did recognize a corporate duty for the provision of curative treatment for those in need of it.[88] During the commission's deliberations, the *British Medical Journal* came out strongly against the medical profession becoming a branch of the Civil Service. This stance was not supported by the British Medical Association, as it expressed no opinion on the idea of a nationally operated medical service. No government action on the poor law system followed the commission's report. When two years later the government proposed a national health insurance scheme for the wage-earning population, it provoked strong opposition from the medical profession, not least over the lack of consultation. The British Medical Association had two major objections, one of which was the intended controlling role in the distribution of finances for the Friendly Societies. However, in the ensuing discussions, the association was able to get the administration of the scheme altered to control by health committees. Overall, four of their six cardinal points were included in the final version of the scheme. Despite this, a majority of general practitioners pledged not to participate, but in the event did not carry out the pledge. Although the medical profession did accept the need for some form of public medical service, their resistance was based on an intense dislike of lay control over the profession's interests. This form of administration had received official status under the New Poor Law in which nonmedical officials had been placed at the heart of the medical system, so that medical authority and independence withered.[89]

Birmingham

Birmingham parish was completely urban in nature, smaller geographically than the Borough of Birmingham and with a population of around three-quarters that of the borough. Both areas increased rapidly in population by about 60 percent in the middle of the nineteenth century; the parish from 133,215 in 1841 to 212,621 twenty years later, and the borough from 177,922 to 296,076 over the same period. Thereafter, both experienced gradual annual percentage increases in the mid-teens until the end of the century. Some of the enlargement of the borough was due to incorporation of adjacent territory whereas the parish retained the same geographical size with a population in 1911 that had almost doubled at 225,447.[90] This study deals only with the parish, as this was the area under the auspices of Birmingham guardians. In the 1890s, the parish was the second most densely populated provincial poor law authority, with eighty-two people per acre, compared with Manchester's eighty-eight.[91] Despite this, it was reported to be "one of the most healthy" among the large towns in the country in 1844, a claim supported by the mortality statistics at that time.[92] However, Birmingham's mortality rate grew to be larger than many similarly large towns by the 1870s.[93]

The town of Birmingham did not receive parliamentary representation and incorporation until 1838. Prior to that, the principal authority in the town was the Street Commission, whose main concern was to keep the streets in good order. However, the Street Commission was not abolished until the Birmingham Improvement Act of 1851, at which time the town council gained full control for the whole of the borough. At that time the council was dominated by small-business owners, who had a vested interest in keeping the rates as low as possible and little in the way of civic improvement was carried out. These so-called Economists were superseded by the later 1850s by large-business owners, ushering in a decade of cautious advance in public provision.[94] Nevertheless, the council remained unprepared and ill equipped to meet the challenges of urban and industrial life, as the older liberal tradition of fiscal frugality remained dominant.[95] Dissenters chose to move to Birmingham, as they were excluded from public civic life in incorporated boroughs and appreciated the openness and freedom of a nonincorporated town.[96] One of the special features of nineteenth-century Birmingham was the strength of nonconformity in the town,[97] and a group of nonconformist ministers who were active in Liberal politics were to lead the civic revolution that began in the 1860s. The most renowned of these was George Dawson, whose teaching focused on the idea of effective moral action and the key role the corporation could play in bringing about practical improvements to the town. He urged the social and economic elite, namely large business and professional men, to take up civic responsibilities and in so doing established the tradition of municipal service, which became known as the Municipal

Gospel.[98] This tradition of municipal service became widely accepted throughout England by the 1880s, especially among members of the dissenting churches. It encompassed a belief in social progress and the moral duty of the individual to the community. This civic gospel movement of municipal socialism is inextricably linked with the name of Joseph Chamberlain.

Chamberlain, a successful businessman and a prominent member of the Unitarian Church of the Messiah in Birmingham, was elected to the town council in 1869. Elected mayor five years later, he rescued the council's ailing finances by buying out the town's two inefficient and competing gas companies and the local water company. For Chamberlain, the purchase was not just a business venture, as he considered that monopolies that were state-aided ought to be in the hands of representatives of the people.[99] He then proposed a scheme of urban development involving slum clearance in the central area, plus the creation of a new street and shopping area that became known as the Great Improvement Scheme. When Chamberlain was elected to Parliament, his philosophy of municipal government continued to influence the council and by 1890, Birmingham was described as the "Best governed city in the world," having gained city status the year before.[100] The city became one of the most influential models for municipal socialism in Europe and North America.[101]

The rapid industrial expansion in the town in the late nineteenth century resulted in a highly diversified economy, which lessened the impact of industrial action in any one trade.[102] Manufacturing was centered on the metal or hardware industries, such as buckles, buttons, pins, and jewelry, known at the time as "toys." The extent of the production of small metal items or trinkets led Edmund Burke, in 1777, to refer to Birmingham as "the toy-shop of Europe."[103] The manufacture of guns, swords, and iron screws were among the other staple industries, while the production of iron and brass bedsteads in England was chiefly limited to the Birmingham neighborhood.[104] The brass trade developed into the chief industry of the town, but the risk of pulmonary disease due to the inhalation of dust from the industrial process was so high that the majority of workers suffered breathing difficulties by middle age.[105] Most of the manufacturing took place in workers' homes, workshops, and small industrial units, and the majority of workers were skilled or semiskilled.[106] Birmingham was unique among the large centers of industry in the country in the number of small, independent manufacturers it supported, the jewelry trade being the prime example.[107] The diversity of trades offered a degree of protection from economic cycles and many workers were able to switch trades within the metal industry. During the seventeenth and eighteenth centuries, Birmingham had few commercial restrictions and gained the reputation as a town of liberal principles with regard to both trade and politics.[108]

The Black Country Towns

In the nineteenth century, Wolverhampton, Bilston, Willenhall, and Wednesfield were in the county of Staffordshire, but are now situated in that part of the West Midlands known as the Black Country, west of Birmingham. Wolverhampton was the largest of the towns with a population in 1831 of 18,380, which doubled by 1851 and almost quadrupled by the beginning of the twentieth century.[109] By comparison, Bilston, which had been designated a market town in 1824, saw an increase of only 66 percent from a base of 14,492. The much smaller towns of Willenhall and Wednesfield, with populations of 5,834 and 1,837 respectively in 1831, experienced huge population increases, in the latter due to the expansion of housing in the area of Heath Town in 1866.[110]

Wolverhampton, like Birmingham, attracted a large number of religious dissenters.[111] It also embarked on a phase of municipal reform from the 1870s in which respect it did not lag behind Birmingham in its achievements.[112] As in Birmingham, the town was managed by commissioners, responsible for streets, markets, public buildings, and sanitary provision, until incorporation in 1848. The political makeup of the initial council was made up of predominately Liberal shopkeepers, later replaced by a dominant group from manufacturing. Although the new council set out to establish its own civic identity, it continually looked to Birmingham for comparison and guidance in all aspects of civic conduct.[113] Nevertheless, the council embarked on its first improvement project before the civic gospel had come to fruition in Birmingham. At the time of inauguration of the council, there was an almost total lack of sanitation in the town and a very high mortality in Wolverhampton East (32.0 per 1,000 population in 1840–50 compared to the national average of 22.4).[114] *The Lancet* described Wolverhampton in 1867 as a "dirty town" where the roads were black with coal dust and "soot begrimes the houses and the people."[115] Because of opposition from the Economists on the council, schemes to put the town's water supply and sanitation under municipal control were not achieved until the late 1860s.[116] In 1877 a street improvement project similar to the one in Birmingham was carried out involving the clearance of around twelve acres in the unhealthiest part of the town with the demolition of over 600 houses. Although adverse comparison with neighboring towns was a factor in promoting municipal developments, Wolverhampton's record compares well with Birmingham, both in the number of projects and dates of completion. Both towns had embarked on the phase of municipal reform from the 1870s and Wolverhampton's rate of progress was equal to Birmingham. Nevertheless, it was the latter town that became the national paradigm.[117]

Of the other smaller Black Country towns that became part of Wolverhampton Union, Bilston's streets were initially controlled by a turnpike trust. An Improvement Act in 1850 set up a local Board of Health to bring about change, and by 1887 the water supply was in public hands, as was the water supply in Willenhall. However, sanitary facilities were rudimentary in both Bilston and Willenhall up to that time.[118] They were the worst in Bilston, where Bilston Brook was the only source of water, but was also used for dumping waste.[119] The town experienced a severe outbreak of cholera in 1832 and ten years later, much of it remained undrained, with pools of green stagnant water throughout.[120] Like many small towns, Willenhall was governed by a combination of justices of the peace and the local vestry until a Board of Health was set up in 1848 to take over the town's affairs.[121] Little information is available for the government and sanitation of Wednesfield as it was a much smaller settlement than the other three. According to the local historian George Barnsby, social conditions throughout the Black Country remained appalling throughout the nineteenth century.[122]

As in Birmingham, the towns that made up Wolverhampton Poor Law Union relied on metal manufacturing as their industrial base. All except Bilston specialized in lock making, although many other small metal items, such as screws, bolts, and guns, were also produced. Wednesfield also specialized in vermin traps and Bilston in shoe buckles and enameled trinkets. By way of contrast, Bilston saw the rapid growth of coal and iron mining in the first half of the nineteenth century. The staple trades of Wolverhampton included tinplate working and japanning, with the production of such articles as trays, coal vases, and tea caddies.[123] Bicycle production began in the mid-nineteenth century and the Sunbeam Company turned to car production in the 1890s.[124] The substantial diversification of trades within the metal industry, typically produced by small family firms, allowed workers to continue in employment when the popularity of particular items declined, so they were less reliant on poor law relief.

The Poor Law in Birmingham and Wolverhampton

A local act of Parliament in 1783 established Birmingham parish as a poor law incorporation under the Old Poor Law and, in 1831, a new local act enabled ratepayers to elect 108 guardians of the poor. After the New Poor Law, Birmingham continued under the local act. The Poor Law Amendment Act did not give the Poor Law Commission the power to dissolve existing corporations formed before 1834. There were about 125 Local Act Unions covering around 10 percent of the population and they acted administratively independently from the New Poor Law. It is doubtful if the central authority's attempts to influence them through the issuing of orders had much effect.[125] As a result, Birmingham guardians had very little contact with the Poor Law Commissioners and continued much as before. Increasing attempts by the central authority to increase its influence throughout the 1840s resulted in the guardians adopting new rules and regulations in keeping with the Poor Law Commission's guidance, but they resisted attempts to send them for the commission's approval. However, by 1850, the guardians were required to consult and defer to the Poor Law Board on a wide range of matters, though relationships remained tense.[126] In 1912, Birmingham parish combined with two adjacent local unions to form an enlarged Birmingham Union.

The first workhouse in Birmingham, said to resemble "the residence of a gentleman," was built in the mid-1730s, at a time when the population of Birmingham was just over 20,000.[127] The earliest recorded number of inmates was 369 on one day in May 1785 and at Easter in 1812 there were 442.[128] At the end of the eighteenth century, 300 children were residing in placements throughout Warwickshire because of lack of accommodation in the workhouse.[129] An Asylum for the Infant Poor was erected in Summer Lane in 1797 to bring them under one roof within Birmingham. The number of inmates in the workhouse itself did not surpass 500 until after 1847. The workhouse was extended twice later in the century, but continued to prove inadequate for the increasing number of the poor requiring indoor relief. Although a larger building was proposed in the early 1780s, it was not built for sixty years.[130] When the new Birmingham workhouse opened in 1852, it had accommodation for 1,610, including 17 officers, 80 tramps, and 310 beds in a detached infirmary.[131] Built in the corridor style on an extensive site, its ventilation system attracted particular attention at the time.[132] Its 1,926 inmates made it the second largest workhouse in a survey of 48 provincial workhouses in the mid-1860s, compared with 3,194 in Liverpool, 1,475 in Portsea Island, and a median value of 215 inmates for all workhouses.[133] In 1870, it ranked seventh among the 1 percent of English workhouses with more than 2,000 inmates, at a time when 93 percent had less than 500 inmates.[134] It continued to expand, housing over 3,500 in 1911 and becoming one of the largest poor law institutions in England with a geographically separate infirmary. In these respects, it was more in keeping with poor law institutions in London than average-sized provincial workhouses of between 200 and 300 inmates. It also resembled metropolitan workhouses in terms of its high institutionalization rate with regard to paupers in general and older paupers in particular.[135]

At a meeting organized by the Poor Law Commissioners in September 1836, Wolverhampton Union was formed by an amalgamation of the townships of Wolverhampton, Bilston, Willenhall, and Wednesfield, all in Staffordshire. Thus, it was typical of a New Poor Law urban union with a medium-sized workhouse in which the infirmary remained integral. The union inherited a workhouse at Wolverhampton, which had been erected in the 1700s, a smaller one at Bilston built in 1828 to accommodate up to fifty inmates, and one on Wood Street in Willenhall, which at that time was in a very dilapidated state.[136] In March 1838, there were 163 inmates in Wolverhampton and 91 in Bilston. All were moved to a new workhouse erected in Bilston Road, Wolverhampton, on October 7, 1839.[137] It was designed as a hexagonal building in keeping with one of the model plans published in the second annual report of the Poor Law Commissioners and could accommodate up to 450 paupers.[138] An auxiliary workhouse was opened in Wednesfield in August 1841, but closed after about fifteen months.[139] The erection of additional buildings at the workhouse could not keep pace with the increasing number of inmates toward the end of the century, and a new workhouse was opened in Heath Town in September 1903 with accommodation for 1,301 paupers.[140] Local and regional studies of provincial workhouses and their infirmaries have managed to cover many geographical areas of England, the one major exception being the urban West Midlands, where the towns of Birmingham and Wolverhampton are situated.

The composition of the boards of guardians in Birmingham and Wolverhampton mirrored that of the local economic structure and the makeup of the council in terms of occupational and political backgrounds. Elections to Birmingham's board were highly politicized and it was not uncommon for the majority on the board to swing from Liberal-Radical persuasion to Conservative in one election, only to be reversed at the next.[141] From the late 1870s the spirit of the civic gospel influenced all local public administration, but it did not prevent the guardians from becoming strong supporters of the crusade against outdoor relief.[142] Most Black Country towns elected Liberals as guardians, but the interests of the ratepayers who elected them exerted a considerable influence.[143] Members of both boards were predominately manufacturers, shopkeepers, businessmen, skilled craftsmen, and those employed in the catering trade, but included a few professional men. There was a considerable overlap in the membership of each board and the local councils. Board chairmen, as well as chairmen of the boards' important committees, tended also to be councilors or aldermen. Women began to be elected from the 1880s and Birmingham always had at least two female guardians from 1882. Birmingham parish and Wolverhampton Union also differed from the majority of unions, which were dominated by the farming community and members of the nobility.[144]

The provision of medical and nonmedical poor law relief has to be seen in the context of the local voluntary and charitable activity. Friendly Societies flourished in Birmingham and the Black Country from the late eighteenth century, although the extent of membership is uncertain.[145] The Birmingham branch of the Charity Organisation Society grew out of the Edgbaston Mendicity Society in 1875, six years after the establishment of the national organization that became the leading institution in the field of organized charity. It supplied hospital tickets as one of its benefits. However, it remained a low-key operation despite the crusade against outdoor relief and was generally rebuffed by guardians and the poor themselves.[146] A place in an almshouse would have been an alternative means of support to admission to a workhouse, but Birmingham had only a few homes run by the Lenches Trust, providing only 224 places in 1816. In general, poor law expenditure was more important in welfare provision than charitable provision. For instance, in 1815 all Birmingham charities spent eleven shillings per head of population compared with six pounds, forty shillings on poor relief.[147] Hospital contributory funds also flourished in the nineteenth century, mostly arising out of craft guilds. The main object was to provide finance for the voluntary hospitals and only later in the century did they provide health benefits to members. One such scheme was the Birmingham Hospital Saturday Fund, but the extent of membership is difficult to determine. The typical subscription rate of one or two guineas was far beyond the means of the ordinary worker.[148]

Birmingham was slow to construct its first voluntary hospital in comparison to similarly sized towns. Championed by a local doctor, John Ash, the General Hospital was not opened until 1779 to provide medical care for the sick poor throughout the borough and beyond the town's boundaries, as the poor law Town Infirmary was available only to those within the parish. The nineteenth century saw the establishment of a second general hospital, Queen's Hospital (1841) and a succession of specialist hospitals: Orthopaedic Hospital (1817), Eye Hospital (1823), Ear and Throat Infirmary (1844), Dental Hospital (1858), Children's Hospital (1861), Women's Hospital (1871), and Skin and Lock Hospital (1881). The first public provision outside the poor law for infectious disease patients took place when the Health Committee of Birmingham Council took over the workhouse smallpox wards in 1874. This was followed by the erection in 1883 of Lodge Road Hospital for scarlet fever patients and Little Bromwich Hospital as the town's main isolation hospital. Lodge Road Hospital was built on the grounds of the Borough Lunatic Asylum, which had opened in 1852. Prior to that time, inmates with mental illness who could not be managed in the workhouse were transferred to a private lunatic asylum at Duddeston or Stafford County Lunatic Asylum, erected in 1818. The latter was also used by the Wolverhampton guardians for unmanageable inmates. There was no voluntary hospital in Wolverhampton or the other Black Country towns until the South Staffordshire General Hospital opened in 1849 with eighty beds. Two specialist voluntary hospitals, Wolverhampton Eye Infirmary and Wolverhampton and District Hospital for Women, followed in the 1880s, as well as Wolverhampton Borough Hospital for fever patients. Although Friendly Societies were plentiful throughout the Black Country, virtually no details of them are available.

Workhouse Medicine

There were important differences in the approaches to the provision of poor law medical services in Birmingham and Wolverhampton. While the former always provided separate facilities for sick inmates and employed nurses and a resident medical officer, discrete sick wards and paid nurses were a later development in Wolverhampton, where medical officers were employed on a part-time basis. Birmingham parish workhouse was established in the early eighteenth century and provided a medical service to the town for almost fifty years prior to the erection of a voluntary hospital in the 1770s. As a result, the practice of poor law medicine in Birmingham could be considered atypical of provincial towns. By way of contrast, medical care in Wolverhampton workhouse was typical of that in New Poor Law urban unions and yet the community in which it was located was similar to that of nearby Birmingham.

The material for this study was drawn from the minutes of the boards of guardians and the boards' committees in Birmingham and Wolverhampton, supplemented by reports from parliamentary papers and local newspapers, and poor law correspondence at The National Archives in London. Despite the massive archive of the poor law administration, it contains little of the views and experiences of sick paupers after the New Poor Law and nothing written by paupers resident in the workhouse.[149] This research has unearthed a few letters written by former sick inmates, providing insight on their perspective of the treatment they received. Thus, the experiences of sick paupers and their medical attendants will be brought to the fore. As a result, a more complex picture of the medical care within the workhouse will emerge, demonstrating that it was an important element of medical care for sick paupers in the nineteenth and early twentieth centuries in England.

The first chapter will consider those inmates who required medical treatment, what proportion they constituted of the total inmate population, the nature of their illnesses, and the medical services provided for them. Despite being the majority of patients, inmates with chronic diseases and disabilities are a group that have been difficult to identify within the workhouse classification system and so have not been studied previously in any depth. However, for those inmates suffering from chronic diseases, the chapter will reveal for the first time the nature and extent of their disabilities and that guardians took a sympathetic approach toward the care they received. However, it will challenge the assumption that the workhouse catered almost exclusively for patients with chronic diseases by showing that it did act as a locus of care for acutely ill paupers. However, to what extent it provided acute treatment for those involved in accidents, how much surgery was carried out, and the nature of the surgery will be analyzed.

One aspect of acute care, namely fevers and infectious diseases, takes up the next chapter, which shows the considerable role the poor law authorities played in providing facilities for such patients and in containing the spread of infection within the community. However, the role of workhouses in the control of epidemics and infectious diseases has not previously been given prominence in the discourse of isolation institutions. The extent of this medical role beyond the workhouse's poor law function has not previously been acknowledged in the secondary literature, and the importance of the poor law institutions to the health of the communities they served has not been recognized. Nor has the degree of cooperation between the poor law guardians and the sanitary and local authorities, as demonstrated in Birmingham, in contrast to the more usual strained relationships that existed over who should provide isolation facilities.[150] The arrangements for the care of smallpox patients in the workhouse are recorded in greater detail than previously, demonstrating how significant they were in containing the spread of infection within the community, in addition to providing care for individual sufferers.

Chapter 3 considers patients likely to exhibit disturbed and challenging behaviors, such as those with mental disorders and disability, usually referred to as lunatics and imbeciles, as well as patients suffering from epilepsy and venereal disease. For these groups of patients, there was no other option than the workhouse as they were usually refused admission to voluntary hospitals and specialist care was sparse. County asylum accommodation was inadequate to cope with demand so that harmless lunatics had to be transferred or returned to workhouses. Boards of guardians had vested interests in retaining lunatics in the workhouse, as the cost of their upkeep was cheaper than in an asylum, but what provision did they make for them within the workhouse? Did the treatment of lunatics in workhouses follow that in asylums in changing from the use of restraint to moral management? With their staff-to-patient ratios lower than those of asylums, how did workhouses cope with behavioral disturbance? To what extent were physical treatments for mental disorders also used for punishing any type of misdemeanor? Patients with epilepsy posed a particular problem for staff as they were at risk of injuring themselves or others during a seizure. Were they still subjected to forms of mechanical restraint after these were no longer used for mental illness? What implications did the development of epileptic colonies in the early twentieth century have for epileptic patients in the workhouse? Dedicated facilities for patients with venereal disease and the types of treatment they received will be analyzed. The chapter will provide evidence for maintaining that both types of patients received appropriate care that was, at times, as good as in specialist institutions.

The day-to-day doctoring and nursing within the workhouse infirmary is currently poorly understood. In chapter 4, what poor law historian Kim Price calls the "reality of poor law doctoring" will be addressed by examining the work of the workhouse medical officers responsible for looking after sick inmates.[151] Their general working conditions and the extent to which their heavy workload affected the level of direct patient care they practiced will be covered. Despite the constraints imposed by guardians, some managed to provide good quality and innovative care. There is no doubt that the practice of conscientious medical officers benefited patients even when staffing levels were low, challenging the assertion that an inadequate number of doctors invariably resulted in low standards of care. By detailing the day-to-day work of medical officers, this chapter reveals what it was like to practice medicine in the workhouse, an aspect that has not been the subject of historical study. It explains why they found it difficult to avoid conflict with guardians who wished to control costs. The context in which charges of medical negligence were made is explored, revealing that the lack of good communication between medical officers and guardians was a critical factor.

The following chapter will illuminate another unexplored area of medical practice in workhouses, namely the wide range of medical treatments that medical officers prescribed. These included medical therapies, such as diet, drugs, alcohol, and physical treatments. However, most medical treatment remained either symptomatic or palliative in nature and the main curative methods were seen as good hygiene, adequate ventilation, and sanitary reform. As medical officers were usually required to pay for drugs they prescribed from their salaries, they stand accused of preferring to order "medical extras," such as extra rations and alcohol, which were paid for by the guardians.[152] Moreover, guardians stand accused of refusing to sanction orders that medical officers regarded as essential for the treatment of a patient.[153] Flinn claims that guardians were reluctant to provide sufficiently for the day-to-day medical care of the indoor sick, while Price is of the opinion that the authorization of medical extras and drugs was always a controversial issue.[154] The exploration in this study of the treatment patients received contradicts the prevailing opinion that inmates were frequently denied standard medical treatments. It will also elucidate whether workhouse doctors were able to provide a standard of treatment comparable to that practiced in voluntary hospitals. The chapter also contains one of the few detailed accounts of the implementation within the workhouse of the same methods of treatment for patients with tuberculosis as employed in sanatoria.

It is generally recognized that nursing was the weakest part of the care provided for patients, and the lack of trained nurses was the greatest handicap for the developing poor law infirmaries.[155] Poor law nurses are usually portrayed in the secondary literature as less efficient, more intoxicated, less well paid, provided with less satisfactory accommodation, and having longer hours of work than those in voluntary hospitals. Nursing duties were initially undertaken by untrained female paupers, but were they as inefficient and unreliable as their reputation suggests? Chapter 6 will show what it was like to work as a nurse in the workhouse infirmary and that it was not dissimilar to nursing in voluntary hospitals. In this first detailed account of the reality of poor law nursing, their reputation of total incompetence in the early days of the New Poor Law is revealed as demonstrably unjust. The high turnover and considerable proportion who failed to complete training were common to workhouse infirmaries and voluntary hospitals, but how similar were working conditions, salaries, and standards of nursing care? Did poor law infirmaries provide nursing staff with less experience of acute medical care and surgery and greater exposure only to patients with chronic conditions compared with voluntary hospitals, leaving poor law nurses with a lesser degree of skill?

Chapter 7 will bring all these aspects together to facilitate an analysis of the overall standards of care provided for sick inmates in Birmingham and Wolverhampton workhouses. It demonstrates that care is multifactorial and its quality cannot be judged solely on the adequacy of medical staffing, as advocated by Price.[156] By demonstrating the positive side of New Poor Law medical care and showing that inmates did, for the most part, receive humane care, workhouse medicine is seen as more complex than previously appreciated and as more important in the lives of sick paupers in the nineteenth and early twentieth centuries than is generally acknowledged.

Chapter One

From Acute Illness to Chronic Disability

The prevailing picture of the Victorian workhouse infirmary is of an institution filled with inmates suffering from chronic diseases and disabilities, a place where almost no treatment of acute illness was practiced. According to welfare historian Samantha Shave, it was the most reviled institution among the British working class.[1] However, we have already seen in relation to the illness of Anne Walford at the beginning of the introduction that it was regarded as an appropriate setting for acutely ill paupers in Wolverhampton in the first decade after the New Poor Law, and this chapter will provide further evidence to demonstrate that acute care was an integral part of workhouse medical officers' work. It will also provide an in-depth analysis of the characteristics of those inmates classified as "aged and infirm," who did make up the majority of patients, but who have been largely neglected within the historiography of the poor laws.

Sick inmates formed a substantial group within the workhouse population, the proportion increasing from 10 percent in 1843 to between 34 percent and 48 percent in the mid- to late 1860s, with the higher figure in London and the lower in provincial workhouses. By the end of our period of study, 32 percent of inmates of poor law institutions in England and Wales were accommodated in sick wards or separate infirmaries.[2] Illness and injury accounted for a substantial proportion of admissions to workhouses; for instance 62 percent of adult males and almost 44 percent of adult females were admitted to Medway Union workhouse between 1876 and 1881 because of sickness.[3] Workhouses had begun to adopt the role of hospitals by 1870 and those in large towns became transformed into "infirmaries for the sick," widely regarded as the first public hospitals.[4] By 1891, the public sector provided about 83,000 beds, compared with only 43,000 by voluntary hospitals.[5] The greater number of sick inmates in poor law infirmaries resulted from the recognition of the benefits of institutional medical care for those who could not be cared for at home, the poor state of health of many paupers prior to illness, and the growing popularity of hospitals among the poor. The policies of the central authority also contributed to the increasing admission of sick paupers.

The Poor Law Commissioners did not initially intend that a test of need should be applied to sick, disabled, and older paupers, but in their Seventh Annual Report in 1841 they extended the principles of less eligibility and deterrence to those seeking medical relief.[6] As a result, paupers admitted to the workhouse because of sickness or disability were subjected to the workhouse test and to the same regime within the institution as all other inmates. Their one concession was a special dietary to provide a better standard of nutrition.[7] In the late 1860s, the Poor Law Board reversed the policy of less eligibility in relation to the sick, and its president, the Conservative politician Gathorne Hardy, declared that the deterrent principle was no longer appropriate. However, the Longley Report in 1874 urged more stringent controls over outdoor relief for the sick and laid down criteria that applicants would have to meet to obtain it.[8] Provincial unions varied in how strictly they applied the workhouse test to sick paupers and some were slow to change; for instance, in Birmingham and Manchester the sick were still subjected to it in 1888.[9] According to Jeanne Brand, the medical care of paupers remained "hedged with a persuasive atmosphere of deterrence" and Jonathan Reinarz and Leonard Schwarz remind us that workhouses "retained both their medical and punitive functions."[10]

The strict exclusion policies of voluntary hospitals, as mentioned in the previous section, were also a major factor in the development of poor law institutional medical care. For instance, Birmingham General Hospital from its foundation refused admission to patients suspected to have "the itch" and only reluctantly admitted patients with chronic leg ulcers, as they were likely to have longer lengths of stay in hospital.[11] For example, in 1903, Margaret Connor was refused admission to the general hospital in Wolverhampton as the regulations prohibited admitting patients deemed incurable. She was subsequently admitted to the workhouse and the guardians expressed surprise that a woman of seventy-four with a fractured thigh could not be cured.[12] Furthermore, when patients in voluntary hospitals were unable to be discharged, they were not allowed to remain indefinitely. This happened in May 1884 to Ann Hackett, who was transferred to Birmingham workhouse from the Queen's Hospital because she was "crippled with rheumatoid arthritis and suffered spinal caries." According to Cornelius Suckling, who was visiting physician at both institutions, her bedsores had improved since admission and were nearly healed at the time of transfer. The hospital pointed out that "it is contrary to the rules of this Institution to allow incurable cases to remain in the Hospital."[13]

Voluntary hospitals also discriminated against older patients; for example, only six patients over the age of sixty years, out of a total of 127, were admitted to the General Hospital in Birmingham in the first three months after it opened. Regarded as chronic cases, older patients would have been admitted to the workhouse infirmary.[14] Claudia Edwards has demonstrated that elderly individuals were overrepresented among admissions to Shoreditch poor law infirmary, compared with their proportion in the local population, whereas the reverse was true at Bristol Royal Infirmary, a voluntary hospital.[15] As a result of these several policies, 80 percent of hospital beds for physical illnesses in 1861 were in poor law institutions, but, perversely, historians' interests have been focused more on the voluntary hospital sector.[16] This disproportionate neglect may have arisen because of the difficulty in identifying medical details within poor law records, particularly relating to sick inmates, who were not identified as a separate group in official statistics until after 1913.[17] Additionally, it is difficult to identify patients in workhouses suffering from chronic illnesses despite them forming a large proportion of inmates. In particular, distinguishing these inmates from healthier older inmates poses quite a challenge. However, Birmingham provided dedicated wards for inmates with disability, labeled "bedridden wards," allowing the more disabled section of the "non-able-bodied" class to be more visible.

The approach society takes toward its less able citizens must be seen within the context of the prevailing view of disability at the time in question. The usual response throughout history was the removal of individuals from the community into an institution. Institutionalization had as its basis the medical model of disability, which regarded impairment as a personal tragedy and a sickness.[18] As a result, disabled people were seen as invalids, incapable of social participation. According to Bill Hughes, a leading academic in disability studies, the medical model has its emphasis on the disabled body, the sight of which has provoked not only pity but also fear in the eyes of those who were not disabled. This resulted in charitable paternalism on the one hand and the demand for segregation on the other.[19] The predominant Victorian response to an impaired body was social exclusion and institutionalization, but the emotional element within that response resulted in the provision of charitable institutions.[20] However, establishments for people with sensory impairments, such as blindness and deafness, and for children with physical ailments predominated, although they developed to a large extent only in the late Victorian period.[21] Less institutional care was provided for those who developed disability later in life, as this was seen as inevitable and incurable or even as divine punishment for past misdemeanors.[22] Furthermore, the concept of chronic illnesses has altered in meaning throughout history and even in the twentieth century, when it emerged as a category of ill health, remained an imprecise term.[23] The recognition of chronic disease as a social problem in the United Kingdom did not take place until after World War II.[24] Prior to the 1980s, historical assessment of disability had come from "outsiders," such as doctors and policy makers, since historians had neglected this area of study, leaving it "unhistorical as a discourse."[25] Major historical studies did not appear until the twenty-first century, most often exploring the transition from the exclusion of disabled people from society to the achievement of fuller rights of citizenship.[26] Although a sizable proportion of workhouse inmates suffered from disability, their relative neglect within the historical discourse may have resulted also from the difficulty in identifying them within poor law institutions, a task made more difficult because those with identical disabilities could be allocated to different categories within the workhouse classification system.[27]

This chapter considers the types of patients who were admitted to the workhouse with physical illnesses, with the exception of communicable diseases, which are covered in the next chapter. It examines whether the provision for both the acutely ill and the chronically sick in Birmingham and Wolverhampton workhouses was different in the two towns and how it compared with the country as a whole. As the number of admissions increased as the century progressed, how did the guardians meet this increasing need for medical care and did the additional infirmary beds merely reflect much longer lengths of stay by patients with chronic illnesses? Jeremy Boulton, Romola Davenport, and Leonard Schwarz have suggested the predominant function of eighteenth- and early nineteenth-century workhouses was the care of those admitted in the end stage of their lives, as the majority of deaths occurred shortly after admission.[28] Was this the case and to what extent did the workhouse perform other medical functions, such as active medical treatment for those with short-term acute diseases? What was the nature and intensity of the illnesses suffered by workhouse patients and how well did the care provided compare with the general standards of medical practice at the time? What were the medical conditions and levels of dependency of inmates with physical disability in the two workhouse infirmaries in the West Midlands? As the infirmaries developed a greater role in treating acute illness, what was the impact on sick inmates who remained in the residual portion of the workhouse?

Poor Law Medical Facilities in Birmingham and Wolverhampton

But before addressing these issues, we need to examine the extent of the provision of medical care both in the Birmingham and Wolverhampton workhouses and in the local voluntary hospitals. Birmingham poor law authorities played a major part in the provision of medical care within the town. An infirmary block had been erected on the workhouse grounds by 1745 to the rear of the main building. In April 1766 it contained forty-eight beds of which twelve were empty and in May 1785 a similar number of patients (thirty-seven) were being treated.[29] However, four years later, the accommodation for sick paupers was felt to be so inadequate that a detached building was approved and erected adjacent to the workhouse in 1793 as the Town Infirmary at a cost of £1,475.[30] By August 1818, 94 patients were being treated in the infirmary, the number increasing steadily to about 233 in 1847.[31] New buildings were also erected in 1835 as the Lunatic Branch of the Town Infirmary. In April that year, the new buildings accommodated 36 "idiotic cases" and patients suffering "mental aberration," who would otherwise have been transferred to a lunatic asylum, but 25 insane women remained in their old apartments. As the workhouse's role in the treatment of mental illness became more important, the number of patients had increased to 78 by 1847.[32] However, when the Borough Asylum opened in 1850, a significant proportion of lunatics were transferred. This contrasts with another huge provincial urban workhouse in Manchester, which in 1841 housed 1,261 paupers with 268 in sick wards, but only 10 lunatics.[33] The first voluntary hospital, the General Hospital, opened in Birmingham in 1779 and the second nonspecialist one, the Queen's Hospital, in 1841, both providing care for the sick poor throughout the borough. By the mid-nineteenth century, the former contained 240 beds and the latter 180.[34]

The infirmary for 310 inmates at the new workhouse in 1852 was described as "one of the finest in the country."[35] Medical cases were divided among a number of separate wards, including those for common cases, convalescent patients, "idiots," and epileptics. Detached buildings were similarly provided for fever, infectious, and maternity cases.[36] In keeping with most workhouses at that time, the erection of extra accommodation was necessitated by overcrowding, as a result of Birmingham parish's population increasing by over one-fifth throughout the 1850s. Illness was also an important factor in giving rise to the need for extended facilities.[37] Cape Hill School was opened with 200 places for boys in 1864, alleviating some pressure on the institution and allowing the old school to be converted into an epileptic ward the following year. A more elaborate extension that same year added a further 340 places to the infirmary.[38] In 1867, isolation wards were augmented when a shed was converted into a smallpox ward, and new wards for 200 old women opened the following year.[39] In 1868, *The Lancet* pronounced it "one of the best managed of all provincial workhouses."[40] The wards were not overcrowded at that time, with the exception of one ward holding 25 insane patients.

However, in later years, overcrowding became so persistent that the guardians decided in 1885 to erect a new separate infirmary building adjacent to the workhouse. It opened four years later with a capacity of 1,511 beds, only 990 of which were in the new pavilion-style building, while the remainder were in some of the old infirmary wards. The new building consisted of nine three-story blocks set on alternate sides of the main corridor, which was almost a quarter of a mile long.[41] The surgical wards and operating room were on the ground floor, while those for patients with chronic conditions were located on the third floor. Separate blocks were constructed to give four wards for 24 patients with infectious diseases. By March the following year, the new infirmary was almost fully utilized, with 1,286 patients accommodated.[42] The development of the infirmary into an acute general hospital has been described by one of its former consultant physicians, George Hearn, although this is a traditional, progressive account written to celebrate the institution's centenary.[43]

By comparison, Wolverhampton's medical service for the poor developed after the setting up of the union. According to Barnsby, no Black Country workhouses had separate infirmaries when they were built and sick paupers were scattered throughout the buildings.[44] Although the new union workhouse in Wolverhampton did not have a separate infirmary, there were infirmary wards and "infectious wards." In 1842, the former could hold 28 men and 25 women and the latter 6 of each sex, accounting for 23 percent of total beds.[45] Thirteen years later, the male sick wards had been enlarged to accommodate 45 patients, but those for women remained unchanged.[46] By 1867, additional sick wards had been built, so that the infirmary consisted of a series of buildings of various ages and "degrees of fitness."[47] When pressure for additional space occurred in the late 1880s, Wolverhampton guardians, following a visit to the cottage homes in Birmingham, decided to erect a similar provision. As a result, 240 children were moved out of the workhouse in November 1890.[48] By this time, the number of beds in the wards for the sick had increased to 273.[49] The equivalent wards in the new workhouse, erected at New Cross in Wednesfield in 1903, could accommodate 196 men and 150 women. Little further information is available in the literature regarding these workhouses or the evolution of the last one to become a general hospital, New Cross Hospital.

Despite being similar industrial towns, there were differences in the structure of their populations that would influence poor law services. For instance, the overall pauperism rate for Wolverhampton was around double that for Birmingham from 1881 for three decades, and did not follow the reduction in the national rate until 1911. By contrast, Birmingham's had decreased sharply by 1891, reflecting Birmingham's stricter enforcement of the workhouse test as part of the crusade against outdoor relief. Indoor relief as a proportion of total relief showed marked differences between the two towns, being much greater in Birmingham than Wolverhampton from 1881, possibly also due to the influence of the crusade. However, James Turner, chairman of Birmingham guardians in 1907, explained that the high institutionalization rate was due to the entirely urban nature of the parish, with an almost exclusively working-class population. The policy of the board of guardians was to provide out-relief whenever a "respectable home" was available.[50] The degree of overcrowding, in terms of the number of people per household, was more severe in Birmingham (30 percent) compared with Wolverhampton (19 percent).[51] This is likely to have contributed to a higher incidence of infectious diseases, including tuberculosis.

Workhouse Classification

The efficiency of the workhouse system depended on stringent classification of inmates to allow complete segregation of all classes and both sexes, although it also imposed a means of psychological deterrence to applicants for relief. To ensure good workhouse management, the Poor Law Commissioners designated seven classes: able-bodied, aged or infirm, boys and girls, all divided by sex, and younger children as one group.[52] Welfare historian Anne Digby draws attention to the fact that the term *able-bodied* was never clearly defined and suggests it included all those over fifteen years of age who could support themselves through employment.[53] Mary MacKinnon is more critical, regarding it as "virtually meaningless," as it could include younger people who were incapacitated by short- or medium-term illnesses or accidents.[54] The non-able-bodied class consisted mostly of older inmates and those with permanent disability.[55] To add to the uncertainty, both central guidance and local workhouse officials were divided in their views over whether sick older inmates should be treated in the infirmary or placed in the ordinary wards of the workhouse.[56] When in 1891 the able-bodied group were divided into those who were healthy and those who were temporarily disabled, it resulted in an increase in the proportion of inmates who were designated as sick.[57] Consequently, inmates who would have been regarded as sick or disabled cannot be easily identified as distinct groups within the workhouse population and are to be found within various sections of the workhouse community.

For instance, non-able-bodied adults admitted to Birmingham workhouse in the 1840s could be found in wards for aged and infirm men and women, in the insane, venereal, itch, lying-in, or bedridden wards. They would also have been present in the various infirmary wards.[58] However, there is also one mention of a ward for partially disabled men, suggesting there may have been subdivision of categories of inmates in smaller wards within the broader classifications.[59] The insane wards were renamed epileptic wards after the new workhouse was built and there were dedicated wards for men with leg ulcers and "consumptive cases."[60] There was less choice in the placement of inmates initially in Wolverhampton Union workhouse with wards for able-bodied men and women, old men, old women, boys, girls, and the infirmary.[61] However, twenty-five years later, dedicated provision had been made for inmates suffering "bad legs, paralysis," itch, and venereal disease.[62] Nevertheless, inmates with illness or disability could still be classified as able-bodied. This happened to a thirty-five-year-old man in Birmingham workhouse who was suffering with difficulty in breathing and who subsequently died from cardiac failure.[63] In Wolverhampton, only a few of the able-bodied men were considered fit to do a "fair day's work" in the mid-1860s and the situation was no different in the early years of the twentieth century.[64]

Medical Activity in Birmingham and Wolverhampton

The point in time at which English workhouses developed a significant medical role is a matter of dispute among historians, although there is agreement that they became increasingly medicalized as the nineteenth century progressed. The debate is hindered by the fact that the medical function of the workhouse and how the medical space within it was used remains undefined.[65] We will now examine this question with relation to the two West Midland workhouses. As early as 1818, Birmingham guardians gave the six visiting surgeons to the workhouse infirmary the authority to admit patients in emergencies without an order from the guardians or relieving officers. Furthermore, patients could be discharged only with the permission of the surgeons. These powers continued after the New Poor

Table 1.1. Admissions, discharges, and deaths in Birmingham workhouse infirmary for selected periods, 1835–44

Quarter of year to end of:	Admissions	Discharges: cured or relieved		Transferred, absconded	Died		Remaining at end of quarter	Patients as proportion of total inmates
March 1835	180	150	47%	3	44	14%	124	32%
June 1835	172	121	41%	10	43	15%	121	34%
September 1835	170	119	41%	3	29	10%	130	37%
December 1835	153	105	37%	4	37	13%	137	38%
March 1836	168	124	41%	2	45	15%	134	35%
June 1836	171	136	45%	5	45	15%	130	37%
September 1836	131	121	45%	1	33	13%	117	35%
December 1836	157	84	31%	0	56	20%	134	37%
March 1837	217	129	37%	0	77	22%	145	50%
June 1837	209	171	48%	0	51	14%	132	31%
September 1837	215	169	49%	0	50	14%	128	28%
December 1837	228	156	44%	0	43	12%	155	33%
March 1840	223	68	19%	22	56	15%	137	45%
June 1840	267	219	54%	14	45	11%	124	26%
September 1840	200	155	48%	10	39	12%	128	28%
December 1840	246	159	43%	16	42	11%	151	30%
March 1841	244	193	49%	13	50	13%	140	27%
June 1841	229	186	50%	15	41	11%	132	26%
September 1841	225	170	48%	12	44	12%	131	31%
December 1841	275	185	46%	9	42	10%	170	38%
March 1842	326	249	53%	9	72	15%	170	32%
June 1842	284	223	49%	16	36	8%	175	35%
September 1842	264	251	57%	11	37	8%	140	26%
December 1842	234	143	35%	16	38	9%	153	30%
March 1844	307	243	50%	11	57	12%	176	31%
June 1844	245	216	51%	11	41	10%	153	29%
September 1844	294	225	50%	23	44	10%	155	31%
December 1844	298	231	51%	19	45	10%	158	29%

Note: The percentages in the discharges and deaths columns are proportions discharged or died of the total of patients in the infirmary at the beginning of the quarter and the number of admissions. The majority of transfers were to an asylum.

Source: BCL, BBG, GP/B/2/1/3–5.

Law until new regulations came into force in 1845.[66] Along with these rights of admission, the guardians required the surgeons to provide a quarterly report of activity in the infirmary. Table 1.1 gives details for the years between 1834 and the time of the new regulations. Admissions varied markedly throughout the period with a small increase toward the end, but the number of patients remaining in the infirmary rose steadily. Discharges of patients "relieved" or cured varied between 41 percent and 48 percent, although it was usually just over 50 percent in the mid-1840s, while deaths remained between 10 percent and 14 percent. After 1840, between half and three-quarters of patients discharged were described as cured, rather than relieved.

On average, there were around eighteen admissions per week and about 125 patients in the infirmary each day in the late 1830s and 160 in the early 1840s. They were under the care of a house surgeon and 6 visiting surgeons, who also attended sick paupers in the dispensary and at home. Sick inmates represented between 26 percent and 50 percent of all those in the workhouse, averaging around a third of the workhouse population. This was greater than the 21 percent of 1,261 inmates who were in the sick wards of Manchester New Bridge Street workhouse in 1841, although an unspecified number were also in the general wards.[67] By comparison, the national average six years later was merely 10 percent.[68] In the 1840s, the infirmary provided a similar number of medical beds as the General Hospital, although it admitted a third fewer patients, and had more beds than the Queen's Hospital.[69] As a result, the wards in the infirmary were extremely overcrowded and described as "offensive and disagreeable," with the floors covered with extra beds. For instance, the ward for "women with loathsome disease" contained 17 patients, but only 14 beds.[70] When plans for the new workhouse and infirmary were being made in March 1849, there were 160 patients with physical illness, plus 95 who were insane, in the old workhouse infirmary.[71] Although the number of patients treated in the infirmary in table 1.1 suggests a steady increase, there was a decline in the early 1850s, before numbers rose again in the middle of the decade (table 1.2). In the new infirmary in 1855, the daily average number of patients had increased to 318, compared with the weekly average of 122 for the Queen's Hospital in 1857–58 and a daily average of 204 for the General Hospital in 1860–61.[72] However, the greater patient turnover in the voluntary hospitals ensured that they treated a greater number of new cases (table 1.3). Nevertheless, the workhouse's contribution was significant in facilitating the hospitals' level of activity by accepting patients from them who required a longer inpatient stay.

In February 1842, Thomas Haney, aged thirty-six years, was admitted to Wolverhampton workhouse because of a bowel disorder, as was William Watts, a miner aged twenty-eight, with fever. Watts required readmission early the following year because of debility, rendering him unable to work. Samuel Highland had been incapacitated due to a fractured leg for three

Table 1.2. Medical relief in Birmingham workhouse for selected weeks, 1851–56

Week ending	Number of inmates	Number on medical relief	Proportion of patients to inmates	Deaths
October 25, 1851	586	112	19%	3
December 6, 1852	628	124	20%	4
January 3, 1852	660	134	20%	3
April 3, 1852	676	139	21%	1
July 3, 1852	662	176	27%	1
October 2, 1852	656	172	26%	3
December 25, 1852	771	154	20%	1
April 2, 1853	798	202	25%	5
July 9, 1853	673	191	28%	2
October 1, 1853	653	166	25%	2
January 7, 1854	940	246	26%	8
April 1, 1854	916	249	27%	9
July 1, 1854	925	246	27%	9
October 7, 1854	893	226	25%	1
December 16, 1854	1,087	280	26%	5
March 15, 1856	1,213	385	32%	6

Note: The transfer of inmates to the new workhouse took place in March 1852.

Source: TNA, MH12/13297–99, 13300.

Table 1.3. New cases of diseases treated in medical institutions in Birmingham in 1876

Quarter ending on	General Hospital	Queen's Hospital	Children's Hospital	Workhouse	Borough Hospital
April 1, 1876	4,883	3,767	3,421	1,074	–
July 1, 1876	5,393	4,256	3,706	824	6
December 30, 1876	5,048	4,940	3,206	3,850	33
Total	15,324	12,963	10,333	5,748	39

Source: TNA, MH12/13326, Medical Officer of Health's Report for 1876.

months before he entered the workhouse in October 1842.[73] Seven subsequent admissions took place over the following eighteen months: Mary Sutherland, aged forty; Anne Langford, aged thirty-five; and Mary Blunt, aged fifty-five, all for debility; John Wittle, a miner aged forty-one, for "disease of the head" from fever; Elizabeth Davies, aged thirty-three, with dropsy; another Elizabeth Davies, aged forty-five, who had been suffering lung disease for two months; and Ann Smallwood, aged fifty-four, with a three-week history of asthma.[74] At that time, there were between forty and seventy patients in Wolverhampton workhouse infirmary and infectious wards, ranging between 11 percent and 16 percent of workhouse inmates.

These early years after the opening of Wolverhampton Union workhouse saw medical admissions increase sharply by 12 percent between 1842 and 1845 (table 1.4). As a proportion of all inmates, those who were sick increased by 4 percent over this period, with roughly an equal number of men and women. When patients in the infectious and insane wards are included, the proportion increased markedly between 1842 and 1843, from 17 percent to 30 percent, and rose further to 37 percent in 1846 (table 1.5). The guardians were concerned about the rapidity of the increase in the number of sick paupers, but concluded that "Not a remedy or a comfort ought to be withheld; the sick and the infirm, the destitute infant and the helpless aged, are our charge."[75] The proportion of sick inmates remained around the one-third level throughout the next three decades, similar to that of Birmingham workhouse, with 588 sick out of a total of 1,781 inmates in 1863.[76] Including those certified as insane in Wolverhampton in the early 1870s, this increased the share of all sick inmates to around half of the workhouse population.[77]

Sixty-five inmates died in Wolverhampton workhouse in 1840, giving a mortality rate of approximately 16 percent, based on the average number of inmates in the year ending in March 1841 of 405. The majority of deaths took place in the age group sixteen to fifty-nine years (45 percent), with only 31 percent in those aged sixty years and above. For the 44 inmates for whom a cause of death was recorded, 13 were due to debility, 5 to tuberculosis, 5 to venereal disease, 3 to liver disease, and only Samuel Lester from fever.[78] Wolverhampton's death rate increased to between 21 percent and 28 percent of admissions in the late 1850s and early 1860s, and was similar to that in Birmingham workhouse in the first half of the 1850s, namely between 18 percent and 28 percent in the first four months of each year (tables 1.4, 1.6). The major cause of death in Birmingham was chronic lung disease, such as asthma and consumption. Most of the deaths occurred in old people, most likely because they were moving into the workhouse as they became frailer.[79] This is supported by the data for Wolverhampton in 1891, where 65 percent of workhouse deaths involved those of sixty-five years and over, but only 26 percent of deaths in the Borough were in that age group. Furthermore, the proportions of those dying between the ages of twenty-five and fifty-nine years were similar (26 percent and 24 percent respectively).[80]

A survey of all workhouses in England and Wales on one day in December 1869 records the number of patients on the medical officers' books plus the nature and cause of their illnesses.[81] Although the total

Table 1.4. Inmates and patients in Wolverhampton workhouse, on selected days, 1842–45

Month, year	Total inmates	Inmates in infirmary			Proportion of patients to all inmates
		Male	Female	Total	
April 1842	354	24	23	47	13%
May 1842	316	20	18	38	12%
June 1842	372	25	20	45	12%
July 1842	415	29	26	55	13%
August 1842	442	34	24	58	13%
September 1842	446	18	21	39	9%
October 1842	337	14	20	34	10%
November 1842	395	17	16	33	8%
December 1842	419	22	12	34	8%
January 1843	485	22	9	31	6%
February 1843	482	28	17	45	9%
March 1843	487	26	25	51	10%
April 1843	469	21	33	54	12%
May 1843	455	26	26	32	7%
June 1843	453	26	26	32	7%
July 1843	512	27	25	62	12%
August 1843	480	28	30	58	12%
September 1843	492	23	33	46	9%
October 1843	456	28	34	62	14%
November 1843	492	27	35	62	13%
December 1843	462	23	34	57	12%
January 1844	454	23	34	57	13%
February 1844	483	26	38	64	13%
March 1844	462	26	38	64	14%
April 1844	436	28	38	66	15%
May 1844	415	26	36	62	15%
July 1844	383	29	28	57	15%
August 1844	368	28	26	54	15%
September 1844	376	26	26	52	14%
October 1844	398	28	29	57	14%
November 1844	431	28	32	60	14%
December 1844	401	26	30	56	14%
January 1845	410	26	32	58	14%
February 1845	444	28	32	60	14%
March 1845	434	28	32	60	14%
April 1845	377	28	32	60	16%
May 1845	346	25	30	55	16%
June 1845	338	25	28	53	16%
July 1845	327	25	28	53	16%
August 1845	314	24	23	47	15%

Source: WALS, Master's Journal, PU/WOL/U/2, 1842–45.

Table 1.5. Sick and total number of inmates in Wolverhampton workhouse for the years 1841–46, 1857–66, 1870–72, and number of deaths in the years 1857–66

Year	All inmates	Sick inmates	Proportion of sick of all inmates	Deaths	
1841–42	1,999	336	17%		
1842–43	2,545	767	30%		
1843–44	2,114	576	27%		
1844–45	2,027	619	31%		
1845–46	2,250	823	37%		
1857–58	570	194	34%	118	21%
1858–59	529	121	23%	128	24%
1859–60	511	185	36%	146	27%
1863–64	575	215	37%	162	28%
1864–65	603	211	35%	169	28%
1865–66	620	220	35%	137	22%
1870	694	219	32%		
1871	659	219	33%		
1872	657	228	35%		

Note: The numbers for 1841–46 are the total admitted to the workhouse in each year, ending at Michaelmas; for 1857–66 and 1870–74, they are the average for the year.

Source: WALS, *Wolverhampton Chronicle*, December 2, 1846; August 14, 1867; November 20, 1872.

Table 1.6. Admissions of sick inmates and deaths in Birmingham workhouse for the months of January to April inclusive, 1850–54

Year	Admissions	Deaths	Mortality rate
1850	346	96	28%
1851	295	55	19%
1852	337	61	18%
1853	427	100	23%
1854	700	134	19%

Source: BCL, Visiting and General Purposes Committee, GP/B/2/8/1/1, April 28, 1854.

number of inmates was very different in the workhouses of Birmingham (2,047) and Wolverhampton (850), the proportion of sick inmates was the same at 35 percent, but larger than that of England as a whole (30 percent). Eight of the provincial workhouses housed more than 1,000 inmates with those who were sick ranging between 22 percent and 52 percent and with

Birmingham close to the average figure.[82] Only six of the twenty-five work-houses holding between 500 and 1,000 residents had a greater proportion of patients than Wolverhampton, with four of them over 40 percent. Within the remainder there was greater variation in the number of sick inmates with over one-quarter housing less than 20 percent. This proportion was also typical of the smaller workhouses where the smallest tended to have fewer sick inmates. Surprisingly, a few of those had a greater proportion of patients suffering acute illnesses rather than chronic diseases; for example, 64 percent of 39 patients at Boston and 77 percent of 61 patients at Reading. By comparison, there were few larger workhouses where patients with acute conditions constituted more than 40 percent of the total sick population. In this respect, Birmingham with 29 percent of patients acutely ill and Wolverhampton with 32 percent were in keeping with the national picture.[83] The question arises as to how representative are data collected on a single day's count. When Dr. Edward Smith, medical officer to the Poor Law Board, visited a selection of provincial workhouses between autumn 1866 and spring the following year, similar proportions of inmates were sick in most of them; for instance, 30 percent in Birmingham and 32 percent in Wolverhampton. His report also gives the opportunity to differentiate levels of sickness between adult inmates and children and, not unexpectedly, children are much healthier. Thus, the proportion of adults who were unwell was over one-third in three-quarters of the workhouses he visited and it was half or more in seven of the institutions, while in Wolverhampton it was 44 percent and in Birmingham 38 percent.[84]

In both of these workhouses the admission of sick paupers increased to around 40 percent of all inmates by the mid-1870s, with the proportion in Wolverhampton declining by half in the 1890s (table 1.7). In Birmingham, those who were ill rose to almost 50 percent in the early 1880s and as high as 60 percent by 1885 as a result of a significant increase in the sick poor in large towns across the country. It prompted the guardians to approve plans for a new infirmary managed separately from the workhouse.[85] The large share of sick inmates remained after the new infirmary opened in 1889, but the subsequent decrease six years later remains unexplained. In a six-month period from the end of 1899 there were on average 96 admissions, 78 discharges, 24 deaths, and 1,167 patients in the wards of the infirmary.[86] One difficulty in making comparisons arises from the varying definitions used to determine sick inmates. The majority of the numbers in table 1.7 are based on inmates in the medical officer's relief books. However, in 1890 and 1896 for both workhouses and in 1885 for Birmingham, they relate to inmates in the "wards for the sick." Birmingham's number of sick inmates in 1896 is

Table 1.7. Sick and total inmates in Birmingham, Wolverhampton, and all England and Wales workhouses, 1867–96

Date	Birmingham			Wolverhampton			England and Wales		
	Total	Sick	Percentage sick	Total	Sick	Percentage sick	Total	Sick	Percentage sick
July 1, 1867	1,692	577	34%	759	168	22%	96,079	23,083	24%
December 16, 1869	2,047	711	35%	805	285	35%	158,576	46,950	30%
January 1876	2,093	861	41%	712	287	40%	125,000	44,755	36%
August 1885	2,268	1,353	60%						
April 1888				1,011	423	42%			
October 1890	2,174	1,330	61%	768	213	28%	176,020	50,308	29%
June–July 1896	2,494	998	40%	951	185	19%	187,000	39,264	21%

Note: The data for England and Wales for 1867 excludes metropolitan unions, but they are included thereafter.

Source: HCPP, 1867–68 (445), *Provincial Workhouses*, 4, 58; 1870 (468–I), *Poor Relief*, 2–3, 19, 21; 1877 (260), *Returns of General Diseases and of Venereal Diseases*, 4, 10–11; 1890–91 (365), *The Number of the Beds in the Wards for the Sick*, 1–18; 1892 (292), *Workhouses (Consumption of Spirits, &c.)*, 4, 16; 1896 (371), *The Number of Sick Persons Occupying the Wards for the Sick*, 4, 26; 1896 (64B.I), *Pauperism (England and Wales). Return (B.I.). Paupers Relieved on 1st July 1896*, 4, 30; BCL, HSC, GP/B/2/3/3/6, January 22, 1878; VGPC, GP/B/2/8/1/9, August 14, 1885; LGB Returns, GP/B/5/1/2, June 6, 1896; WALS, *Wolverhampton Chronicle*, December 29, 1875; April 4, 1888; WBG, PU/WOL/A/22, April 6, 1888; Williams, *From Pauperism to Poverty*, 159–60.

calculated from all those in the infirmary plus those in the workhouse who were "temporarily disabled."[87] Which inmates were designated as sick may also have depended on what affliction they suffered.

Details of the diseases suffered by paupers in the workhouses of England and Wales in December 1869 are included in a parliamentary return, allocating one diagnosis per inmate.[88] Acute medical illnesses accounted for 32 percent of patients in Wolverhampton, 21 percent in Birmingham and 17 percent nationally; acute surgical conditions were less common, with only 8 percent; 0.4 percent and 6 percent respectively. Acute infectious diseases accounted for less than 10 percent in both towns and the country as a whole, while old age was given the most frequent diagnosis, in around one-fifth of patients. The most frequent causes of illness in Birmingham were bronchitis and emphysema (8 percent), rheumatism (7 percent), and paralysis (7 percent), all of which matched the national proportions. This is surprising as the workers in the brass trade, the major industry in Birmingham, experienced high levels of respiratory distress. Epilepsy was also a common diagnosis (9 percent), but in Wolverhampton, it was recorded in 43 percent of patients.

The very high number of epileptic patients (121) is at variance with other figures recorded in the guardians' minutes, although there is no record for this same year. Nevertheless, it is obvious that the large number of epileptics in the parliamentary paper is either a clerical error or an incorrect diagnosis on the part of the medical officer, since the national figure for epilepsy is only 3 percent. Ulcers of legs or other sites on the body were also more frequent in Wolverhampton at 11 percent, compared with 7 percent in Birmingham and 6 percent nationally.[89] Leg ulcers were also one of the most common afflictions affecting patients in voluntary hospitals in the eighteenth century, for example 22 percent of inpatients in Birmingham General Hospital in the 1780s and 1790s and between 40 percent and 50 percent of surgical admissions in several voluntary hospitals in the early years of the nineteenth century. Surprisingly, almost half of sufferers were under the age of thirty.[90] Leg ulcers were one of the main reasons for inmates spending more than five years in workhouses in July 1861, accounting for 11 percent of those given a specific diagnosis for "Bodily Disease," only 3 percent less than for rheumatism, although there were no such patients in either Wolverhampton or Birmingham at that time.[91] However, in January 1861, Thomas Ferris applied to Birmingham guardians to have his leg amputated because of an "enormous" leg ulcer, which had been present for twenty-five years. The guardians deferred making a decision for one month, but the eventual outcome is not recorded.[92]

At the turn of the century in Wolverhampton workhouse, the proportion of those under the care of the medical officer, with the exclusion of "imbeciles and epileptics," was only 23 percent (table 1.8), although 3,257 patients had been attended in 1899.[93] However, in August 1903, the month before the new workhouse opened, only 9 men and 8 women were both able-bodied and in health out of a total of 880 adult inmates. Of these, 230 were in the infirmary undergoing medical treatment, plus "40 were imbeciles" and 50 epileptics.[94] After the move to the new workhouse, the medical workload remained much as before, a similar number to the 2,496 patients admitted to Wolverhampton and Staffordshire General Hospital in the year 1902–3.[95] In Birmingham, the proportion of those under medical care continued between 40 percent and 50 percent of inmates. Returns to the central authority were divided into those in the infirmary and those in the workhouse (table 1.8). Infirmary inmates represent those with more acute illness, but those with chronic diseases in the workhouse have been estimated from the "able-bodied temporarily disabled" group. However, this would exclude non-able-bodied adults under the medical officer's care and they will be now considered.

Table 1.8. Sick and healthy inmates in Birmingham and Wolverhampton workhouses on selected day, 1899–1900

Category of inmate	Wolverhampton, January 1, 1900				Birmingham, December 30, 1899			
	Male	Female	Total	Percentage of total inmates	Male	Female	Total	Percentage of total inmates
Ordinarily able-bodied adults: in health	44	23	67	7%	107	164	271	10%
Temporarily disabled	76	59	135	14%	456	344	800	31%
Children under 16 years of age			51	5%			189	7%
Not able-bodied adults	456	192	648	65%	757	586	1,343	52%
"Insane" persons	41	58	99	10%				
Total inmates	617	323	1,000		1,320	1,094	2,603	
Inmates under care of medical officer, excluding "insane"	136	90	226	23%				
Adults in infirmary							1,083	42%
Total in infirmary							1,171	45%
Total in infirmary plus able-bodied temporarily disabled in workhouse							1,263	49%

Note: Age breakdown is not available for children in Wolverhampton workhouse and those under the medical officer's care exclude "imbeciles and epileptics." The Birmingham returns do not differentiate between health and sickness for non-able-bodied inmates in the workhouse.

Source: BCL, LGB Returns, GP/B/5/1/4, December 30, 1899; WALS, WBG, PU/WOL/A/28, February 9, 1900.

Chronic Disability

Inmates suffering from chronic diseases with varying levels of disability formed a majority within the sick workhouse population and this section will concentrate on this important, but previously neglected, group. One extreme example was Manchester workhouse, which had become overcrowded in 1850 because of so many inmates with chronic diseases that the guardians erected a new building to accommodate the able-bodied.[96] Edward Smith, medical officer to the Poor Law Board, in a survey of provincial workhouses in the late 1860s, found that among those in workhouse infirmaries whom he regarded as sick "in the hospital acceptation of the term," the majority suffered from diseases "of a chronic character, mainly chest complaints and debility."[97] A survey of workhouses in England and Wales in 1869 confirmed this pattern with 77 percent of inmates on the medical officers' books assessed as having a chronic disorder.[98] Birmingham and Wolverhampton were just below the national average (71 percent and 68 percent respectively) in the survey. However, some workhouses were much higher; the most extreme being Bath Union workhouse with 96 percent. Smith considered the medical officer's cases there as "totally unlike those at a general hospital."[99] Even among those diagnosed as having a surgical disease, chronic conditions were more common than acute illness, averaging 63 percent of all surgical cases in England and Wales and 50 percent in Birmingham.[100] This situation persisted into the next two decades, as can be seen from the description of a female surgical ward in Birmingham workhouse in 1885:

> The female surgical ward is another big ward. Here 69 beds, closely arranged side by side, hold their suffering occupants, most of them old and decrepit. It is impossible to enter these long wards and see, amongst the old and infirm, younger women suffering from some affliction requiring medical and surgical treatment . . . without pitying their condition. (*Birmingham Daily Mail*, August 5, 1885)

Nationally, 43 percent of sick inmates in the 1869 survey were aged sixty years and over and 21 percent of them had "old age" recorded as the main disease, assuming that no one under sixty years would be given that designation as a diagnosis.[101] The *Report of the Royal Commission on the Aged Poor* (1895) confirmed that the majority of older inmates in the late 1800s suffered chronic infirmity.[102] The proportion of older paupers among adult inmates in Birmingham workhouse increased markedly between 1841 and 1871 and then rose more slowly to 1911, when it was more than double the 1841 figure (table 1.9). A number of factors were responsible for this change, including Birmingham parish's high rate of older pauperism and reliance on institutionalization rather than outdoor relief, even when compared to London.[103] The proportion of older inmates in Wolverhampton workhouse in 1841 was much higher than Birmingham and generally remained at the same level throughout the century, demonstrating the important part the workhouse played in the care of older paupers as early as the middle of the century (table 1.10). As older people formed the majority within the disabled population, old age has been promoted as an easily measured parameter of disability.[104] However, age alone cannot predict precisely how many inmates were disabled. For instance, on one day in September 1903, the medical officer of Wolverhampton workhouse assessed 81 percent of inmates aged sixty years and over as being unable to "take care of themselves" due to physical

Table 1.9. Birmingham workhouse population by age group, 1851–1911

Year	Birth to 15 years		16–59 years		60–79 years		80 years and over		Total	Percentage of older inmates of:	
	Male	Female	Male	Female	Male	Female	Male	Female		Total inmates	Adult inmates
1841	166	158	125	145	77	70	11	8	760	22%	38%
	22%	21%	16%	19%	10%	9%	1%	1%			
1851	178	135	80	107	63	58	11	5	637	22%	42%
	49%	21%	13%	17%	10%	9%	2%	1%			
1861	244	225	262	357	260	134	7	4	1,493	27%	40%
	16%	15%	18%	24%	17%	9%	0.5%	0.3%			
1871	293	219	227	307	377	252	49	37	1,761	41%	57%
	17%	12%	13%	17%	21%	16%	3%	2%			
1881	180	126	457	506	635	330	68	39	2,341	46%	53%
	8%	5%	20%	22%	27%	14%	3%	2%			
1891	90	73	547	458	656	447	83	56	2,410	52%	55%
	4%	3%	23%	19%	27%	19%	3%	2%			
1901	87	119	585	440	747	545	76	104	2,703	54%	59%
	3%	4%	22%	16%	28%	20%	3%	4%			
1911	119	68	593	413	915	435	72	78	2,693	56%	60%
	4%	3%	22%	15%	34%	16%	3%	3%			

Note: Numbers for 1851 include children in the Infant Poor Asylum, built to take children, as accommodation was not available in the old workhouse. They were transferred to the new workhouse in 1852.

Source: Census Enumerator's Books, 1851–1911.

or mental illness.[105] This compared with 42 percent in Birmingham and the national average of 61 percent. The difference between the two workhouses was due to all inmates aged seventy-five years and over in Wolverhampton needing care. Only 51 percent in Birmingham were dependent, with one-third more women unable to care for themselves than men.

Few workhouses had dedicated wards for more dependent inmates; only three in London did in 1866, but only Lambeth provided them for both men and women. Smith was critical of the practice of "congregating the bed-ridden together," as at Lambeth, because of the detrimental effect on the sanitary arrangements.[106] However, he did suggest that older inmates who were incontinent of urine should be placed in separate wards, classing them as "Offensive and Disagreeable."[107] In his report on 48 provincial workhouses, Smith indicated that Birmingham provided 159 beds in the bedridden wards, 31 percent of total beds. The only other union designating wards as bedridden was Cheltenham, with 18 beds, or 23 percent of total capacity. Bath

Table 1.10. Wolverhampton workhouse population by age group, 1841–1911

Year	Birth to 15 years		16–59 years		60–79 years		80 years and over		Total	Percentage of older inmates of:	
	Male	Female	Male	Female	Male	Female	Male	Female		Total inmates	Adult inmates
1841	31	35	30	31	42	24	3	4	200	37%	54%
	16%	18%	15%	16%	21%	12%	2%	2%			
1851	66	58	100	95	62	32	10	5	428	25%	36%
	20%	14%	23%	22%	14%	7%	2%	1%			
1861	86	113	107	109	120	35	14	24	608	32%	47%
	14%	19%	18%	18%	20%	6%	2%	4%			
1871	119	86	114	150	167	56	15	9	716	35%	48%
	17%	12%	16%	21%	23%	8%	2%	1%			
1881	157	126	153	160	204	83	24	18	925	36%	51%
	17%	14%	17%	17%	22%	9%	3%	2%			
1891	17	15	197	179	273	113	17	12	823	50%	51%
	2%	2%	24%	22%	33%	14%	2%	1%			
1901	34	21	199	152	349	175	43	28	1,001	59%	63%
	3%	2%	20%	15%	35%	17%	4%	3%			
1911	51	37	221	180	312	107	34	19	961	49%	54%
	5%	4%	23%	19%	32%	11%	4%	2%			

Source: Census Enumerator's Books, 1851–1911.

provided 114 beds (27 percent) for invalids and Manchester, Bridge Street Workhouse, 15 beds for "old helpless women" and 91 for "helpless sick men" (a total of 13 percent). Dependent patients might not always be placed with sick inmates. In York Street Workhouse in Nottingham in 1841, 3 men suffering from paraplegia or spinal and hip disease were in the sick wards, while 3 with paralysis and 1 with spinal disease, plus 4 women with paralysis, were in wards in the workhouse.[108] In Battle workhouse in Reading, Berkshire, in 1873, half of the 189 inmates classed as "infirm or disabled" were in the infirmary and the others in the main workhouse building.[109]

Bedridden Wards in Birmingham Workhouse

As Birmingham had specific wards for those with disability, designated bedridden wards, identification of the more disabled section of non-able-bodied adults is possible. However, detailed recording of the medical condition of these inmates did not take place, but their proportion and the levels and nature of their disabilities can be determined. The first reference to these wards was in a list of appointments in April 1842, when Mary Ann Raven was appointed as nurse in No. 9 ward, the women's bedridden ward, at an annual salary of eight pounds. Dependent patients were also present in the women's infirm ward, where many were in a "helpless and weak state" and required as much attention during the night as in the daytime.[110] The men's bedridden ward did not have a designated nurse until 1848, with the appointment of Ann Brittain at a salary of ten pounds per annum, although she left two years later. The guardians recognized the need for the care of the bedridden, whom they considered "very helpless creatures" requiring a responsible person to assist them, and ensured that one nurse was appointed for each ward.[111] At that time, neither the guardians nor the medical officers regarded those in the bedridden wards as sick. In their recommendation in 1849 as to the maximum number of inmates the workhouse could accommodate, bedridden inmates were included among those in health. The bedridden wards consisted of seventy-three beds, making up 11 percent of total accommodation with 17 percent for those designated as healthy paupers; in addition, there were 160 beds for sick inmates and 95 for lunatics.[112]

Eight years after the opening of the new workhouse in 1852, accommodation in the bedridden wards proved insufficient and unoccupied children's dormitories were used to accommodate some of these patients. Overcrowding in the wards had more impact on male patients, with 36 in a ward meant to accommodate only 30.[113] The situation had deteriorated to such an extent that in May 1865, all 83 bedridden men were scattered throughout the workhouse with none of them in the appropriate ward. By contrast, all 63 bedridden women were in their designated ward, with seven beds vacant.[114] The following year, 141 (29 percent) of the 481 patients in the infirmary were described as bedridden. The medical officer was satisfied with the quality of the nursing care in the bedridden wards, pointing out that only 1 woman was suffering from "bed-sores" and these had been present on admission. The patient suffered from paralysis and had been provided with "water-cushions."[115] By the early 1870s, accommodation had been increased to 212 beds (98 for men and 114 for women), which were only 87 percent occupied, so that the bedridden patients made up 17 percent of all those in the infirmary.[116] However, severely disabled patients were to be found in other departments and not included in the bedridden numbers; for instance, the commissioner in lunacy had noted that 13 men in the wards for epileptics and lunatics were bedfast and, on another visit, 20 inmates in the same department were confined to bed.[117]

Table 1.11. Number of patients in the bedridden wards in Birmingham workhouse, 1865–1911

Year	Men	Women	Total	Comment
1865	83	63	146	31% older inmates
1866	77	64	141	29% sick inmates
1873	97	109	206	31% older inmates
				17% sick inmates
1885	134	154	288	21% sick inmates
1891	60	66	126	
1911	30	103	133	

Sources: BCL, VGPC, GP/B/2/8/1/4, May 22, 1865; GP/B/2/8/1/5, March 23, 1866; HSC, GP/B/2/3/3/3, June 3, 1873; VGPC, GP/B/2/8/1/9, August 14, 1885; HSC, GP/B/2/3/3/13, December 8, 1891; WMC, GP/B/2/3/6, June 16, 1911.

In 1885, the guardians discussed which inmates would need to be transferred from the workhouse to the proposed new infirmary. They suggested that the 288 patients in the bedridden wards should remain in the workhouse, as they required mainly nursing care and were not "classed under the head[ing] of sick."[118] The medical officer disagreed, assessing half the patients as requiring acute care and 144 beds were allocated for them in the infirmary. The guardians later decided that those patients who never or only occasionally required medication should be retained within the wards in the workhouse.[119] The 288 bedridden patients constituted 21 percent of the 1,353 inmates in the sick wards in the workhouse, but after the acute cases had been transferred to the infirmary, their number decreased to 126 by 1891.[120] They remained at this level into the twentieth century, but with a preponderance of female patients; for instance in 1911, there were 103 women but only 30 men. Until this time, there had been generally an equal number of bedridden patients of each sex, in contrast to the much greater number of men in the aged inmates' wards. Three years later, similar proportions (35 men and 112 women) continued to occupy the bedridden wards. However, there were also 84 men in the male chronic ward in the workhouse, plus 61 patients of unrecorded gender in the convalescent ward. Most of the patients in these two wards were "crippled" or suffering from cardiac or respiratory disease.[121]

Disabled patients in poor law institutions were usually included under the umbrella term of *infirm*, making it difficult to identify the extent of their disability.[122] Birmingham's designated bedridden wards were occupied by patients exhibiting varying degrees of dependence. In 1866, one-third were reported as able to "leave their beds and their rooms."[123] In 1891 it was planned to introduce the Brabazon scheme to give light work for old and infirm inmates. Of the 127 inmates considered unable to do the ordinary work of the house, in 65 men and 22 women it was due to age, in 16 men and 4 women to blindness, and in 6 men and 14 women to infirmity. Some of the 126 bedridden patients (60 men and 66 women) were able to do light work; one man was occupied in carving frames and 4 women who could knit and sew were able to do a share of housework.[124] The census of April that year recorded 11 men and 5 women as blind among the 1,184 inmates in the workhouse. Three of the men were in their forties or fifties and another 3 men and 2 women were over seventy years of age.[125] Blindness was a common cause of admission to the workhouse. For instance, in a study of residents of Herefordshire suffering from disability in 1851, Christine Jones found that the majority of those who were blind were receiving either indoor or outdoor relief. Ten years later, only 32 percent of blind adults were in work.[126] In 1873, there were 9 women in the "Blind Womens Room" in Birmingham, although only eight beds were provided.[127] By 1911, the levels of dependence had increased significantly as 68 of 71 women in two of the wards in the female bedridden department were described as "actually bedridden."[128] By the turn of the century, the bedridden wards in Birmingham could include younger disabled adult inmates, such as "chronic cripples and paralytics," as the medical officer considered that it was no longer the age of sixty years that determined whether "a man was able-bodied or infirm" but his physical condition. The change was prompted by the issue of a Local Government Board order relating to the dietaries of the various classes of inmates, in which the classification of inmates according to age was superseded by one based on their physical condition.[129] Following his appointment as medical superintendent in 1913, Dr. Frederick Ellis devised a scheme to improve the classification in the infirmary and workhouse, based mainly on physical ability. Inmates unable to work because of infirmity were classed as "The Infirm," but men between sixty and sixty-six years were allocated to this group only if "so physically crippled to merit infirm." "The Bedridden" group contained those who found it necessary to be in bed part of the day or at least part of some days during the week, as well as those who were in bed continuously and had no hope of improvement or where skilled nursing was unnecessary.[130]

The majority of inmates in the sick wards in the mid-nineteenth century suffered from chronic diseases such as consumption, bronchitis, paralysis, and debility.[131] The nature of the medical condition of the inmates in the workhouse infirmary prompted the *Birmingham Daily Mail* to comment, following a visit in 1885, "there are comparatively few really sick. It is not so much disease as decrepitude that has to be treated here; and not so much physic as food and nursing that is required." The article includes a description of the patients in one of the bedridden wards:

> Take for example the largest of female bed-ridden wards. It is a long apartment with 81 beds in it, 80 of which are now occupied. No measurement can give any idea of it, but imagine a room, not over lofty, with 81 beds as close as they can possibly be packed to allow room to pass between them, all filled with decrepit, withered, and haggard specimens of humanity in all stages of senile helplessness. Some are lying in their beds asleep, with the clothes drawn over their faces, inert and seemingly lifeless. Some are sitting crouched up in bed poring over scraps of periodicals. One or two are creeping about the room, getting about a bit.
>
> In this ward the beds run in four rows, with a low wooden partition between the two centre rows, and here are these people herded close together, with nothing to do but to gaze at one another, to grow callous to one another's sufferings, to see one by one their fellow inmates grow stiff and cold in their beds, and speculate upon whose turn it will be next. (*Birmingham Daily Mail*, July 20, 1885)

One reason for the increasing dependency levels was that the guardians had agreed that patients could be transferred from the infirmary to the workhouse for convalescence.[132] However, this resulted in the chronic and convalescent wards taking patients with severe disability and the workhouse medical officer commented in 1893 that these wards "were practically the same as the bedridden wards."[133] This arrangement did not prevent the female surgical wards becoming "chronically congested" at times with patients awaiting transfer.[134] Patients transferred to the convalescent wards suffered similar conditions to those already present in the workhouse, namely paralysis, blindness, deafness, and bronchitis.[135]

In the 1890s, Ebenezer Teichelmann, resident workhouse medical officer, spent a considerable part of his time treating women in the bedridden wards.[136] In 1906, Mr. Herbert, a Local Government Board inspector, urged the Birmingham guardians to transfer the bedridden patients to the infirmary as he felt their quality of life would be improved by the more highly skilled infirmary nurses.[137] Five years later, the Workhouse Management Committee was concerned that some of the bedridden cases required the attention of two nurses and would be better served by the nursing care provided in the infirmary.[138] Despite their concerns, the bedridden wards remained in the workhouse and were no longer considered part of the medical provision. In a national return of inmates occupying the wards for the sick in June 1896, Birmingham guardians declared 917 sick and bedridden patients in the separate infirmary, but none in the workhouse. However, there were 818 non-able-bodied adults in the workhouse at that time and some of those would have been in the bedridden wards, as they had not been transferred to the infirmary.[139] Nevertheless, it is clear they were no longer regarded as requiring medical care, an attitude that prevailed elsewhere. The medical officer at Battle workhouse in the first decade of the twentieth century attributed overcrowding in the infirmary to the number of infirm inmates who needed attention, but not medical treatment or skilled nursing.[140] This viewpoint was also reflected in the decision by the Birmingham guardians to change the designation of officers employed in the workhouse wards from nurses to attendants. However, they were forced to rescind this a few months later because of the difficulty in retaining sufficient staff.[141] The bedridden wards remained in the workhouse and, from early in the twentieth century, the movement of patients was from the infirmary to the workhouse, where the chronic and convalescent wards became occupied by inmates who suffered from severe disability. At times, the infirmary was required to take bedridden patients from the workhouse when it was overcrowded, but always on the understanding they would return in due course.[142]

In Ellis's scheme for classification of the indoor poor in 1914, he considered it essential for the economic administration of the infirmary that "chronic cases" not requiring medical or nursing skill should be removed to the workhouse. He gave examples of patients with leg ulcers and chronic sores. There were three male and three female wards in the infirmary for chronic cases, where patients could receive treatment for a "fair length" of time, namely for several months. He estimated that up to fifty-five of such patients could be transferred at that time.[143] The transfer of chronically disabled patients from acute hospitals and infirmaries became standard practice nationally. According to Weisz, as hospitals became more medicalized, they frequently denied admission to "chronics" on the grounds that there was nothing medically that could be done and beds should be reserved for those who might benefit from medical treatment.[144] Poor law infirmaries could not refuse admission to paupers and so needed to make transfer arrangements. For example, Leicester poor law infirmary at North Evington transferred patients to the local workhouse, despite the infirmary having infirm wards for patients not requiring "sick nursing." Bedridden patients and those suffering for paralysis were among those sent to the workhouse, where the medical officer described their move as inappropriate.[145] One of the reasons in defense of this practice given by the chief medical officer in 1930 was that the continued presence of such patients in a hospital would lower medical and nursing standards throughout the institution.[146] This policy cemented Birmingham workhouse's role as the provider of care for older patients and those with chronic illnesses and disabilities and led to its development into a specialized geriatric hospital in 1948.[147] In that year, the Birmingham Chronic Hospital Survey reported that nearly half of the male patients and just below two-thirds of the women in the hospital were bedridden.[148] According to Weisz, poor law institutions such as Birmingham workhouse became seen "as a dumping ground for indigent elderly and chronically ill people."[149] The practice of removing long-stay patients from the acute hospitals gave rise to the division in British hospital medicine between a voluntary sector that dominated acute care and a public sector in which the older, "chronic" patient was located.[150]

Dependent Patients in Wolverhampton

The ability to identify severely disabled patients in the Birmingham poor law records has aided the understanding of the establishment of chronic hospitals within the National Health Service, but it has been more difficult to determine how smaller workhouses, such as Wolverhampton, managed these patients. In Wolverhampton, the wards, as recorded in master's journal in 1842, were for able-bodied inmates or old men and old women, plus infirmary wards.[151] However, the guardians' minutes contain a reference to an "aged infirm women's" ward and, ten years later, to male and female infirm wards, but it is uncertain how dependent inmates in these wards were.[152] Around this time, Mr. Dunn and his children were allowed to leave the workhouse, but his wife, who was paralyzed and partially disabled, remained as she was in constant danger of falling into the fire. He was unable to earn sufficient money to pay for a nurse to take care of her at home, but he agreed to a weekly payment to the guardians of two shillings and six pence.[153] Bedridden patients were first mentioned by the workhouse medical officer in 1863 when he transferred them out of the cottages in order to use these buildings for patients with smallpox.[154] As in Birmingham, the workhouse was overcrowded in 1866, when there were around 260 sick and infirm inmates (36 percent of the total), of whom 200 were considered by the medical officer to be chronic cases, unlikely ever to leave the workhouse.[155] The lack of sufficient accommodation may have been the reason for 10 "crippled or infirm" men residing in the able-bodied ward.[156] When a correspondent from *Wolverhampton Chronicle* visited the sick wards twenty years later, a man aged over eighty years of age had been an inmate for more than forty years, while some of the very old women were bedridden.[157] When Edward Smith, medical officer of the Poor Law Board, visited the infirmary in 1867, there was an eleven-bed ward for "aged and incurable" females, and two similar-sized wards for paralytic males and females.[158] However, the occupants of these wards get no mention in the guardians' records.

In 1882 around 850 (about 90 percent) inmates were incapable of work with 12 men partially disabled and 106 "actually bedridden."[159] Toward the end of the century, 83 of the 225 patients in the infirmary were described as requiring "everything done for them" and 16 children were included in that number. The following year, 149 of the 233 patients required "special attention" by medical and nursing staff and 18 were "quite helpless." One reason for the high levels of dependency was that a large proportion of patients had been sent from other institutions to the workhouse as incurable.[160] One of those may have been Mary Ann Wilkes, an illegitimate child of thirteen years, suffering from "Spinal Caries" and hip joint disease. At the medical officer's instigation, the guardians agreed to her transfer to the Royal Alexandria Children's Hospital in Rhyl and pay eight shillings weekly toward her keep.[161] In the new workhouse in 1903, wards for partially able-bodied and older adults could accommodate 440 inmates (66 percent of the accommodation for non-sick inmates). The infirmary had 280 beds for surgical, medical, and chronic cases out of a total of 502.[162] However, the "mental and epileptic wards" contained sick and bedridden patients, who were to receive diets similar to those of patients in the infirmary.[163] In 1912, Mr. L. W. Riley successfully applied for the admission of his "paralysed wife" to the infirmary, contributing ten shillings and six pence for her keep.[164] The guardians obviously considered her admission appropriate, at a time when such patients were thought inappropriate in Birmingham infirmary. There is no further information on patients with chronic diseases in the new workhouse and Wolverhampton workhouse appears typical of most poor law institutions in not facilitating identification of this particular group of inmates. With no separation between infirmary and workhouse, the institution developed into a single general hospital.

Acute Medical Care

Where a geographically separate infirmary was established, two distinct institutions evolved in the early twentieth century. Brian Abel-Smith has made the point that in urban areas, patients were divided into those with acute illnesses, who went to the infirmary, and the chronic sick, who went to the

Table 1.12. Number of "casualty cases" admitted to Birmingham infirmary, 1904–10

Year	1904	1905	1906	1907	1908	1909	1910
Number	78	135	177	248	271	364	480

Source: BCL, Infirmary Management Committee, GP/B/2/4/4/5, January 24, 1910; GP/B/2/4/4/6, January 9, 1911.

workhouse.[165] By the early twentieth century, Birmingham infirmary had adopted the role of a general hospital, becoming the institution for acute medical care, admitting patients with such conditions as pneumonia, typhoid, and rheumatic heart disease. However, as Otto Kauffman, visiting physician, admitted, the majority of patients continued to have chronic conditions, particularly tuberculosis.[166] The medical superintendent's scheme in 1913 to transfer patients with long-term conditions to the workhouse after an initial stay in the infirmary was designed to emphasize the infirmary's role as an acute-care facility.[167] By giving preference to acute illnesses and excluding older and disabled patients, he attempted to emulate the policies of the voluntary hospitals.

To emphasize its acute role, the infirmary admitted an increasing number of patients involved in accidents across the first decade of the twentieth century (table 1.12).[168] Of the 480 accident cases admitted in 1910, 295 were discharged on the same day and 184 detained as inpatients. The accidents had occurred at home, at work, or in the street in 359 cases, while the police had brought in the remaining patients.[169] In 1907, Henry Manton, a Birmingham guardian, described it as a "casualty hospital," as it could not refuse to admit those who had suffered accidents, given its position in the center of the city and surrounded by factories. Three-quarters of admissions were admitted directly to the infirmary, rather than via the workhouse, and many were not paupers. Manton cited the example of a lady who sustained an accident while riding her bicycle and was admitted for three weeks. Her husband made a voluntary financial contribution for her care.[170]

However, patients involved in accidents had been brought directly to the workhouse before the early twentieth century. For instance, among inmates involved in accidents admitted to Leicester workhouse in 1873 were one with a fracture of the thigh, one with fractured ribs, and four with fractures of the arm.[171] In the 1840s, Thomas Wilshaw was brought to Wolverhampton workhouse having fallen from the shafts of a van, which had then passed over his body. Although the medical officer was in immediate attendance, he died in less than an hour after arrival. A week later, another man was brought after being run over by a vehicle and received attention from the medical officer.[172] A few years earlier, Samuel Highland had been admitted after fracturing his leg.[173] George Roberts was admitted in 1855 after having cut his throat, which required suturing and bandaging.[174] Paupers also suffered injuries, both accidental and deliberate, while resident in the workhouse. In Wolverhampton workhouse, Thomas James Lovatt was scalded while taking a bath and died two days later from "shock," while Martha Forrester, aged eighty-four years, fell on the old women's ward, fracturing her thigh.[175] A similar occurrence happened in Birmingham workhouse to an old man, Edward Heap, who was pushed over, dislocating his hip, while eighty-four-year-old James Potter was injured by a tile falling from the roof of the aged men's ward.[176] In 1886, sixty-eight-year-old William Peters, who suffered from mental illness, managed to obtain a knife, with which he deliberately cut his abdomen, showing the need for careful supervision of such patients as they were prone to attempt suicide and self-harm.[177]

Surgery

The practice of surgery was revolutionized in the middle of the nineteenth century with the development of inhalation anesthesia and antiseptic techniques, which have been hailed by some as the greatest innovations ever made in medical theory or practice.[178] Although they made more complex surgery possible, the most commonly performed surgical procedures were amputation, setting fractures, and treating wounds. In the period up to World War I, surgery has been designated localistic, with the emphasis on resection of tumors, inflammations, and injuries.[179] The operations carried out in Birmingham workhouse are an accurate reflection of this period, although more complex surgery took place from the 1880s (table 1.13). The common perception that surgeons in the preanesthetic era were limited in the number of procedures they could undertake and in the time available to perform each operation has been challenged by Peter Stanley in his history of British surgery.[180] However, Brand and Price maintain that surgical operations were performed in the workhouse in many unions without anesthesia despite the fact that anesthetics were in use in hospitals from the 1860s.[181] This was made possible since the Local Government Board did not approve their use in the treatment of inmates until the 1890s. However, anesthesia is recorded as being used during surgery in Birmingham workhouse as early as 1858.[182]

A few instances of minor surgery in Wolverhampton workhouse have been recorded. In 1855, Richard Nugent lanced Arthur Belcher's lumbar abscess and applied poultices. When George Roberts was admitted having cut his throat, Nugent sutured and bandaged it, later applying poultices with astringent lotions.[183] Later surgery involved the removal of "gravel" in the bladder of four-year-old Henry Weckman in 1861 and "shot" from the abdomen of Samuel Perks in 1900.[184] There were few surgical patients in Wolverhampton in the decades after the New Poor Law, with only one out of a total of 285 sick inmates on one day in mid-December 1869. This contrasts with Birmingham, where there were 55 acute and 56 chronic surgical patients, each type corresponding to 8 percent of total patients, compared with the national figures of 6 percent and 10 percent.[185] A similar position occurred in Reading Union workhouse, with 4 acute (5 percent) and 8 chronic (10 percent) surgical patients out of a total of 79. This was despite a ruling by the guardians the year previously that all paupers with fractures and all emergency cases should be directed straight to Royal Berkshire Hospital, for which purpose they increased their annual subscription from six to ten guineas.[186]

Birmingham guardians required the medical officer to seek their consent for inmates to have surgery and preferred them to be transferred to the General Hospital for the operation. This ensured that the decision to carry out surgery was approved by more than one surgeon.[187] When amputation of Mary Norton's leg because of "disease of the knee" was recommended to the guardians in 1851 and of the arm of the "man, Trafford" for a diseased elbow in 1854, they suggested further surgical opinions.[188] The guardians' position was challenged by one workhouse medical officer, Redfern Davies, when he amputated Edward Waite's leg in the workhouse without permission, although he eventually had to concede he would do so again only in an emergency (table 1.13).[189] However, Davies had performed other surgical procedures in the workhouse prior to that time and published details in medical journals. The following decade, Davies's successor, Edmund Robinson, declared that there were hardly any surgical cases in the workhouse and "capital operations" did not take place there.[190] However, he found it necessary to amputate John Walsh's leg for malignant disease in the workhouse in 1867, as he was too ill to be transferred to hospital (table 4.8). By the mid-1880s, the number of operations in the workhouse had increased, but after the opening of the new infirmary at the end of the decade, details of the surgery performed there are mostly available from published case reports, which contain the more difficult and rarer cases, rather than routine surgical procedures.[191] Nevertheless, Dr. Stuart, assistant surgeon, performed forty-five major and ten minor operations over a three-month period in 1913.[192] At that time, the surgeons had the benefit of X-ray apparatus, which proved invaluable in confirming a suspected kidney stone in a man admitted with vague abdominal symptoms. Jordan Lloyd successfully removed the stone and the patient was discharged cured. Another successful removal was possible after X-ray confirmed the exact site and extent of tuberculous disease in the bone of a patient's foot. The machine was also useful in the diagnosis of the large number of cases being admitted with suspected fractures.[193] Wolverhampton workhouse medical officers did not publish case reports, but Woodward Riley, while acting as deputy to Henry Gibbons, did so in 1870. He repaired successfully a small femoral hernia in David B., a ninety-year-old inmate, after attempts at reduction had failed. He administered chloroform himself as he was "rather pressed for time."[194] In all the operations listed in table 1.13, anesthesia was used in the form of chloroform or ether and was administered by an assisting surgeon. However, it was not without risk to the patient. Edwin Loach, a seventy-five-year-old inmate in Birmingham workhouse in 1888, died during the administration of chloroform prior to a proposed amputation for necrosis of the bones of his left thumb following an injury.[195]

At the beginning of the twentieth century, the infirmary in Birmingham took on more acute medical work and became more akin to a general hospital. For the twelve months to May that same year, 1,137 surgical cases had been admitted, representing 34 percent of all admissions.[196] The number of operations carried out in Wolverhampton workhouse at the beginning of the twentieth century can be estimated from the record of payment to a second surgeon for administering anesthetics. It increased from 4 in 1901 to 42 in 1902, but decreased to 14 in 1903 as the appointment of a resident medical officer for the workhouse in that year allowed the anesthetic to be given by him without additional payment.[197] Although surgical operations were uncommon in both workhouses in the mid-1880s, this form of medical care gradually increased in frequency and importance into the twentieth century.

A Visit to the Workhouse Infirmary

Poor law historian Kim Price has claimed that workhouse infirmaries provided a level of care that was almost half a century behind that practiced in voluntary hospitals.[198] However, there have been no direct comparisons, but what we do have is the opinion of a surgeon to a voluntary hospital during a visit to the workhouse infirmary in Birmingham. Beatrice Martha Webb was a medical student at Birmingham University, graduated in medicine from the University of Edinburgh, and carried out a research project to gain her medical doctorate from Birmingham in 1908. The following year she

Table 1.13. Operations performed in Birmingham infirmary, 1859–92

Date	Surgeon	Patient	Operation	Outcome
June 1858	Redfern Davies	Henry Bagotts 8 years	Removal of glandular enlargement in neck	Breathing improved
December 1858	Redfern Davies	Male 17 years	Compression of varicocele	Radical cure
February 1859	Redfern Davies	Patrick Coyne 32 years	Drainage and repair of hydrocele	Radical cure
June 1859	Redfern Davies	Edward Waite	Amputation of leg	Patient died
December 1860	Redfern Davies	E.S. (female)	Repair of prolapse of uterus	Successful
January 1867	Edmund Robinson	John Walsh	Amputation of leg for disease of knee	Successful
May 1872	Adam Simpson	Richard Windsor 57 years	Repair of strangulated hernia	Patient died
June 1887	Jordan Lloyd	B. (female) 47 years	For acute intestinal obstruction due to incarcerated loop of bowel	Complete recovery
May 1889	Jordan Lloyd	Catherine B. 38 years	For subacute intestinal obstruction due to cancer of colon	Colostomy; tumor inoperable
January 1891	Ebenezer Teichelmann	A.R. (female) 22 years	Removal of ruptured pyo-salpynx and ovary	Complete recovery
May 1892	Jordan Lloyd	M.A.H. (female) 40 years	Colpo-hysterectomy for cancer of cervix of uterus	Successful

Note: The outcome is as defined by the surgeon.

Sources: BCL, BBG, GP/2/1/23, June 8, 1859, VGPC, GP/B/2/8/1/6, May 10, 1872; Davies, "Birmingham Workhouse Infirmary" (1858), 284; Davies, "Birmingham Workhouse Infirmary" (1859), 677; Davies, "On the Radical Cure of Varicocele," 60; Davies, "Remarks on the Operative and Mechanical Treatment of Prolapsus Uteri," 407; Lloyd, "On Acute Intestinal Obstruction and Its Treatment by Abdominal Section, with Illustrative Cases," 996, 844, 1891; Anonymous, "Birmingham Workhouse Infirmary: A Case of Peritonitis Following Parturition," 1276–77; Lloyd, "Reports on Medical and Surgical Practice in the Hospitals and Asylums of Great Britain, Ireland, and the Colonies: Birmingham Workhouse Infirmary," 16.

was appointed honorary surgeon to the Birmingham Lying-in Charity and Women's Hospital. On a visit on September 27, 1908, to one of her research patients who had been admitted to Birmingham infirmary, she recorded her impression of the care delivered, giving us a glimpse of life on the ward:

My Tuesday pat. [patient] was in the Workhouse Infirmary, a place I have often wanted to penetrate into. Our pat. is there not because we operated on a fibroma but because she has some paralysis of her left side and she comes of a class that finds the workhouse or the infirmary the fitting place for its useless members. She is an unmarried woman in early middle life and for such there is not cover when earning powers are gone. Just now she is in the infirmary rather than 'the house' because she has developed a cardiac condition. It is a huge place, the main corridor, down which one looks from end to end, is ¼ mile long and from it all the pavilions go off. It is a three-storey building and in a very compact space it has 1800 beds, five times as many as at the General. The H.P. [House Physician] to the physician in charge of this ward (Dr Short, I regret to say) met me and took me through the building. He has about 150–200 beds in hand but I was delighted to see that he really did take notes and I understand from Sister that it was so all round (I am afraid I had suspected him of taking them because I was coming) and indeed another chance bed I walked up to had equally good notes. Sister showed me her ward, open windows, open fires, bed quilts, pictures, plants, flowers, every thing pretty much as in a rather economical hospital and not more than 38 beds in the wards as compared with our 26. But the class of pat. is different, mostly wrecks. It was tea time and a very large number were sitting at a table (and having jam as a treat). In cotton gowns and red shawls. They are the homeless, or they are not wanted, those not likely to earn a living again, the elderly who have given up the fight, and they are not looking forward to getting well and going out, for there is little if anything in the way of home to go to, and going out may only mean going across the grounds into 'the house.' You feel at once how different from the hosp. where everyone has a home and is going back to it. Visiting day can't be the joy it is in hosp. when the visitors are probably the people who ought not to have let you go to the infirmary—or so you think—and a visiting day a fortnight, which sounds a harsh rule, may meet the case. Sister says they come in starving and yet they grumble at the food. But of course they do, for the nearer you live to the starvation line the more your money goes on fried fish and pickled onions, tinned lobster and chip potatoes, and how should you appreciate Irish stew with oatmeal porridge, boiled pots and bread and dripping. I took my pat. a substantive plum cake of Pattinson's and Sister was very nice about it and would see she had it, with her neighbours. The poor soul was pathetic, a dull stupid patient woman who would just have got along somehow in her factory but for the paralysis which came on shortly before her op. Sister was a pleasant woman of the ordinary hosp. type and I am sure she tries to keep her difficult charges content. (Royal College of Physicians of London, MS84, "Medical School Letters," 6:20–24)

The Medicalization of the Workhouse

Sick paupers were not identified as a distinct group within the poor law system before 1910 and not separated out in official statistics until 1913. Thus, information regarding acutely ill inmates is difficult to obtain from government publications so the extent of medical activity within workhouses remains unclear. This chapter has revealed that a substantial amount of medical treatment of paupers took place in Birmingham workhouse's Town Infirmary prior to the New Poor Law and in the years immediately following it. Although the proportion of sick inmates in Wolverhampton workhouse was half that in Birmingham in the early years after the New Poor Law, patients with a range of acute conditions were treated and the proportion matched Birmingham's by the mid-1840s. In the early decades after the New Poor Law, both workhouses contained a higher proportion of sick inmates than most similar-sized workhouses, possibly due to the industrial nature of the towns, as workhouses with higher percentages of patients were usually urban manufacturing towns or seaports. Surprisingly, the average share of sick inmates in the counties for Wolverhampton (Staffordshire) and Birmingham (Warwickshire) was almost as high as in the towns themselves despite the rural nature of many parts of the counties. However, within each county there was a wide variation between workhouses that did not appear to be related to the local economy. Indeed, welfare historian Hilary Marland found great variability between similar types of union within the West Riding of Yorkshire. By 1870, Wakefield Union had made great progress toward establishing an effective medical relief service, while Huddersfield guardians were reluctant to take on the responsibility for providing a hospital service.[199] Despite this, around one—quarter of inmates in both unions' workhouses were sick, although three times as many in Wakefield were acutely ill.[200] The variability, both between and within regions, remained unchanged into the twentieth century when there continued to be "every possible variety in the character and efficiency of their [urban unions] provision for the sick."[201]

The workhouse also played a major role in caring for those suffering from chronic illnesses similar to those experienced by patients in long-term institutional care today and with a similar wide range of disability levels. However, Birmingham and Wolverhampton guardians differed in how they managed arrangements for their welfare within the two workhouses, contradicting the traditional interpretation of the history of disability as one of a single process gradually progressing toward increased social participation.[202] Many disabled inmates remained in the workhouse for long periods of time;

for instance, 7 percent of Birmingham workhouse's inmates had spent more than five years in the institution in 1861.[203] The relative neglect of those in the bedridden wards in the guardians' records needs to be seen in the context of the medical model of disability. Chronic diseases did not arouse the interest of the medical profession to the same degree as acute illnesses, nor did they improve the profile of the infirmary as much as acute care.[204] Nevertheless, disability historian Deborah Stone has suggested that disability as an administrative category arose from the classification system of the New Poor Law with the "sick, aged and infirm" classes giving rise to today's concept of disability.[205] Furthermore, workhouse medical officers were responsible for the assessment and allocation within the classification system and for determining inmates' ability to work. This poor law medical practice explains how the concept of disability became associated with clinical medicine and how medical practitioners became "gatekeepers for disability verification" in the twentieth century.[206]

Despite the increase in the number of inmates in Birmingham and Wolverhampton workhouses as the century progressed, it is difficult to ascertain a point in time at which they had become significant medical spaces. There is a consensus that an extensive system of poor law health care had developed in provincial England by the end of the nineteenth century. However, exactly when the workhouse became more medicalized is disputed by historians. Some maintain that a well-established medical service was in place by the eighteenth century, while others take the contrary view that, under the Old Poor Law, there was only a rudimentary medical service for the poor.[207] Indeed, Crowther suggests that the provincial workhouse was hardly ever used as "a centre for the sick" before 1834.[208] The lack of appreciation of this function of the workhouse has been challenged by Siena with regard to London. He asserts that workhouses in the capital provided a significant level of institutional health care by the early eighteenth century.[209] He cites St. Margaret's workhouse in London, which increased its provision of sickrooms substantially within two years of its erection in 1725.[210] He is supported in this view by Boulton, Davenport, and Schwarz, who estimated that around 20 percent of inmates in St. Martin's in the Fields workhouse were sick in 1817–18. However, London's response to the poor laws was different from that in the provinces, with its greater reliance on institutional care. Furthermore, the development of the majority of its workhouses occurred in the eighteenth rather than the nineteenth century.[211] The situation outside the metropolis remains uncertain, but the proportion of sick inmates (17 percent) in the urban workhouse in Birmingham in the third quarter of 1818 equates its medical role with that of London workhouses.[212]

Thus, Birmingham was providing a prominent medical service in its poor law institution in the early nineteenth century and it maintained it into the first decade after 1834.[213]

This chapter has contributed a rare positive view of the character of medical practice in the workhouse and of its role within the medical provision for local communities. It has shown that urban provincial workhouses were medicalized earlier than has previously been recognized. Although there is no doubt that workhouses and their infirmaries took on more medical work as the nineteenth century progressed, it was not a steadily progressive development and a significant medical role occurred at different times in different workhouses. This will become more apparent as we address in the next chapter the role that workhouses played in the management of patients with communicable diseases.

Chapter Two

Segregating Fever Patients

Nineteenth-century Britain was characterized by epidemics and the wide-spread prevalence of infectious diseases. They were the most common causes of morbidity and mortality and with the exclusion of bronchitis and pneumonia accounted for 33 percent of deaths in the years 1848–72 in England and Wales.[1] When these respiratory diseases are included, infection was the cause of 48 percent of deaths nationally in 1851–60.[2] Communicable diseases were more prevalent in areas wherever people were crowded together and rapid urban growth occurred in the early nineteenth century, and its associated problems of sewerage and water supply multiplied the risk of infection. Thus, urban environments became more unhealthy and allowed diseases to become endemic.[3] According to Anne Hardy, there grew up within these areas "fever nests," from where the Victorians feared that epidemics could escape and spread to the rest of the population.[4] For example, Whitechapel was considered the "nucleus of the metropolitan fever field," while Southwark held the same status within the cholera field in London.[5]

The mortality rate from infectious diseases declined markedly in the second half of the nineteenth century, both in absolute terms and in relative importance among all causes of disease. In 1901–10, they accounted for only 19 percent of all deaths.[6] This mortality decline was accompanied by an epidemiological transition, with degenerative diseases such as cardiovascular disease and cancer replacing pandemics of infection as primary causes of morbidity and mortality.[7] This shift in disease patterns, with a progressive decline in infectious diseases, began in the mid-eighteenth century, but a more marked fall in overall mortality rate in England and Wales took place from the middle of the following century. The reasons for the mortality decline have long been a contentious issue among historians and epidemiologists. Abdel Omran, who first proposed the theory of "epidemiologic" transition, ascribed the decline of infection in western European societies to socioeconomic factors, augmented by the sanitary revolution in the late nineteenth century.[8] The work of Thomas McKeown has been influential in stressing the primary reason as the improving nutritional status of the population.[9] However, Simon Szreter argues that preventive public health provision and services were more important in explaining the mortality decline.[10] Hardy's view is that no one factor was of overriding importance in reducing death rates, but the measures taken by the preventive authorities made a fundamental contribution.[11] In a recent reinterpretation of the epidemiological transition, historian Andrew Mercer emphasizes the role of preventive measures and public health interventions in the virtual elimination of the major epidemic diseases. He also argues that the original concept of the transition as one of replacing one group of distinct diseases by another is an oversimplification due to the interrelationship between infection and chronic diseases.[12]

An integral component of preventive policy to combat infectious diseases was the development of fever and smallpox hospitals to provide facilities for isolation. Indeed, the historiography of infectious diseases is most often set in the context of the general development of the public health movement, rather than in terms of their impact on local communities. The Sanitary Act of 1866 empowered sanitary authorities to build hospitals and the Public Health Act of 1875 permitted compulsory isolation of patients in institutions. However, the development of isolation hospitals by local authorities was slow and only one-fifth had made any provision by the 1890s, although the smallpox epidemics gave a degree of impetus.[13] An important policy development that promoted isolation in the late nineteenth century was the notification of certain infectious diseases. For instance, after notification was implemented in Birmingham, the number of admissions for scarlet fever in 1890–93 was as great as in the preceding fifteen years.[14] A further stimulus to hospital development was provided by the Isolation Hospitals Act of 1893, enabling local governments to build their own isolation hospitals from public funds and to remove forcibly patients with infectious diseases to these hospitals. Nevertheless, the geography of hospital provision remained very uneven across the country.[15] Additionally, until the 1880s, fever hospitals were small, usually containing around seventy beds.[16] Thus, the task of coping with patients with infectious diseases fell to the poor law authorities and this provides the theme for this chapter. As Edmund Robinson, medical officer at Birmingham workhouse, succinctly put it in 1866, "the workhouse as a matter of course is the receptacle for all classes of disease."[17]

The chapter will consider the arrangements for admitting paupers with infectious diseases to either the workhouse infirmary or the local isolation hospital and will explore the extent of cooperation between the guardians and the sanitary authorities or town councils. On the basis of mortality data, it has been suggested that workhouses must have been efficient at preventing the admission of paupers with infectious diseases.[18] However, this study demonstrates that poor law medical facilities were an essential component of the management and treatment of communicable diseases in the nineteenth and early twentieth centuries in the prevention of the spread of infectious diseases within the local community. As such, the medical role of the workhouse provided a service to the community beyond its poor law function. The workhouse's role in managing infectious diseases will be considered from the standpoints of the impact of a number of childhood infections; the outbreaks and epidemics of cholera, typhoid, and smallpox; and the prevalence of endemic diseases, such as typhus and puerperal fever. In each case, the contribution of the workhouse infirmaries in Birmingham and Wolverhampton was substantial. Any attempts by guardians to prevent admission or seek alternative institutions for paupers were based mainly on the concern that infection introduced into the workhouse might affect the incumbent inmates. Workhouses had a reputation as contagious spaces, but whether spread of infection within them due to overcrowding and unhygienic conditions took place is, according to Ruth Hodgkinson, "a moot point," but she gave one example of a serious outbreak of cholera in Leeds workhouse in 1834, at a time where there were few cases in the town.[19] Before turning to individual diseases, we must first consider the arrangements for accommodating fever patients.

Fever Wards

The most striking manifestation of infectious diseases was fever, which remained acceptable as a diagnosis as late as the end of the nineteenth century. The distinguished eighteenth-century Edinburgh physician William Cullen identified the three stages of fever as debility, chill, and heat, and defined it as a disease in itself when it was not associated with another identifiable disease process.[20] In the 1860s, it was classified clinically according to the temperature pattern into acute, intermittent, or continuous types, while the presence of a rash would aid a more precise diagnosis.[21] In English and Welsh workhouses in 1869, a one-day survey of inmates under the care of medical officers revealed that 12 percent of sick inmates suffered from an infectious disease and 25 percent of those were identified by the type of fever only.[22]

From the early eighteenth century some workhouses set aside special wards for inmates with infectious diseases. However, it was not until the mid-nineteenth century that guardians of provincial workhouses felt the need to provide detached buildings for the isolation of inmates with infective conditions.[23] For example, Battle workhouse in Reading, erected in 1867, could accommodate fever cases in a small, detached building, which was enlarged three years later to hold twenty-four patients. An additional isolation facility, the "Infectious Hut Hospital," was erected in 1881, consisting of two wards, each with three beds.[24] Two workhouses in Warwickshire erected temporary fever wards or sheds during the 1847 typhus outbreak and two others either planned new isolation facilities or identified properties for isolation during the 1871 smallpox epidemic.[25] However, the significant role of provincial workhouses in caring for patients with infectious diseases and in providing additional facilities to cope with epidemics has been largely neglected. The historiography of institutions for infectious diseases is sparse and has concentrated on isolation hospitals, especially those established in London, following the Metropolitan Poor Act in 1867. The act set up the Metropolitan Asylum Board to manage isolation hospitals and lunatic asylums, rather than local boards of guardians, and provided centralized funding from the capital's poor rates. This system of care for infectious diseases remained unique to London and consequently provincial English isolation hospitals have been neglected within historical accounts and workhouse histories contain only brief reference to isolation facilities.

In the early 1840s, the medical officer of Wolverhampton Union's workhouse called for a detached building to isolate inmates with infectious diseases, as he was apprehensive that typhus fever affecting a woman in the lying-in ward might rapidly spread throughout the workhouse.[26] Although new fever wards were provided, they had become so overcrowded five years later that beds had to be pushed together to allow three inmates to sleep in two beds. This followed a marked increase in the number of "fever patients" admitted, for instance, in the midsummer quarter in 1847, patients suffering from fever constituted 66 percent of the 593 patients admitted.[27] As a result, sheds were converted with canvas curtains as walls instead of board to be used as fever wards. However, three months later the master reported that the "sheds were full of fever cases" and the guardians decided that temporary sheds covered with calico could be erected if fever cases were admitted. Clearly, the guardians were committed to responding to outbreaks of infectious diseases by providing additional space to accommodate sufferers. A larger building accommodating between 40 and 50 patients with infectious diseases was needed twenty years later.[28]

In the spring of 1847, the medical officers in Birmingham workhouse also requested immediate separate provision for fever cases because of

Table 2.1. Inmates in fever wards in Birmingham workhouse on one day in various months in 1847

Month	Total inmates	Sick inmates		Sick inmates with fever	
March	644	186	29%	55	30%
May	684	229	33%	69	30%
June	753	345	46%	130	38%
September	689	233	34%	69	30%

Source: BCL, BBG, GP/B/2/1/5, March 8, May 10, and October 12, 1847.

overcrowding so that in some instances, two patients occupied the same bed. At that time, there were 55 patients out of a total of 186 suffering from "contagious fever" and the majority were Irish. The admission of fever patients peaked over the next few months (table 2.1). Interestingly, at the height of the epidemic, nearly half (46 percent) of all inmates were suffering from some form of ailment. The guardians responded initially by converting nearby premises to provide 35 places; then sought permission to convert property they had already purchased to give an additional 120 places. Because of continuing overcrowding and the urgent need for separate provision for fever cases, they shortlisted three possibilities to open as a "Fever Hospital": White Lead Works, New Town Brewery, Dr. Church's late residence. Unfortunately, we don't know which they chose. The likely cause of fever was typhus as 125 of the 500 deaths in the workhouse in 1847 were attributed to "Irish fever." In addition, one district surgeon, three nurses, seven pauper assistant nurses, and the schoolmaster died of the infection.[29]

Detached buildings for the admission of patients with fever and infectious diseases, separate from the main infirmary, were included in the plans for the second Birmingham workhouse erected in 1852.[30] However, twelve years later, the workhouse medical officer declared these wards inadequate "according to the advanced state of sanitary science," as they were too close to the general infirmary and had to be accessed via the workhouse. He suggested two wards built "side by side" to give efficient ventilation and these provided fifty beds for each sex when built two years later.[31] When the second workhouse in Wolverhampton opened in 1903, it also had two wards for twenty patients of each sex with infectious diseases within the infirmary buildings, which were designed in the pavilion style. There was an additional "Isolation Hospital" with two two-bed wards, two nurses' rooms, and three single bedrooms.[32] However, little information is available on the arrangements for infectious patients in the separate infirmary built on the site of the Birmingham workhouse in 1889, although the "infectious wards" were allocated a larger area per patient than the general wards.[33]

Childhood Infections

In the mid-nineteenth century 60 percent of deaths of children aged between one and four years old resulted from airborne infectious diseases.[34] Susceptibility to these infections was accepted as an inevitable part of childhood in Victorian Britain and institutional care would rarely have been considered necessary for the management of the disease process. Nevertheless, children did get admitted to workhouses because of childhood infections, although it was more likely that these diseases were contracted after admission for other reasons, either orphanhood or with their whole family. The infections that were responsible for most of childhood morbidity and death in nineteenth-century Britain were measles, whooping cough, scarlet fever, and diphtheria. They were highly transmittable diseases by personal contact with infected individuals or by airborne droplets, had high fatality rates, and were common in crowded conditions, such as schools and workhouses. The most contagious was measles, a viral infection that almost always produced clinical disease in those infected.[35] Secondary bacterial infection was responsible for 80 percent of deaths and could result in long-term disability in those who survived. The mortality rate was highest in the first two years of life and remained unchanged throughout the century.[36] Little action was taken to reduce the death rate until the 1880s, but even then, it was unaffected by preventive services. It was also highest in large towns, as the disease required a certain density of population to become established as endemic. Its prevalence and severity in any one community also may have been related to the degree of overcrowding and the level of malnutrition.

Birmingham guardians were concerned that Bridget Hunt's children, who had been admitted to the workhouse with their mother in 1856, were suffering from measles, despite being detected by the workhouse medical officer prior to admission. They urged that "infectious cases" should be managed on outdoor relief, no doubt fearful of rapid spread of the infection within the institution.[37] However, an outbreak of measles occurred in the workhouse with 24 cases in October 1876. They had to be managed within the inadequate workhouse accommodation, as the borough isolation hospital could not accept admissions of patients with measles.[38] Thereafter, a small number of cases were usually present up to 1911, even though the majority of children had resided in Marston Green Cottage Homes from 1880 (appendix

A). However, the year before they were transferred, there were 40 cases of measles on one day in March among the 621 children in the workhouse.[39] In four months in early 1886, 30 children contracted measles and in the first half of 1907, there were on average 6 cases in the infirmary.[40] There were greater numbers of cases occurring in the Lady Day and Midsummer quarters in the late nineteenth and early twentieth centuries, reflecting the peak incidence of the disease in the spring. For the year ending on May 31, 1910, 19 cases of measles were admitted to the infirmary out of a total of 3,338 patients.[41] In contrast, the presence of measles in Wolverhampton workhouse was only noted when three inmates suffered from the disease in February 1864 and a similar number in March 1891.[42] Yet, the disease was prevalent in the Borough of Wolverhampton. For example, between 1884 and 1889 reported cases varied between 300 and 1,100, with a median mortality rate of 6 percent, slightly higher than the national rate of around 4.5 percent.[43] Similarly, only 2 cases were recorded in any of the workhouses in the county of Worcestershire between 1834 and 1871 and both occurred in Droitwich, 1 in 1859 and the other ten years later.[44] The reason why sufferers from measles were not often found in these smaller workhouses may have been because poor parents rarely sought medical attention for their affected children, whereas the situation was different in Birmingham with its higher population density.[45]

The other highly contagious infection that was regarded as an almost universal experience in childhood was whooping cough, now known as pertussis. As a result, it was not subject to substantial preventive action throughout the nineteenth century.[46] It was the next most frequent cause of infant mortality after measles. The infection began with a catarrhal period, during which airborne transmission made it highly contagious. Thereafter, paroxysms of coughing developed, ending with a stridulous inspiratory "whoop."[47] When John Edwards, his wife, and six children applied to enter Wolverhampton workhouse in 1843, the medical officer confined them to the receiving ward so that they could be considered for out relief. The children had been diagnosed as having whooping cough and he wished to prevent it from spreading throughout the institution.[48] Whooping cough was a significant cause of death among infants in Wolverhampton in the 1890s, most frequently accounting for around 1 percent of deaths in children less than six years of age in the first quarter of each year, although in some years mortality could be as high as 9 percent.[49] Despite this, there is only one record of children being admitted, when in October 1893 eight were accommodated in one room without a fire.[50] The disease also gets no mention in the Birmingham guardians' records, despite being the most common childhood infection in the infirmary and being prevalent for the whole of the period covered in appendix A. The only recorded cases in Worcestershire workhouses were twelve children affected in an outbreak in Droitwich in 1868.[51] As with measles, parents did not feel the need to seek medical attention for the condition and the preventive authorities did not promote isolation in institutions. Nevertheless, like measles, sufferers were admitted to Birmingham workhouse.

One of the other great killers of very young children was scarlatina, or scarlet fever.[52] It was one of the most difficult diseases to diagnose clinically in its early stages and there was no diagnostic test.[53] Different strains of the bacteria have varying degrees of virulence and a more virulent strain became prevalent after 1830, leading to eight epidemics in the subsequent five decades.[54] Severe local epidemics, which occurred frequently, were usually associated with transmission due to infected milk.[55] A milder strain reappeared toward the end of the century, but epidemics continued into the next, occurring in 1901, 1907, and 1914. Nevertheless, the fatality rate fell by almost 50 percent—from 49 percent in the ten years after 1895 to 26 percent in the next decade.[56] In the epidemics in the 1860s and 1870s, the greatest number of deaths occurred in London, northern industrial cities, and the Black Country.[57] The mortality rate in England and Wales fell dramatically in the 1860s and had reduced by 81 percent by 1891.[58] The reduction was due to a combination of reduced virulence of the organism and measures to control the spread of infection. The disease was one of the first to have an active preventive policy applied to it in the form of institutional isolation, especially after the development of infectious disease hospitals from the 1870s.[59] Beds in these hospitals came to be dominated by scarlet fever patients by the end of the century; for example, they were the largest group in the City Fever Hospital, Edinburgh, between 1888 and 1892 and again in 1904, when the 942 admissions, with a fatality rate of just below 3 percent, constituted 33 percent of all patients.[60] However, the decline in mortality was mainly due to a decrease in the virulence of the organism.[61]

Wolverhampton guardians took measures to prevent outbreaks in the workhouse by restricting visiting when scarlet fever was prevalent in the town in the 1870s and 1880s.[62] Although 20 children were admitted in November 1877, they all recovered and no more cases occurred within the workhouse.[63] In the mid-1890s, they arranged for cases to be admitted to Wolverhampton Borough Hospital for infectious diseases for a payment of two shillings and six pence per patient per day.[64] Thereafter, children with scarlet fever were usually admitted to the hospital, which treated 1,215 patients between 1888 and 1892.[65] However, an outbreak took place in the children's ward of the workhouse infirmary in 1895, with at least 9 children affected. Isolating the sufferers proved difficult because of overcrowding in the infirmary wards.[66] Birmingham guardians took a different approach in 1889, allowing the town's health committee to use a building, previously employed as a test workhouse for able-bodied men, to accommodate children convalescing after a bout of scarlet fever, as they would no longer be infectious. The move released thirty to forty beds in the town's isolation hospital.[67] Over the years 1877–80 and 1894–1911, only one case of scarlet fever was recorded in the workhouse (on June 29, 1895), but the numbers are one-day counts on only a few days in the year and may not represent the overall prevalence for those years. In addition, the isolation hospital in Lodge Road had taken on the role of admitting patients with scarlet fever from 1875, with 424 admissions that year. In 1882 they increased to 627 and, in the four years from 1888, they treated 7,206 patients, including 2,525 in 1890.[68] However, some children with scarlet fever continued to be admitted to the workhouse infirmary; for instance, six cases in a four-month period in 1886 and five in the twelve months to May 31, 1910.[69] It was difficult to avoid admitting infected patients, as the disease may not always become apparent until after admission. Such an instance occurred in 1902, when a child was admitted via the workhouse and the infection only developed once in the infirmary. The Infirmary House Subcommittee suggested that all further suspected cases should be kept in the workhouse for a few hours in order not to infect both institutions.[70] In summary, the cooperation between the guardians in both towns and the sanitary authorities ensured that as few patients as possible with scarlet fever were admitted to the poor law institutions.

As scarlet fever waned in virulence toward the end of the century, diphtheria took its place as a major killer of young children. It had only become recognized in England as a distinct disease entity in mid-century after an epidemic of throat disease in 1858. Prior to that time, it had been included in mortality statistics under scarlatina.[71] The disease results in inflammation and severe swelling in the upper airways, which can cause obstruction and death by respiratory failure. It is spread by droplet infection following direct contact with cases or carriers. The main form of management was strict isolation in hospital to limit the spread of infection, but this had little effect on the mortality from the disease. By the middle of the 1890s, the organism could be isolated from throat swabs, aiding accurate diagnosis, and antitoxin was available to counteract the systemic effects on the heart and nervous system.[72] However, to be effective, antitoxin had to be administered within the first four days of the illness, when symptoms were not pathognomonic of diphtheria. Furthermore, it was expensive and not provided free of charge by the sanitary authorities in Birmingham until 1902.[73] Nevertheless, throat swabbing and antitoxin helped to check the spread of the disease and contributed to the rapid reduction in mortality, although a decline in virulence may also have occurred. It was the only disease in the nineteenth century that was affected by the germ theory and that preventive measures linked laboratory investigations, clinical practice, and public health action in a coordinated way.[74]

The incidence of diphtheria in Birmingham had declined markedly after 1873, but a sudden increase in deaths occurred in 1895, more than three times that of the previous year, although notified cases only doubled.[75] However, admissions to the workhouse did not take place until five years later and continued sporadically through the 1900s (appendix A). In addition, there was an outbreak in the female epileptic wards in 1912.[76] According to F. B. Smith, Birmingham had the reputation as a "notoriously bad" diphtheria town.[77] A large increase in cases also occurred in Wolverhampton in 1895, by over four times the number in the year before, although the fatality rate fell by half. The mortality rate among children under six years old, which had been 2 percent or less in the first half of the 1890s, increased to between 6 percent and 11 percent after 1894.[78] In October 1895, a child with diphtheria was admitted to the workhouse having contracted the disease prior to admission.[79] In contrast, an outbreak occurred in Wolverhampton workhouse in December the following year, with the disease affecting eight boys, one of whom died, and nurses Hilton, Riley, Whittaker, and Wright over the following three months. The boys were isolated in a ward away from other children and the nurses in their rooms. The medical officer raised concerns over the condition of the lavatories attached to the wards where the disease had begun and requested measures to improve the drainage.[80] It is surprising that the disease was being linked to sanitary issues at that time, as the bacterium had been discovered in 1883 and the toxin had been in use in Britain since 1894. However, Hardy comments that bacteria were not fully accepted as the cause of the disease in England until the mid-1890s.[81] The medical officers of health for Birmingham and Stoke Newington believed at that time that unsanitary conditions were a predisposing cause of the disease due to the release of sewage gases.[82] A more enlightened approach was taken by the members of the Workhouse Visiting Committee in Wolverhampton at that time when they instructed the medical officer to send throat secretions to London for examination if more cases of diphtheria arose.[83] He did not do so during that outbreak, but the following year he sent secretions from the throat of Nurse Rogers for analysis and the charge of five shillings and

Table 2.2. Prevalence of communicable diseases in Britain in nineteenth and early twentieth centuries

Disease	Prevalence
Measles	Endemic, with epidemic in 1807–8; highly contagious; mortality unaltered
Whooping cough	Endemic; mortality unaltered
Scarlet fever	Endemic; more virulent strain from 1830 to 1880, with epidemics in 1840, 1844, 1858–59, 1863–64, 1868–71; milder from 1890s, with increased prevalence in 1901–14 with lower mortality
Diphtheria	Endemic after epidemic in 1858–59; mortality declined in the twentieth century
Typhus	Epidemics in 1817–18, 1837–38, 1846–47, 1869–70; endemic in urban areas; mortality declined after 1870; disappeared by the end of the nineteenth century
Typhoid	Separately identified as a disease in 1869; endemic; mortality declined in the 1880s
Cholera	Epidemics in 1832, 1848–49, 1853–54, 1865–66
Smallpox	Endemic; epidemics in 1817–19, 1825–26, 1837–40, 1871–72, 1884–85 of *Variola major*; milder strain, *Variola minor*, with epidemics in 1892–93, 1901–2
Tuberculosis	Endemic; mortality declined toward the end of the nineteenth century

nine pence was approved.[84] At that time, laboratory testing remained concentrated in the capital and no facilities for the detection of diphtheria were available in large cities such as Birmingham.[85]

Childhood infectious diseases occurred in workhouse infirmaries to a variable extent, but measles and whooping cough were rarely absent, as was diphtheria from the end of the century. In the main, they were managed in the workhouse without difficulty and so are mentioned in the records infrequently. It was in the early years after the New Poor Law that guardians were concerned that childhood infection might spread throughout the workhouse because of a lack of appropriate isolation facilities. In the majority of outbreaks, the guardians and medical officers took steps to manage the situation appropriately. Scarlet fever was a different matter, where guardians in Wolverhampton and Birmingham sought to make arrangements for admission to the local isolation hospitals. However, isolation facilities were not in place until later in the century and until then, workhouses had to shoulder the burden of caring for sufferers from infectious disease. In Wolverhampton in 1891, the lack of an isolation hospital meant that all cases of infectious diseases were treated at home, except for two patients with scarlet fever, who were admitted to the workhouse.[86] Until isolation policies were introduced, children would not usually have been admitted to medical institutions primarily because of their illness if they could have been looked after at home. Although it is more likely that infection was coincidental to their admission with their parents or contracted while in the workhouse, some children were admitted because of their infection, especially in Birmingham.

Puerperal Fever

Puerperal fever was the major single cause of maternal death after childbirth, with a fatality rate of between 35 percent and 80 percent; the earlier the onset of the condition, the higher the mortality. The disease reached epidemic proportions in lying-in institutions in the nineteenth century, although sporadic cases also occurred.[87] The most common causative organism was *Streptococcus pyogenes*, discovered by Louis Pasteur in 1879. The bacterium gained entry via the traumatized birth canal, resulting in local infection, including peritonitis, which could spread into the bloodstream, causing septicemia. Symptoms usually began a few days after delivery, with shivering, headache, vomiting, abdominal pain, and high fever.[88] One of the earliest physicians to publish evidence of the contagious nature of the disease and of its transmission by midwives and doctors was Alexander Gordon in 1795, following an outbreak near Aberdeen. According to Irvine Loudon, Gordon's "brilliant treatise" was neglected and forgotten because it could not be linked to generally accepted knowledge at that time.[89] Further evidence in support of the contagious theory was provided by Oliver Wendell Holmes in America in 1843 and Ignaz Semmelweiss in Vienna in 1847, the latter significantly reducing maternal mortality in hospital by instituting hand washing using a solution of chloride of lime. However, both met with formidable opposition from the medical establishment, most likely due to the inference that doctors spread the disease. However, Loudon suggests that by the 1850s, it was difficult for doctors to plead total ignorance of the part played by contagion.[90] For twenty years from the mid-1860s, the contagious versus miasmic nature of puerperal fever attracted considerable attention by the medical press, but by the end of this period, most British lying-in hospitals had adopted Joseph Lister's methods of antisepsis, with a subsequent decline in maternal mortality.

In spite of the fact that the disease was widespread in institutions, there is only one recorded outbreak in Wolverhampton workhouse. It occurred in the lying-in ward in February 1842 and separate accommodation needed to be provided to prevent patients not affected from catching the infection.[91] By comparison, more frequent outbreaks took place in Birmingham workhouse, the first in 1854 causing the death of one woman and possibly a second woman and resulting in the closure of the lying-in ward.[92] Five years later, two women caught the disease and separate accommodation had to be found for new admissions.[93] No further cases were reported for twenty-four years, but in 1874 Nurse Freeman was given leave and a gratuity due to attending an infected patient.[94] A series of outbreaks took place in the lying-in wards throughout the 1880s. The first resulted in the deaths of two women, but a third sufferer appeared to be making good progress. On this occasion, arrangements were made for the isolation of infected patients; a new midwife was appointed; and the resident surgeon replaced by a locum to attend lying-in women.[95] In 1885, patients in the lying-in wards had to be transferred to the female infirmary and then to the vacated girls' school because of puerperal fever.[96] Continuing transfers to various buildings were necessary and by December, the lying-in wards were in the Test House, previously used for unemployed men. Patients subsequently underwent a further transfer to the "old cottages" in July the next year, while new lying-in wards were opened in the workhouse for new admissions under Nurse Tibbins and Dr. Mitchell, the assistant medical officer.[97] The following month, Emma Lee in the "Lock ward" contracted puerperal septicemia and a year later, Emma Allsop was admitted with the same condition.[98] After the new infirmary opened in 1889, patients continued to contract puerperal fever into the twentieth century, albeit infrequently.[99]

Diarrheal and Dirt Diseases

Workhouses were the obvious locus of institutional care for paupers suffering from diseases associated with poverty and guardians responded to the demand by adopting varying strategies to cope with the influx or to divert it to other facilities. Typhus and typhoid fever are linked as so-called dirt diseases since they flourish in conditions of poverty, overcrowding, uncleanliness, and poor personal hygiene.[100] Typhus, often referred to as "spotted fever," is transmitted to humans from body lice and is contracted by the inhalation of contaminated dust, resulting in fever, headaches, and a purpuric rash with a case fatality rate between 20 percent and 45 percent.[101] However, louse transmission was not demonstrated until 1909 and medical men remained in total ignorance of the nature and origins of typhus throughout the nineteenth century.[102] Nevertheless, by the 1860s, it was accepted as a contagious disease associated with destitution and overcrowding.[103]

Consequently, typhus was endemic in urban areas, but two major epidemics, which were less dependent on domestic and working conditions, occurred in the nineteenth century in the years 1837–38 and 1846–47. The first caused the deaths of 75 individuals in Birmingham in the second half of 1837 and 45 in Wolverhampton.[104] The latter one reached England from Ireland at the time of the famine and was referred to as the "Irish fever." Over 17,000 people died in England and Wales from typhus in that year, following which the number declined to under 1,000 by 1878 and less than 250 by 1886. By the end of the century, it had virtually disappeared. The decline of the disease has been attributed to rising living standards, improved sanitary conditions, and better personal hygiene, as well as the isolation in hospital of infected families, which allowed the opportunity of disinfecting their homes.[105]

It was liable to cause outbreaks in crowded institutions, hence its pseudonyms of "jail fever," "hospital fever," and "workhouse fever," the last because of its prevalence in eighteenth-century workhouses.[106] For instance, an outbreak occurred in Bromsgrove Union workhouse in May 1844. The matron was the first to suffer with diarrhea and fever and the infection quickly spread to the inmates. Those affected were separated from the other inmates and the worst was over by mid-July, but not before three guardians died of the infection.[107] After its appearance in Birmingham workhouse in 1847 as mentioned earlier in the chapter, there were usually a few cases present over the following decade (appendix B). A few infected patients were admitted in Wolverhampton workhouse in 1842, one of which caused the lying-in ward to be closed for a month. Two years later, Ann Morris was brought to the workhouse in an open cart suffering from typhus, with "high state of fever and delirium," so the medical officer detained her in the receiving room rather than admit her to the infirmary.[108] On one day in December 1869, the only patients in the workhouse with infectious diseases were twenty-five with typhus and they constituted 10 percent of all patients. By contrast, no patients in Birmingham workhouse suffered from the disease on that day and only 325 did so in all the English and Welsh workhouses.[109] It is surprising that so little is recorded about infection with typhus in the workhouse, as admission of infected paupers in the 1860s usually led to severe outbreaks within workhouse infirmaries in London.[110] It is possible that the practice of removing the clothes of inmates and subjecting them to bathing on admission may have limited the spread of body lice to other inmates.

Typhoid, a type of enteric fever, was not identified in annual registration reports as a separate disease distinguishable from typhus until 1869, although the clinical differentiation between the two had been widely accepted in Britain by the medical profession following Edward Jenner's studies of the disease in the 1840s.[111] Like typhus, it presents with fever, headache, a rash, and diarrhea.[112] The disease is contracted by ingestion of food or water contaminated by human feces, hence its reputation as the "filth disease" due to its association with fecal pollution. Despite this, it affected all social classes as the houses of the wealthy had private wells and poor drainage, as was the case in Birmingham.[113] The responsible bacterium was discovered by Karl Eberth, a German bacteriologist, in 1880.[114] However, acceptance of the organism as the definitive cause of typhoid was not universal in Britain until the emergence of a diagnostic test in 1896 and a vaccine the following year.[115] Although endemic in England, outbreaks took place in the 1820s, 1840s, and 1870s. Mortality from typhoid declined substantially from 0.85 per 1,000 of the population at that time until the early 1880s (to 0.21 out of 1,000) and continued to decline slowly until the end of the century.[116] For instance, in Birmingham Registration District, it was halved between the decades 1871–80 and 1901–10, falling from 788 deaths and a death rate of 0.33 per 1,000 to 351 and 0.15 per 1,000 respectively; figures similar to the national picture.[117] The major factors in achieving this change were improved domestic water supply and better individual hygiene, but the more stringent hospitalization of patients was also important.[118] The medical officer of health for Birmingham attributed the decline in cases of enteric fever predominantly to the provision of isolation accommodation.[119]

An outbreak of typhoid occurred in a house in Oxford Street, Wolverhampton, in 1869 and the eleven sufferers who survived were admitted to the workhouse. They joined five existing patients with the disease, causing the female fever wards to be fully occupied.[120] However, typhoid does not appear in the poor law records of Wolverhampton and Birmingham until the 1880s. An outbreak occurred in the town of Bilston in the Union of Wolverhampton in 1885, and the guardians arranged for infected paupers to be admitted to the local isolation hospital. Despite this, two inmates died from typhoid in the workhouse the following year, as well as four in the General Hospital.[121] In 1892, when Elizabeth and Ellen Brooks arrived at the workhouse suffering from typhoid, it was the General Hospital that the guardians turned to for their admission, agreeing to meet the cost of their care.[122] Despite this, patients with typhoid continued to be admitted to the workhouse, as there were four present three years later in March and one in November, as well as one in the same month in 1895.[123] A small number of inmates with typhoid were also present in Birmingham workhouse throughout the 1870s, 1880s, and 1890s (appendix A). Prior to 1882, they were being treated in the general sick wards, but in that year, the guardians decided they should be isolated from other patients and agreed to convert the room over the "old swimming bath" for this purpose.[124] Three years later, the bed provision for typhoid patients was eight for men and, surprisingly, none for women, although they would have been able to reside in the twelve-bed, female infectious ward.[125] The following year the guardians asked the Town Council if patients with typhoid fever could be admitted to the borough isolation hospital. However, the medical officer of health declined on the grounds that there was a serious risk that these patients would become infected with smallpox or scarlet fever if admitted.[126]

Only one inmate is recorded as having typhoid after midsummer 1899 (appendix A), but as the figures are based on one-day counts, it might reflect the reduced prevalence of the disease rather than its nonexistence in the workhouse. However, there were no cases of typhoid between October 1906 and the same month two years later. The opening of a second isolation hospital in the city at Little Bromwich in 1895 may be a further reason for the lack of patients admitted to the workhouse. Despite this, patients with typhoid were present in the infirmary in the early twentieth century. Jordan Lloyd, visiting surgeon to the infirmary, complained in 1908 that two or three cases of the disease had been transferred from the workhouse into his wards and he believed that the visiting physician had had the same experience.[127] In the same week, Miss Emma King, assistant matron of the workhouse and a qualified nurse, contracted the disease, was admitted to the nearby City Fever Hospital, but died ten days later.[128] These occurrences are suggestive of an outbreak in the workhouse at that time, but no cases of typhoid were recorded in the returns to the Local Government Board for that month. Epidemics within workhouses could result in high fatality rates, such as the outbreak of enteric fever in Bridgewater parish workhouse in the winter of 1836–37, which killed one-third of inmates.[129] From the available literature, it appears that, in contrast to Birmingham and Wolverhampton, workhouses had very few if any inmates suffering from typhoid. However, inmates with severe infective diseases were more likely to die within the first month of admission.[130] Their relatively short length of stay in the workhouse makes it likely that statistics collected on one-day counts may underrepresent how many inmates had been admitted with infectious diseases associated with a high fatality rate. This would also be the case for the other diarrheal disease, cholera.

Asiatic cholera first arrived in England from India in 1831 at Sunderland and spread throughout the country over the next eighteen months, highlighting the unsanitary conditions of industrial Britain.[131] Further epidemics arrived in 1848, 1853, and 1866, although the virulence of the organism varied on each occasion.[132] Bilston was one of the "worst hit" places during the first epidemic in 1832, with 3,568 cases out of a population of 14,500 and a fatality rate of 21 percent. On the other hand, Birmingham surprisingly escaped with only 31 cases reported.[133] The second outbreak arrived in Wolverhampton Union in August 1848 once again at Bilston Brook, causing 550 deaths in a population of 22,000 within the first month.[134] Like typhoid, it is spread by drinking water or eating contaminated food and can lead to rapid dehydration and death in about half of those affected.[135] The account of John Snow's epidemiological observations of the spread of the disease in Soho during the 1848 and 1853 outbreaks, leading to his "waterbourne theory," is one of the most familiar in medical history. Although Robert Koch first isolated the bacillus in 1882, it did not gain immediate acceptance as the definitive cause of the disease among British medical opinion.[136] Strict isolation of the sufferers, with careful disposal of their excreta, was the most important preventive measure instituted after the first epidemic.[137] Subsequent improvements in sanitation later in the century and the development of a vaccine in 1893 greatly reduced the impact of the disease.

When 267 cases were recorded in the Wolverhampton Union's districts in one week in August 1849, the guardians considered converting the vagrants' wards as isolation accommodation, but instead bought land to erect a cholera hospital in cooperation with the Committee for Health of Wolverhampton.[138] One woman who tried to escape from the "contagion raging there" by walking from Bilston to Birmingham was admitted to the latter's workhouse infirmary with the affliction.[139] By the end of 1849, the epidemic had subsided and the guardians ordered the cholera hospital to be demolished. They agreed on a joint plan with the town council in 1853 in anticipation of further outbreaks. The main emphasis was on attempting to keep cholera victims at home rather than admitting them to a cholera hospital, providing houses of refuge for healthy relations and organizing dispensaries to give out antidiarrheal medicines.[140]

Before the arrival of Asiatic cholera, the term *cholera* had been used to denote any disease characterized by intense diarrhea and abdominal pain.[141] Such a disease in infants was known as infantile cholera and in adults, English cholera, both of which were associated with unsanitary domestic conditions.[142] When a case of "choleraic diarrhoea" occurred in Bilston during the last epidemic in 1866, the medical officer was able to reassure the guardians that it was the English type.[143] Diarrheal diseases formed a substantial proportion of admissions with infectious conditions in the 1850s (appendix B) and it is not surprising that outbreaks of diarrhea took place from time to time within workhouses.[144] For instance, several cases of dysentery occurred in Wolverhampton in 1901, requiring the employment of additional nurses.[145] Many Birmingham inmates were affected by an outbreak of diarrhea in one night in July 1865. Only adults were afflicted: ninety-six in the old men's wards, forty-six in the old women's ward, twenty-four able-bodied inmates, two in the probationary ward, eight epileptic men, and thirty-three pauper nurses.[146] Edmund Robinson, workhouse medical officer, put the cause of the outbreak down to miasma from the unsatisfactory drains. However, the clinical pattern of many inmates affected at the same time for a short period, plus patients in the infirmary and children, who would have had a different dietary, being unaffected, suggests the culprit was a mild form of food poisoning. This is the only recorded incident of a major outbreak within either institution, and one presumes that many more must have occurred without being mentioned in the records.

Smallpox

Smallpox was the only one of all the major epidemic diseases that was controlled by means of medical discovery and a successful public health campaign.[147] References to a disease presumed to have been smallpox have been traced as far back as antiquity, but the disease appears to have been more virulent in the early modern period, resulting in several epidemics across Britain in the nineteenth century. It is spread mainly by droplet infection and the disease is contracted when in the immediate vicinity of an infected person, even after the death of the sufferer.[148] There is no sign of illness until a week after infection, when symptoms of headache, fever, and backache commence, and a rash appears as the fever abates. The patient is infectious from just before the rash until the last scab drops off, as the virus is shed from the rash. The average fatality rate is 25 percent, but many who recover are left with pockmarked facial scarring due to destruction of the sebaceous glands and a few with blindness. The disease confers lifelong immunity.[149] A new species of smallpox appeared in the late nineteenth century, producing a milder disease with a fatality rate of only 1 percent.[150]

Inoculation into the skin of pus or powdered scab to give immunity to the disease had been practiced in England from the early eighteenth century, but had a 1 percent to 3 percent risk of death.[151] Following the work of Edward Jenner toward the end of the century, vaccination using cowpox or vaccinia virus to produce a mild infection was a safer procedure, but as it did not provide lifelong protection, revaccination after a few years was necessary. In the 1860s, the procedure was commonly performed by vaccinators using the arm-to-arm technique, taking lymph from pustules on a previously inoculated person.[152] The early developments in smallpox prevention have been well documented, but, according to Hardy, the nineteenth-century history of smallpox has been neglected by historians.[153]

In susceptible communities, smallpox causes large epidemics, but following the decline in prevalence can remain endemic in cities. The early nineteenth century witnessed a quiescent period until the epidemic of 1837–40, which resulted in 35,644 deaths in a three-and-a-half-year period in England and Wales, mainly among infants and young children. In Birmingham, 284 deaths from smallpox were registered in 1838, but only 55 the following year.[154] However, there is no mention in the poor law records for Birmingham or Wolverhampton of admissions to the workhouse at this time. The epidemic of 1837–40 brought about the first piece of legislation against smallpox in England, with the Vaccination Act of 1840, which provided free vaccination for children if their parents wished it. A further act, thirteen years later, made it compulsory in infants before they were four months old, financed by the poor law rates under the responsibility of the guardians. In the years following the epidemic, smallpox remained prevalent in the country and isolated cases occurred; for instance, a man with "virulent smallpox" admitted to Wolverhampton workhouse in 1845 was promptly transferred to a room on his own, under care of a dedicated nurse.[155] Between 1863 and 1865, the number of smallpox patients present in the workhouse at any one time ranged between none and nine, with a peak in May and June of 1864. In November 1863, the workhouse master transferred inmates from isolated cottages to enable them to be used for smallpox patients, as they were the only buildings away from the main hospital.[156] The guardians considered extending facilities for paupers with infectious diseases on the grounds that it was better to admit them than to treat them at home in order to increase their chances of recovery, thereby accepting a medical role for the poor law.[157] In May 1864, Birmingham guardians arranged fifteen patients on outdoor relief and ten from the workhouse to be transferred to the General Hospital.[158] As it was unusual for voluntary hospitals to accept patients with infectious disease, it was no surprise that later in the year there were forty-one cases of smallpox and ten of fever in the workhouse, which was so crowded that inmates were moved between departments to accommodate the infectious patients.[159]

The next great epidemic took place in 1871–72, resulting in 42,084 deaths in England and Wales in those years and afflicting mostly youths and adults.[160] The increased virulence of the virus resulted in a fatality rate that was much greater, at 66 percent in the first year and 77 percent in the second, and also it affected those who had already been vaccinated. According to Hardy, it was the worst of the century.[161] On this occasion, both workhouses in Birmingham and Wolverhampton were deluged by admissions of small-pox sufferers (see tables 2.3 and 2.4). The guardians in Birmingham found it necessary to appoint a temporary medical officer, Mr. Edward Burton, to care for smallpox patients in the workhouse and prevented him from see-ing private patients unless they had smallpox. Eliza Matthews and Elizabeth Fellon were appointed as additional nurses for patients with the illness.[162] When the medical officer commenced duties on December 19, 1871, there were 21 patients in three wards, but, by May 10, the next year, this had increased to 75 patients in seven wards and the time spent treating them had increased from two-and-a-half hours per day to between four and five hours.[163] By the time his services were no longer required on February 8, 1873, he had treated 982 patients.[164]

William Sharp, master of Birmingham workhouse, provided the guardians with a detailed report on the epidemic. The first case to arrive on March 11, 1871, was a servant girl from Hockley, followed on April 27 by four chil-dren from London and later by four more. He considered that the disease had not displayed "much of an epidemic nature" at that time, but the number of admissions increased rapidly after Christmas, for instance, 109 admissions in January 1872 compared with 21 in the month before (table 2.3a).[165] The greatest number of patients in the wards at any one time was 94 on one day in April and two days in June. The borough sanitary authorities were responsible for arranging 60 percent of admissions. The mortality rate of 15 percent was well below the average of 77 percent for the country as a whole. The patients had been nursed by an inmate under the supervision of the nurse in the female infirmary initially until the two paid nurses were appointed. Visiting by rela-tives and friends was strictly prohibited, even when the patient was dying, to ensure complete isolation. The workhouse master praised the conduct of offi-cers and inmates who were required to attend the patients, as well as that of the patients themselves for "submitting so readily to the regulation." Only one man had absconded and another patient had misbehaved. Finally, the con-cern that the health of the inmates already present in the workhouse would be endangered proved unfounded as only twelve contracted the disease.[166] This was not an irrational fear as Lancaster infirmary found that smallpox spread from the walled-off fever wards to the rest of the hospital during the epidemic in 1876.[167] Although the number of patients declined after the epidemic, admissions with smallpox continued. By June 1873, there were only 15 patients in the 103 beds available in the smallpox wards, which were reduced within five months to 30 beds, occupied by 21 patients.[168] However, the reduction in admissions in early 1873 was only a brief respite before a further increase occurred in the early months the following year (table 2.3b).

Table 2.3a. Number of patients with smallpox admitted and died by month, Birmingham workhouse, October 1871–January 1873

Year and month	Admissions			Deaths		
	Male	Female	Total	Male	Female	Total
1871						
October	3	2	5			
November	11	4	15	2		2
December	16	10	26	4		4
1872						
January	68	41	109	10	3	13
February	37	33	70	5	5	10
March	53	41	94	7	5	12
April	70	48	118	12	3	15
May	64	49	113	10	6	16
June	62	37	99	9	3	12
July	44	50	94	8	6	14
August	32	37	69	3	6	9
September	15	16	31	6	5	11
October	33	30	63	7	5	12
November	20	12	32	4	2	6
December	14	14	28	3	2	5
1873						
January	8	8	16	2	2	4
Total	550	432	982	92	53	145
Percentage	56%	44%		17%	12%	15%

Source: BCL, House Sub-committee, GP/B/2/3/3/3, January 28, 1873.

Table 2.3b. Number of patients with smallpox admitted, died, and discharged, Birmingham workhouse, first third of 1872, 1873, 1874

Year and months	Admissions	Deaths	Discharges
January–April 1872*	390	56 (14%)	334
January–April 1873	91	12 (13%)	79
January–April 1874	455	66 (15%)	389

* The figures for January–April 1872 are not exactly the same as those given in table 2.3a. They were provided by two different people (the workhouse master and the medical officer) to two different committees.

Source: BCL, Visiting and General Purposes Committee, GP/B/2/8/1/6, May 22, 1874.

Table 2.4. Number of smallpox cases in Wolverhampton workhouse and union district, 1871–72

Date	Workhouse	District	Date	Workhouse	District
1871			**1872**		
October 27		199	March 1	6	74
November 10	9	196	March 8	6	61
November 17	6	209	March 15	5	75
November 24	12	197	March 22	5	59
December 1	12	199	March 28	4	52
December 8	18	215	April 5	3	43
December 15	22	246	April 12	5	42
December 22	20	248	April 19	3	34
December 29	25	225	April 26	3	31
1872			May 3	5	24
January 5	30	220	May 10	6	22
January 12	26	171	May 17	3	15
January 19	18	170	May 24	2	23
January 26	15	135	May 31	6	26
February 2	16	142	June 7	5	27
February 9	8	113	June 14	5	25
February 16	5	100	June 21	6	21
February 23	5	77			

Source: WALS/WBG/PU/WOL/A/14, October 27, 1871 to A/15, June 21, 1872.

Smallpox patients were present in Wolverhampton workhouse at the time the first patients arrived in Birmingham in March 1871, although Henry Gibbons, medical officer, subsequently declared it free from smallpox one month later. The guardians directed Mr. Gibbons to revaccinate all inmates who had not been vaccinated within the previous five years.[169] July that year saw five cases occur among inmates in the workhouse, with one death. By October, an increasing number of cases of smallpox was being reported by the district medical officers, with a resultant increase in admissions to the workhouse (table 2.4). The number of infected paupers peaked around December that year and January the next, a few months earlier than in Birmingham. Mary Ann Salt was engaged in November as an additional nurse to care for the smallpox patients for a period of two months.[170] In December, Mr. Humphreys, the nurse for the male wards of the infirmary, contracted the infection, but recovered within a few weeks.[171]

The next epidemic in 1884–85 was less severe, resulting in only 5,043 deaths in England and Wales in those years.[172] A case of smallpox was reported to the guardians in Wolverhampton Union's district in the autumn of 1882, when they appointed a temporary attendant for the smallpox wards and stopped workhouse visiting. However, only four patients with smallpox were in the workhouse at that time.[173] An outbreak occurred in October the following year, resulting in sixty-seven patients being admitted in the ensuing six months with six deaths. Forty-one of the patients lived in Bilston, where the borough commissioners had failed to provide isolation facilities. Seven further cases were admitted over the next three months and one inmate who had been in an adjoining room to the smallpox wards also contracted the disease. The guardians decided to forbid the admission of patients with "infectious epidemic disease" from June to give the local sanitary authorities time to establish places for isolating patients and the workhouse infectious wards became free of smallpox cases by the end of July, the temporary nurse being given notice to leave.[174] Birmingham also experienced an outbreak of smallpox in the workhouse prior to the epidemic in 1884 and all visits and leaves were stopped.[175] Neither institution appears to have admitted smallpox sufferers during the epidemic. By that time, alternative arrangements were in place, in association with the local health boards, for admission for isolation, which was a central plank in the program to eradicate the disease. However, sporadic cases occurred in Birmingham infirmary in the early 1890s. In April 1893 Jordan Lloyd, visiting surgeon, reported that two patients in his department had contracted smallpox, probably from the visitors' clothing. Prompt action had been taken with the isolation of the patients and then their transfer to the Fever Hospital. Revaccination was carried out on all fit and willing patients as well as nursing staff and all visits to the infirmary were stopped. Over the following year a few more patients became infected, but by June all quarantine measures were terminated. Smallpox appeared for the first time in the lying-in ward in February 1895. The woman affected had contracted it after admission and succumbed due to the severity of the disease.[176]

The vaccination program in England became less effective after this epidemic as the number of cases decreased, the virulence of the virus declined, and the antivaccination lobby gained prominence. The fear of catching the disease from vaccination or being infected with syphilis and the risk of scarring in young children created reluctance among the general public to agree to vaccination.[177] The disease was recognized as highly contagious throughout the nineteenth century, but in the 1870s, opinion became polarized between the anticontagionists, who believed it resulted from miasma, and the proponents of the new germ theory, who believed a specific infectious agent was the cause.[178] The antivaccinationists gained the upper hand resulting in the Vaccination Acts of 1898 and 1907 that allowed parents to decline protection for their children by stating conscientious objection.[179]

Consequently, 33 percent of unvaccinated children died in the 1893–94 epidemic in Birmingham, compared with only 0.5 percent of vaccinated children.[180] However, partly due to a decline in virulence of the virus, later epidemics in 1892–93 and 1901–2 were mild.[181]

Isolated incidents occurred in Wolverhampton workhouse in the 1890s and 1900s, unrelated to the times of the epidemics. A man from Willenhall was admitted in February 1893 because of the need for urgent isolation. He had contracted the disease while working in Derby and, once back home, was sleeping in the same bed as his wife and newborn child. As Willenhall did not have an isolation hospital, the only appropriate facilities were in the workhouse.[182] The guardians had contracts with the sanitary authorities in Wolverhampton and Bilston, but not in other districts of the union. They had been paying Wolverhampton fifteen shillings per week for the maintenance of paupers with infectious diseases. However, two years previously, the sanitary authority offered to admit paupers without charge as part of its duty to contain the spread of infection. After advice from the Local Government Board that the care of such patients was the responsibility of the sanitary authorities, the guardians gave notice to Bilston Sanitary Authority that they would rescind the contract to pay for paupers admitted to its isolation hospital.[183] When the master reported an outbreak of smallpox in the workhouse in February 1896, Esther Gubby was transferred to the Borough Hospital and Ellen Faulkner, another infected inmate, was transferred the following month.[184] In the winter of 1902–3, two cases of smallpox arrived in the casual wards.[185] The tramp wards in Birmingham also were the locus for an outbreak in January 1893 at the time of the epidemic. It spread within three months to the infirmary and six months later to the workhouse, as a result of which all visiting was suspended.[186] During the epidemic in 1902, five patients were admitted to the infirmary suspected of having smallpox as they all lived in a lodging house where the disease had been present, but they had been misdiagnosed. However, the next year John Russell was found to have the infection after his admission to Birmingham infirmary by the workhouse medical officer, who claimed there had been no sign of smallpox when Russell was examined in the ambulance.[187]

Hardy makes the point that guardians were reluctant to admit smallpox patients into the main workhouse or additional buildings during epidemics.[188] However, they often had little alternative, as few public isolation facilities were available until the 1890s. During the 1872 epidemic, Wolverhampton guardians considered erecting a new building as a smallpox hospital, but deferred it in preference to using the recently built receiving wards for convalescent smallpox patients and utilizing the old receiving wards for their previous purpose. Three months later, the guardians agreed to a request from Wolverhampton Town Council to accept nonpauper patients in the infectious wards of the workhouse on a payment-per-case basis.[189] Conversely, during the epidemic in the early 1880s, arrangements were made for pauper patients to be admitted to the infectious hospital in Bilston for payment of three shillings per removal, fifteen shillings per week and the cost of the funeral. When the Local Government Board questioned this arrangement, the guardians responded that it was the duty of the sanitary authorities to provide isolation facilities in order to keep the workhouse from the danger of a large number of smallpox sufferers in the infirmary wards.[190] Ten years later during the next epidemic, Willenhall Local Board of Health was informed that the isolation wards at the workhouse were not for the admission of nonpaupers.[191] In April the following year, the guardians went further by forbidding the admission of sufferers of smallpox or "other infectious epidemic disease."

The arrangements for the isolation of smallpox sufferers in Birmingham involved greater collaboration between the guardians and the Town Council. Admissions of paupers with contagious diseases, including smallpox, into the workhouse only took place after 1864.[192] Because of the threat of cholera around that time, two straw sheds and several stone-breaking sheds at the rear of the workhouse had been converted into wards and they had subsequently been used for smallpox cases. During the 1871 epidemic, they became overcrowded within ten months of the first admission. In cooperation with the borough authorities, an additional ward was to be built, but before it was ready, there were more than enough cases to fill it, so a further one was agreed with the same result. The two buildings to hold 30 acute cases were completed and occupied within one week, although several of the workmen contracted smallpox. In addition, two wards for convalescent smallpox patients were erected.[193] The guardians requested payment from Birmingham Corporation for the maintenance of 599 cases sent to the "smallpox hospital" by the Sanitary Commission between December 7, 1871, and February 8, 1873, an amount totaling £1,388 for 11,101 days at two shillings and six pence per day. However, they also requested that no further cases be sent.[194]

The following year they agreed to let the buildings containing the smallpox wards to the Town Council, who decided to build additional wards for patients with infectious diseases on land in the workhouse grounds.[195] However, over the next ten years, there was continual haggling over the length of tenure of the lease and for the majority of the time it remained on annual renewal, despite the guardians agreeing in 1878 that it would be for seven years. In the ensuing discussion, the Health Committee requested an extended tenure of the smallpox hospital and declared it would be impossible to find another site for it within Birmingham Borough if the lease was not renewed. The committee pointed out that the hospital needed "extensive rebuilding." The committee had purchased a piece of land from the Asylum Committee for the erection of wards for scarlet fever cases as they had come to the conclusion that it was absolutely necessary to separate cases of smallpox from scarlet fever. Consequently, the building in the workhouse grounds would be used only for smallpox. If the lease was not renewed, the guardians would therefore need to provide their own building for paupers with scarlet fever.[196] The guardians agreed the corporation could purchase the smallpox buildings and have tenancy of the land as long as it was required. However, they requested that paupers requiring admission should have priority over all others.[197] In 1888, the Town Council demolished several of the wooden buildings used for smallpox as they had become "unfit for human habitation."[198] However, the epidemic in 1893–94 was more severe in Birmingham than the one in the previous decade and consequently the Town Council had to request the use of the stone yard sheds at the workhouse for treating smallpox cases.[199] Six months later, they were asked to vacate the buildings as soon as possible as the guardians felt that the proximity of the sheds to the workhouse constituted a "great danger" to the inmates.[200] Anxiety over the danger to the public of isolation hospitals as the foci of infection had been growing from the 1870s and protest over the siting of these hospitals was more forceful in London, where every locality voiced opposition to their erection.[201] A challenge by local residents resulted in intermittent closure (1872–75 and 1879–82) of the Metropolitan Asylum Board's first infectious disease hospital in Hampstead and a decision to stop admitting smallpox patients in 1884.[202] When the Birmingham Health Committee requested a renewal of the lease for the smallpox hospital in 1896, they indicated that they would no longer use it for smallpox patients, who would be admitted to the Borough Hospital in Lodge Road.[203]

By that time, smallpox prevalence had declined nationally and locally. In the Birmingham Registration District, deaths had fallen from 1,042 in the 1870s to 253 in the 1890s, with only one person dying from the disease between 1901 and 1910.[204] The last outbreak of *Variola major* in England occurred in 1901–2, confined mainly to London, and endemic smallpox disappeared from England in the 1930s. The World Health Organization declared its eradication worldwide in 1979, the only disease where this has been achieved by immunization.[205]

Shared Responsibility

The need for additional facilities for isolation during epidemics meant that cooperation between the responsible authorities was essential. This was particularly true in the case of smallpox. Poor law facilities were used extensively in Birmingham to cope with smallpox epidemics, and to a lesser extent in Wolverhampton, during the epidemic of the early 1870s. In both towns, access by nonpauper patients to workhouse accommodation was permitted. Until the end of the nineteenth century, institutional provision for smallpox patients in Birmingham was in poor law buildings and on workhouse land, leased by guardians to the corporation. It was not unusual for workhouse infirmaries to be utilized in this way, as the development of isolation hospitals by local authorities was slow until the 1890s and those that were built were too small to cope, especially during epidemics. John Pickstone notes that arrangements for fever in the Manchester region other than provided by guardians were present only in Manchester, Preston, and Lancaster in the 1860s. Elsewhere in the region, guardians resorted to pressuring local authorities to take responsibility for the isolation of infectious patients, but with limited effect. In most cases they had no option but to admit infected nonpaupers into the workhouse wards. In Salford, a degree of shared responsibility did exist. Nevertheless, the guardians had to erect sheds for all smallpox sufferers during the 1870s epidemic. When there was still no public isolation hospital by 1875, they issued an ultimatum to the local authority by refusing to take nonpaupers. Salford Council eventually opened facilities the following year, but the guardians, on the advice of the Local Government Board, continued to admit those who were destitute. The council refused to collaborate in the provision of a single isolation hospital, causing the guardians to build their own smallpox accommodation. However, the following year, the use of a single hospital for all smallpox patients was agreed.[206] More often the conflict between the guardians and their local authorities over which one was financially responsible for nonpauper patients with infectious diseases remained unresolved. As a result, it was still possible for smallpox patients to be admitted to general workhouse wards until the 1890s.[207] Even when guardians agreed that nonpaupers with infectious diseases could be admitted to workhouse fever wards, patients were not always cooperative. A nonpauper girl aged twenty-five with smallpox refused admission to Battle workhouse in Reading in 1876 because of the stigma of pauperism.[208]

An isolation hospital in the Borough of Wolverhampton was erected in 1891, accommodating around thirty-six patients, although some beds had been available for the previous ten years. However, the lack of isolation facilities in all districts making up Wolverhampton Union meant that poor law accommodation continued to be utilized. Wolverhampton guardians collaborated with the local health committee in the town in the late 1840s over the building of a cholera hospital and in the development of a joint plan to tackle the disease. Similarly, joint action was agreed to for typhoid patients from Bilston in the 1880s. However, the question of who should pay for paupers admitted to isolation hospitals within the union did create conflict between guardians and sanitary authorities at times. When Annie Birch was admitted to the infectious diseases hospital in 1912, the guardians accepted liability for the charges, but warned that in future, they would do so only if they had requested the admission.[209] In many ways relationships in Birmingham were more harmonious with close cooperation over the handling of smallpox and scarlet fever arrangements in the 1870s and 1880s. The borough infectious hospital, built in the early 1880s, had 300 beds, but buildings still needed to be leased from the guardians to provide for a further 100 patients. From 1888 to 1892, they were used to treat 89 patients with smallpox and 1,217 with scarlet fever in the earlier year and 7,206 in the last one.[210] The extent of cooperation between the poor law and sanitary authorities in Birmingham, with joint management of facilities for infectious diseases, was exceptional. The part workhouses played within these joint arrangements was important in isolating patients with infectious conditions and greatly assisted in preventing the spread of infection within their communities. However, the control of infection within the workhouse demanded strict co-operation from patients. The next chapter will consider those patients whose behavior was difficult to control.

Chapter Three

Controlling Disorderly Behavior

This chapter is primarily concerned with certain groups of patients whose behavior was challenging or difficult to control within the institution. For those with mental illness or epilepsy, it was beyond their control. Patients who contracted venereal disease did so as a direct result of their actions, but they were prone to misbehave when residing in the workhouse. However, mentally ill patients were not completely absolved of blame for their condition because of the links between insanity and bodily disturbance; for example, one strongly held theory by many doctors was that it was caused by masturbation and other acts that were regarded as immoral.[1] A number of questions will be addressed in relation to these groups of paupers and the workhouses in the two towns. As the treatment of mental illness in asylums changed throughout the nineteenth century from the widespread use of mechanical restraint to moral management, what effect did this have on the treatment of lunatics in workhouses? With their lower staff-to-patient ratios than asylums, how did workhouses cope with behavioral disturbances? To what extent were physical treatments for mental disorders also used for punishing any type of misdemeanor and how frequently were workhouse staff at risk of sustaining injury from disturbed patients? Patients with epilepsy posed a particular problem for staff as they were at risk of injuring themselves during a seizure. How frequently were they subjected to forms of mechanical restraint after these were no longer allowed for mental illness? How disturbing was the frequency of epileptic fits to both sufferers and other inmates? What implications did the development of epileptic colonies in the early twentieth century have for epileptic patients in the workhouse? A significant proportion of inmates with mental disability suffered from epilepsy, and as a result lunatics and epileptics were usually accommodated in the same wards in the workhouse. So it is not always possible to identify them discretely, although attempts will be made to do so as much as is possible. Workhouse provision and dedicated facilities for patients with venereal disease will be covered in respect of the scarcity of specialist care. The types of treatment they received will be analyzed and the extent to which they were subject to discrimination on moral grounds will be explored. The chapter will provide evidence for maintaining that these patients with behavioral problems received appropriate care that was, at times, as good as in specialist institutions.

Mental Illness Institutions

The late eighteenth and the first half of the nineteenth century saw a dramatic transition in the care and treatment of sufferers of mental illness. The main facets of this revolution were the increasing numbers admitted to specialized institutions and the replacement of coercive methods of treatment by a regime based on discipline that would encourage socially acceptable behavior through psychological means.[2] These changes were accompanied by mental illness becoming an essentially medical problem and by the resultant emergence of a specialized branch of the medical profession, whose members styled themselves alienists. Furthermore, the asylum came to be regarded as the officially approved response to the management of those with mental illness and the state assumed responsibility for mental health care. Thus, as Andrew Scull, one of the foremost historians of mental illness, has succinctly put it, "The Victorian age saw the transformation of the madhouse into the asylum into the mental hospital: of the mad-doctor into the alienist into the psychiatrist; and of the madman (and madwoman) into the mental patient."[3]

For most of the seventeenth and eighteenth centuries, those with mental illness existed within their community, while a minority were accommodated in small private madhouses, typically with less than ten residents. In the 1760s, charitable institutions specifically concerned with the insane began to emerge, but along with them arose a private, profit-oriented "trade in lunacy." The "unsavory" reputation of this industry led to legislation in the form of the 1774 Private Madhouses Act, which required licensed premises and appointed inspectors for madhouses in London. However, it "proved little more than a token gesture."[4] The responsibility for licensing and inspection in the provinces was given to local magistrates. Continued allegations of mistreatment of the mentally ill, or lunatics as they were referred to at the time, led to the setting up of a parliamentary Select Committee in 1807 and the County Asylum Act the following year. The act granted magistrates the

power to raise finances to provide asylum accommodation for pauper lunatics. Because the act was only permissive, take-up was slow and only nine had
been erected by 1827.[5] Nevertheless, it laid the legislative basis for the first
generation of county asylums and signaled direct intervention by the state in
health provision.[6] Inspection of metropolitan madhouses was strengthened
by the Madhouse Act (1828), which set up a new commission to provide
supervision and increased the number of inspectors, now referred to as commissioners in lunacy. After fourteen years, this was extended to provincial
institutions with the appointment of two itinerant commissioners. However,
the number of these asylums remained small, with twenty-one counties having made no provision for an asylum on the grounds of expense.[7] The growth
of the public asylum system received impetus from the 1845 Lunacy Act,
under which every county and borough had a statutory obligation to provide
adequate asylum accommodation out of the local rates. Within the following
two years, sixteen of fifty-two counties had erected an asylum.[8] The act also
reformed the Lunacy Commission, creating a powerful national inspectorate
on a permanent basis to ensure that asylum inmates were not abused. It laid
down regulations regarding the certification required to confine a pauper in
an asylum. This process included medical certificates by both the poor law
doctor and an independent practitioner.

The lunacy problem that the various acts sought to solve revolved around
the fact that the majority of lunatics were indigent, often as a result of their
infirmity. The proportion of paupers among the lunatic host was around 80
percent in 1844, rising to around 90 percent in 1890.[9] It is unsurprising
that many would drift into workhouses or only be maintained in the community with outdoor relief. Despite this, mental health historian Leonard
Smith considers that the significance of the workhouse in "the tapestry of
care" for mentally disordered people in England has been underestimated
by historians.[10] Under the Old Poor Law, lunatics usually mixed with other
inmates within the workhouse and rarely were they provided with special
accommodation. The only reference to the mentally ill in the Poor Law
Amendment Act (1834) was a clause determining that they should not be
detained in workhouses for longer than fourteen days. Probably because of
this, the model plans for workhouses issued by the Poor Law Commissioners
the following year did not allocate geographical space for their accommodation, nor were they included in the classification system. Guardians were
not encouraged to provide dedicated accommodation as it was expected that
all lunatics would reside in the workhouse only on a temporary basis. As a
result, only 10 percent provided separate insane wards in 1859.[11] However,
the transition in attitude toward the mentally ill in the early nineteenth

century had resulted in the differentiation of the insane from the wider category of the merely indigent and transformed it into a condition diagnosed only by medical experts.[12] Furthermore, as county asylums began to suffer overcrowding from the mid-1850s onward and were increasingly unable to receive lunatics from workhouses, guardians were required to provide specific accommodation in the form of lunatic or insane wards. The difficulties that arose in the transfer of these patients both from the workhouse to the asylum and in the opposite direction will be analyzed later in the chapter.

The terminology used throughout will be that of the time, namely *lunatic*, for those with any mental illness, and *idiot* and *imbecile* for those who would now be seen as suffering from learning difficulties. The term *insane* will cover all of these three categories. Further definitions were introduced in the late nineteenth century such as *weak-mindedness*, and these will be elucidated as appropriate. However, many of these terms were never satisfactorily defined and cannot be regarded as equivalent to modern terminology. Provision of facilities for these groups of patients was limited. As they were usually refused admission to voluntary hospitals and asylum accommodation was limited, there was little alternative but admission to a workhouse, especially when their illness led them into destitution. Harmless lunatics were considered appropriate to be transferred or returned to workhouses, but considerable disagreement arose between workhouse medical officers and the commissioners in lunacy over the question of whether individual lunatics were harmless. Boards of guardians were suspected of having vested interests in retaining lunatics in the workhouse as the cost of their upkeep was cheaper than the sum they had to pay to the asylum, but was this the main reason for retaining patients in the poor law institution? Because of the need to retain lunatics, guardians provided dedicated wards in the workhouse to a greater or lesser extent and this aspect will be explored in Birmingham and Wolverhampton.

Accommodating Pauper Lunatics

As Wolverhampton Union workhouse was built according to the hexagonal model plan of the Poor Law Commissioners, it is not surprising that there were no dedicated wards for lunatics. Within a few years, the need for such had become obvious and the master was drawing the attention of the board to "our want of proper idiot wards."[13] Around that time there were 13 male and 9 female lunatics and idiots and 59 patients in the infirmary out of a total of 368 inmates.[14] The commissioners in lunacy, on a visit on February

10, 1846, found all insane persons "quiet and comfortable" with the two who were ill and in bed receiving "every care and attention."[15] However, it took a further six years before the guardians agreed to provide two wards for female lunatics and two for men, one for each sex "set apart" as a receiving ward until the medical officer determined whether they required transfer to an asylum or could be retained in the workhouse.[16] The commissioners in lunacy were not so impressed by the conditions on the wards when they visited in 1857. On this occasion, the twenty-two men and twenty women were found to be "dirty in their person and dress" and in many their clothes were "ragged." Several of the "bed-ticks" were soiled or wet with urine and the new wards appeared "more cheerless" than the previous ones. A more serious allegation involved the finding of three knives in one of the ventilators in a room that accommodated a young woman suffering from "melancholia," who had previously attempted to cut her throat. This state of affairs was not peculiar to Wolverhampton. The commissioners were highly critical of the conditions in almost all the workhouses they visited with separate lunatic wards. They found the rooms crowded, the ventilation imperfect, the yards small, bedrooms also used as dayrooms, and a lack of classification by type of illness. They expressed strong opposition to the introduction of separate wards, while also decrying mixing lunatics with other inmates because of the inability to provide specialized care. Their ideal solution was direct admission of all lunatics to asylums.[17] Wolverhampton guardians did make improvements to the accommodation and diet following the criticisms. In 1859, the commissioners reported that one-quarter of the insane were idiotic and helpless, while the others helped with tasks, and considered "all to be more appropriate for residence in the workhouse rather than an asylum."[18] In the mid-1860s, there were thirty epileptic patients in Wolverhampton workhouse, comprising 4 percent of total inmates and 19 percent of lunatics, similar to the national proportion of 4 percent of patients in workhouses suffering from epileptic seizures in 1870.[19]

The number of lunatics in the workhouse increased markedly throughout the next three decades, although as a proportion of total inmates, it was highest in the early 1870s (table 3.1). However, the increasing admissions made it difficult to accommodate them all in the insane wards. For instance, only 28 of the 61 in March 1860 were appropriately placed, although this improved in the December of the following year with 34 lunatics out of 45 in the insane wards. Over that period, 92 lunatics had been admitted and 50 had been transferred to Stafford Asylum.[20] Over half of admissions moving to an asylum contradicts the prevailing view of historians that guardians attempted to retain as many lunatics as possible in the workhouse because

Table 3.1. Number and proportion of lunatics in Wolverhampton workhouse in selected months, 1860–1900

Date	Number of lunatics			Number of all inmates	Proportion of lunatics
	Male	Female	Total		
March 1860	22	17	39	517	8%
December 1861	23	22	45	754	6%
February 1863	13	23	36	653	6%
July 1866	28	27	55	607	11%
December 1867	35	32	67	817	9%
October 1872	–	–	102	629	16%
September 1873	–	–	117	643	18%
December 1875	57	60	117	712	16%
June 1881	52	72	124	991	13%
June 1882	51	78	129	947	13%
January 1900	52	66	118	1,305	9%

Source: WALS, WC, March 28, 1860, to June 28, 1882; WBG, PU/WOL/A/28, 2 February 1900.

of financial economy.[21] A greater majority of lunatics were to be found in the appropriate wards thereafter (85 percent by 1866). In April 1877, 5 of the 53 male lunatics were in the infirmary, 1 in the fever ward and 4 in the body of the workhouse; 4 of the 57 women were in the infirmary, 1 in the fever ward and 6 in the main workhouse. However, as 9 were ill and in bed, misplacement was not simply due to lack of beds in the insane ward.[22] Nevertheless, the greater number of lunatics in the early 1870s posed staffing problems and the commissioners pressed for the appointment of an additional assistant as the superintendent of the male insane ward could not "take proper care of" all of the patients.[23] At that time, there were 108 (16 percent) insane inmates, plus 219 (33 percent) classified as sick, out of a total of 659 inmates.[24] On one occasion, the superintendent had to sit with a sick inmate for three days and nights, as he needed "constant watching." The patient was a blind man suffering from "brain disease," who subsequently died. The superintendent took this action as he felt he would have been held responsible for anything that happened to the patient and despite having 51 other patients under his care.[25] The fact that almost half of the patients on the lunatic wards were epileptic throughout the 1870s and 1880s would have implications for staffing levels.[26]

The situation in Birmingham was very different as there were no asylum facilities available locally until 1850, the guardians having to send patients to Droitwich Asylum in Worcestershire and subsequently to Stafford Asylum from 1828.[27] When a private asylum was opened at Duddeston Hall in Birmingham in 1835, the guardians contracted to send dangerous lunatics there and receive them back when they had become calmer.[28] The first record of dedicated provision for lunatics was not until 1834, when one of the surgeons reported that there were twenty-eight men and eight women in the two wards in the new buildings, while twenty-five women remained in the old building. The patients were either "idiotic cases" or suffering "mental aberration," but were "perfectly manageable"; otherwise they would have been transferred to an asylum. Despite their arrangements with local asylums, the guardians applied for a license for the "reception of insane paupers" in what they now termed the Lunatic Branch of the Town Infirmary.[29]

The conditions on the lunatic wards were heavily criticized in a special report in 1844 to the Poor Law Commission by Samuel Hitch, medical superintendent of Gloucester County Asylum. At the time the twenty-seven epileptics in the wards were thought to make up an "unusual proportion" at 38 percent among the seventy-one residents and several were described as "idiots."[30] The male and female wards faced each other across a courtyard and on the male side there were five single rooms with no windows for refractory patients. Bathing and washing facilities were inadequate and the wards generally not fit for accommodating insane patients. However, it was noted that patients were kindly treated and some of the women were knitting.[31] The following year, the commissioner in lunacy was still not satisfied with conditions in the Lunatic Branch, particularly regarding the inadequate arrangements for segregation of the sexes and suggesting transferring the women out of the new building. He recommended that one of the surgeons should supervise the lunatics and Thomas Green agreed to take on sole responsibility for medical care in the "lunatic department."[32] Five months after his appointment, he realized the "labour and responsibility" were greater than he expected, with daily or at times twice daily visits to the wards. Time was also taken up with obtaining a history from the patients' friends of their condition prior to admission, which he considered essential to their "proper treatment." Since his appointment there had been 83 admissions, of which 27 had been cured, 4 sent to an asylum, 17 discharged to friends or other parishes, and 5 had died.[33] He kept a casebook with a detailed record of all 666 admissions until he resigned in 1850 to take up the post of medical superintendent at the newly opened the Birmingham Borough Lunatic Asylum. The increase in the number of patients over the next few months amounted to nearly double the capacity of the wards, which Green felt were ill adapted for the treatment of "different forms of insanity" and did not allow any kind of classification by diagnosis to be

Table 3.2. Epileptic and insane patients in Birmingham workhouse, by gender, 1845–50

	Patients with epilepsy only		Patients with epilepsy and mental disorder		Total of patients in lunatic wards	
	Male	Female	Male	Female	Male	Female
1845	19	14	4	5	82	42
	23%	19%	5%	12%		
1846	12	8	7	4	75	63
	16%	11%	11%	6%		
1847–50	29	33	32	17	223	212
	13%	15%	15%	8%		

Source: BCL, Register of Insane, MS/344/12/1.

Table 3.3. Diagnosis for patients with mental illness in the lunatic branch of the Town Infirmary, Birmingham, 1845–46

Diagnosis	Number of males	Number of females	Total
Mania	56	20	76
Dementia	26	23	49
Melancholia	21	14	35
Melancholia + dementia	4	1	5
Mania + dementia	1	3	4
Imbecility	4	7	11
Partial insanity	3	5	8
Moral insanity	–	2	2
Puerperal mania	–	5	5
Hysteria	–	4	4
Dementia senilis	1	1	2
Other conditions	9	12	21
Total number of patients	125	97	222

Note: The diagnostic label of dementia in the nineteenth century was not synonymous with current usage, but was used to denote a delusional and hallucinatory form of insanity, similar to today's schizophrenia. Conditions related to what we now call Alzheimer's disease would be labeled *Dementia senilis*.

Source: BCL, Register of Insane, MS/344/12/1, 1845–46.

affected. As a result, the guardians converted a court of seven small houses in the nearby street as a men's insane ward. At that time, there were forty-four men and forty-three women in the insane wards, comprising 21 percent of all inmates.[34] When the Borough Asylum opened in 1850, the majority of the insane patients were transferred, leaving two men and twelve women in the workhouse.[35]

Table 3.4. Number and proportion of lunatics in Birmingham workhouse in selected months, 1844–1900

Date	Number of lunatics			Number of all inmates	Proportion of lunatics
	Male	Female	Total		
April 1844	38	40	78	567	14%
April 1847	41	37	78	573	14%
April 1849	45	40	85	684	14%
October 1851	2	12	14	–	–
May–June 1860	45	46	91	1,078	8%
May 1865	–	–	152	2,006	8%
October 1870	86	94	180	–	–
December 1874	115	126	241	–	–
March 1892	119	140	259	–	–
February 1899	75	66	141	2,960	5%
January 1900	71	68	139	3,122	4%

Source: BCL, HC, GP/B/2/3/1/1, 1844; BBG, GP/B/2/1/5–6, 1847–49; TNA, MH12/13297, 1851 and MH12/13297, 1892; VGPC, GP/B/2/8/1/3–4, 1860–65; HSC, GP/B/2/3/3/2 and 2/3/3/4, 1865–74; LGB Letters, GP/B/1/2/1/6, 1899–1900.

The lunatic wards were renamed epileptic wards when the second work-house opened in 1852, no doubt because the borough asylum was operational by then. However, the wards still contained the same mix of lunatics and epileptics, some of whom were not insane. They continued to be over-crowded due to the increasing number of admissions and new wards had to be erected within ten years. Nevertheless, a varying proportion (between 8 percent and 18 percent) of those with "unsound mind" remained scattered in other wards of the workhouse throughout the remainder of the century. On his visit in February 1888, the commissioner in lunacy found 168 males and 148 females "classed of unsound mind," of which a large number (70 and 57) were epileptic. Many were in advanced years and 89 were in bed when he visited. The others were described as "clean and neat in person and dress" and half of the women were "usefully employed." He felt they were all suitable for treatment in a workhouse. Five months later, the 319 lunatics comprised 12 percent of the workhouse population.[36] By then the guardians had added a dining hall and a recreation room in the epileptic block.[37] At the turn of the century in Wolverhampton workhouse, 118 "lunatics, insane persons and idiots" (52 male, 66 female) resided in the special wards for lunatics and comprised 12 percent of the 1,015 inmates. However, they were around one-third of patients under the care of the medical officer, a similar proportion to a number of other workhouses in England (table 3.5).[38]

Table 3.5. Imbeciles and epileptics as a proportion of inmates under the medical officer in selected union workhouses on January 1, 1900

Union workhouse	Number of inmates under medical officer	Number and proportion of imbeciles and epileptics	
Bristol	1,220	428	35%
Bath	268	84	31%
Walsall	164	26	16%
West Bromwich	362	134	37%
Wolverhampton	344	118	34%
Dudley	317	120	38%
Stourbridge	180	73	41%
Worcester	146	16	11%

Source: WALS, WBG, PU/WOL/H/28, June 8, 1900.

"Dangerous Patients"

Which lunatics were appropriate for care in a workhouse and which required transfer to an asylum remained a contentious issue between guardians, medical officers, and the commissioners in lunacy throughout the nineteenth century. In the early years of the century when asylums were regarded as primarily curative institutions, commissioners were keen that virtually all lunatics should be admitted to them as early as possible after the onset of their illness. However, as the asylums took on a more custodial role accommodating increasing numbers of chronic cases in the 1850s, the transfer policy became based on the concept of dangerousness or harmlessness. The interpretation of how dangerous a patient was varied greatly, but was not related to the possibility of cure and lunatics could be kept in the workhouse and transfer to an asylum delayed until they were completely unmanageable.[39] Another factor involved in the controversy over transfer was the preference to maintain lunatics in the workhouse, where the cost of their care was cheaper. However, this chapter does not confirm Hodgkinson's assertion that guardians refused medical officers' request for the transfer of dangerous lunatics because of the expense.[40]

The Wolverhampton medical officer recommended the removal of three lunatics to Stafford Asylum in 1842 and the request was placed before the magistrates, who at that time had the authority for admission. Later in the year, the master reported William Walter, an idiot, whose fits of violence had grown in ferocity. He had risen from his chair and kicked William Biddle so badly he was in bed for several weeks and also hit Eli Hawkins without provocation in "a very savage manner." Henry Swift required several men to hold him when he became violent and the other inmates were so terrified of him, they slept in fear. All were assessed by the medical officer as fit for an asylum, though there is no record of transfer taking place.[41] Once the commissioners in lunacy had oversight of provincial institutions, they constantly challenged the continuing placement of particular individuals within the workhouse, especially if they considered them dangerous, as in five cases in the 1850s. On the other hand, Dr. Bowers of Stafford Asylum complained of too many of Wolverhampton's paupers being inappropriately accommodated in the asylum as most were "merely idiots" or epileptic patients. The guardians arranged their transfer to the workhouse, but three years later requested that 50 or 60 lunatics and idiots be admitted to the asylum from the workhouse.[42] In October 1873, the commissioner in lunacy regarded many of the 129 inmates of unsound mind as very troublesome, especially among the 60 epileptics, and Elizabeth Pearson, who was both violent and obstructive, was sent to the asylum.[43] Thereafter, those queried by the commissioner were moved to the asylum, except in the cases of Sarah Meakin and Mary Watson, where the medical officer did not agree with the commissioners that they were dangerous to themselves or others.[44] He also disagreed over the case of William Howell, "a melancholic in low desponding condition," pointing out that he had been returned from the asylum as a "proper subject" for workhouse treatment.[45]

Although Birmingham guardians did not have ready access to a local public asylum, sixteen transfers took place in 1843 and forty-eight in 1844 to private institutions, the majority because of disturbed and violent behavior. In the metropolitan commissioner in lunacy's visit on September 29, 1843, several of the twenty-seven epileptics among the seventy-one lunatics were idiots who were excessively violent after their fits and some were "maniacal." Two women had strong suicidal tendencies and one had attempted suicide. Subsequently, two men and nine women were transferred to Haydock Asylum, ranging in ages from twenty-two to sixty-two years: seven idiots, two epileptics, and two lunatics.[46]

After he had taken charge of the lunatic wards, Thomas Green described the difficulties that disturbed patients posed in his casebook. In his first two years in charge, twenty-six men and eighteen women were considered dangerous, including three epileptic men and three women. In many, this designation was based on their history prior to admission and still applied even if they had been well behaved while in the wards. Nor was it applied only to patients who attacked others, but also for those who attempted self-harm. For instance, Elizabeth Hurd, aged forty-nine years, tried to jump through a window and Sarah Cooke, forty-eight with mania, was "violent, screaming and tearing her hair." On the other hand, Lucy Jacob, thirty-three with partial insanity, had sudden fits of excitement when she threatened and attempted to injure other inmates; George Noble, an eighteen-year-old epileptic, kicked another patient; and M. A. Spencer, an epileptic woman of twenty years, would strike or kick anyone who displeased her. These last three were transferred to an asylum, whereas Hurd and Cooke were not, presumably the decision being made on the basis of protecting other patients.[47] In 1846 seven men and three women were dangerous, nine men generally quiet, but could be violent at times. Two of the men who had been very violent were improving rapidly and almost convalescent. The twenty-six males and thirty-five females who were harmless were easily excitable and could become dangerous without proper management. Arrangements were made for some to go to Camberwell Asylum.[48]

In 1871 the commissioner in lunacy challenged the appropriateness of the placements of one idiot, Walter Tully, and three epileptics. Tully, aged twenty years, kicked and scratched on occasions, but the medical officer considered he was "not in the way" in the summer months and neither he nor the three epileptics required removal to an asylum. Downes Ireland, aged thirty-two, had been admitted in January 1870 and transferred to the asylum on two occasions, returning back to the workhouse for the second time in December. He was having fits about once per month, was ill tempered, used bad language, but had no delusions. Although fit to be discharged from the workhouse, he was unable to get work. Eli Ensor, a twenty-eight-year-old woman admitted in November 1867, was subject to fits about every seven days, was sometimes morose, but appeared contented. Elizabeth McGuire's fits had occurred every seven to ten days since her admission in November 1870 and, although the thirty-two-year-old was sometimes noisy, she could not be regarded as dangerous. The remainder of patients with unsound mind were found by the commissioner to be "free of excitement."[49] Toward the end of the century and into the twentieth, there were few reports of dangerous behavior by lunatics and no concerns on the part of the commissioners in lunacy over the lack of transfer to asylums in both Birmingham and Wolverhampton.

Withdrawing Restraint

Mechanical restraint was almost universal practice in both charitable and private asylums in the eighteenth century mainly for controlling disturbed behavior, but it was also used to punish any form of nonadherence to the institutions' regulations. The variety of implements in use included chains and straps to confine patients to a chair or bed, the coercion chair, and the straitjacket, although other means of coercing patients such as forcible streams of cold water were employed. They were considered as both therapeutic and a prerequisite for curative treatment.[50] Although mechanical restraint began to be regarded as cruel and inhumane, it remained in general use throughout the 1820s and 1830s. However, by the end of the latter decade, many asylums had introduced moral treatment. The care of lunatics in workhouses did not necessarily follow what was happening in asylums, especially as the moral treatment approach demanded higher staffing levels to provide greater supervision of patients. The presence of lunatics and other inmates who could not or would not abide by the rules of the institution—"this concentration of deviants" as Scull has called them—could cause disruption to the smooth running of the institution. Even a single mad inmate could threaten the order and discipline of the workhouse.[51] According to Hodgkinson, mechanical restraints were still widely used in workhouses in the 1850s.[52] Even after the abandonment of restraint, some form of containment for disturbed or violent behavior remained necessary, usually as some form of seclusion such as the padded room.

Restraint was required to contain violent behavior in two patients in Birmingham workhouse in 1844. The attendants were afraid to leave Martha Gould, a lunatic, without either confining her to her bed with a strap round her arm or "close watching" because of her occasional outbursts, although the medical officer considered she showed only "slight indications of decided insanity." Nevertheless, he recommended transfer to an asylum, but did not in the case of Emma Bailey, an idiot. She suffered incurable epilepsy and was restrained at night to prevent injuring herself, but she had never tried to injure others.[53] In the two years after Green took over the lunatic department, 37 of the 275 admissions required some form of restraint. George Proctor, aged seventeen years, was prone to violent fits, which he had had from childhood, and wore a pair of boots at night, which were secured to the bedstead. William Roper, aged twenty, was one of seventeen epileptic patients who were secured at night with a strap, which went over the top of the bedclothes and was fastened to the sides of the bed. He and Frederick Wade, aged twenty-five, also wore boots at times as well as the strap. In the case of Fanny Docker, aged seventeen, the strap was used to prevent her falling out of bed. It was tied to one side of the bed only when used for Emma Oxford, who had been having continual episodes of fitting for one week with seizures, which were always very violent. However, Hannah Hoskins, whose fits occurred at intervals of one to two weeks, required only slight restraint after some attacks. Venesection was used to good effect initially on forty-two-year-old James Benham, who had been epileptic for twenty-five years. When his fits returned after two months with greater violence, a further sixteen ounces of blood was taken from his arm, but the result is not recorded. Frederick Wade's fits had become less violent than at the time of admission in 1843. However, in April 1846, he became more violent again after fitting. He was noted to be deaf, have increasing enlargement of the "glands of the neck," and was treated with one milligram of iodine, presumably as the swelling was thought to be a goiter.[54] The clinical picture would be in keeping with a diagnosis of hypothyroidism.

Relatively fewer patients without epilepsy required restraint, only 20 out of 202, used mainly for those with mania and more frequently at night. Joseph Gure, aged thirty-five years and considered dangerous, was restrained in bed at night for preventing "self destruction." Charles Powell, also aged thirty-five, was also restrained in bed as he had jumped out of a window and injured a leg. Sarah Henrick, a twenty-three-year-old melancholic, also injured herself jumping out of a window in the middle of the night, spraining her ankle and bruising her back. Several patients were disturbed at night and would keep getting out of bed. Jane Smith, aged thirty-eight with acute mania, also would tear both her own clothes and the bedclothes. She was continually restless at night despite a warm bath on one occasion and a dose of opiate on another. She was eventually required to wear a belt and gloves for a few nights. Thereafter, she continued settled after being prescribed hyoscyamus every four hours. Another patient who pulled her clothes off and was unsettled at night was Ann Griffiths, aged twenty-eight and suffering melancholia. She required restraint on some nights, but eventually also became calmer on treatment with hyoscyamus. However, she subsequently had to be restrained by day as she was attacking the old women. Restraint was used on two of the women as they had tried to strangle themselves.[55]

In January 1852, Wolverhampton guardians decreed that any nurse or wardsman should use only restraint in the presence of the master, matron, or surgeon. Nevertheless, the commissioners in lunacy repeatedly attempted to curb the use of restraint and in May recommended that straps and "all other means of coercion" should be removed for use by the attendants and kept locked up and the guardians complied with their request.[56] Five years later, they questioned why several women were being "habitually restrained" in the epileptic wards of Birmingham workhouse. They were informed that the women were in a "helpless physical condition" and in danger of falling out of bed. Thus, the master did not consider it to be restraint.[57] He also defended the use of a straitjacket for M. Russell when he went out in the yard on the grounds that it prevented him eating stones and dirt. However, the commissioners felt it could be discontinued "with proper supervision" and if not, he should be sent to an asylum.[58] Thereafter, the commissioners did not find any use of restraint. However, there was in place a cell "used for punishment of refractory inmates" and the guardians instructed the medical officers that it required the consent of two of them for any form of restraint or seclusion to be used. An exception was made when a patient required urgent admission to the padded room, but consultation had to occur within fifteen minutes of the use of seclusion.[59] When the commissioner came across one woman in Wolverhampton workhouse in 1881 who was tied to her bed by a "pocket-handkerchief" on each wrist, he refused to accept the excuse that her disposition was to get out of bed when left alone. He reiterated that restraint of any kind was not countenanced by the authorities.[60] However, means of restraint were still available in the workhouse for occasional use. The "long-sleeved jackets" in Wolverhampton workhouse were usually in the keeping of the master and were justified on the grounds of being needed for the transfer of patients to the asylum.[61]

One of the consequences of the introduction of moral treatment was the increased difficulty for attendants in controlling disturbed behavior and the number of incidents of assault in asylums increased, both by staff on patients and by patients on other residents. However, this "period of turmoil" was a temporary phenomenon as staff learned new methods of management.[62] Pauper Undernurse Woolley was removed from her position in the epileptic wards in Birmingham in 1877 after using "undue violence," resulting in an inmate's arm being broken. The following year, nurses Ankers and Harris were found guilty of gross cruelty for tying an aged inmate to her bed because of her inclination to wander about the ward.[63] When, in 1876, an inmate in the lunatic wards in Wolverhampton workhouse, John Grainger, was found to have bruises, the guardians were satisfied that they had resulted from necessary force exerted in compelling him to take food and medicines. However, they did find the ward attendant guilty of beating Grainger with a pillow and removed the attendant from the ward. John Evans attended a meeting of the Wolverhampton Board of Guardians in 1875 complaining that his brother Joseph had been ill treated in the insane ward. Although the guardians concluded that no member of the workhouse staff had used undue violence toward Joseph, they did direct the medical officer to carefully examine all lunatics on admission and issued rules on confining patients in the padded room.[64]

When John Harbour, an imbecile, was subjected to ill treatment, the attendants Johnson and Clinton reported that another patient had struck him in self-defense. On further inquiry into the allegation that the attendants had mistreated Harbour, they were exonerated and retained the confidence of the board.[65] Conversely, attendants were at risk of injury from patients' behavior. In 1862, Charles Smith was admitted to the epileptic ward in Birmingham workhouse with an attendant to keep a close watch on him. However, at five o'clock in the morning, he knocked the man over, kicked down a door, picked up a table, and attempted to strike the attendant with it. Smith was transferred to the asylum, but at the time there was no padded room available in the men's ward to contain his behavior.[66]

Workhouse staff found it even more difficult to manage epileptic patients during a fit and the trouble pushed them to breaking point at times. In Birmingham in 1844, Abel, one of the underkeepers in the men's insane ward, brought a complaint for assault against Weare, the keeper. At the time, many of the twenty to thirty men in the insane ward were troubled with fits, following which some would go into "a raving state." According to Abel, one of them became "outrageous" and in the attempt to put on the "strait jacket, boots and cuffs," Weare struck the patient several times even when he was on the floor and strapped him "in a crib till morning." Apparently, Weare had informed the underkeepers that striking patients was not allowed, but if done on the abdomen would not be able to be detected. The other underkeeper, Hollyoak, confirmed Abel's account, whereupon Weare admitted the assault and was dismissed.[67] Some patients were prone to develop a state of "raving madness, known as epileptic fever," immediately after the fits ceased and in this state could resort to excessive violence that could lead to "many fearful homicides."[68] Although supervision during the day could be just adequate, it was a different proposition at night. One solution proposed by the commissioner in lunacy when visiting Wolverhampton was that sane inmates should sit in the wards during the night. He would have preferred paid night attendants, but the guardians chose the cheaper option.[69] By way of contrast, night attendance by paid staff was in place in the insane wards in Birmingham workhouse at the latest by 1849. In the mid-1870s, all the epileptic wards had paid night attendants (within ten years they were being designated night nurses) and early in the twentieth century, epileptic patients were being checked every fifteen minutes during the night.[70]

Epilepsy

The Hippocratic Corpus included a treatise on the "The Sacred Disease," as epilepsy was known in the ancient world. However, it was not until the later part of the nineteenth century that the nature of the epileptic process was elucidated by Hughlings Jackson, a London neurologist who is regarded as "the father of modern epileptology."[71] His definition of the epileptic seizure as a manifestation of a paroxysmal disturbance of brain function remains the one in current use.[72] The most striking form of seizure is the grand mal fit, with sudden loss of consciousness and muscle spasm, followed quickly by muscular jerking. The onset of a fit may be heralded by an aura, most often an auditory hallucination. In the immediate aftermath, known as the postictal state, a period of confusion may ensue when psychotic behavior is possible. This usually passes off within about fifteen minutes, but may last for several hours. According to Thomas Smith Clouston, one of the most eminent of Scottish psychiatrists of the late nineteenth century, the majority of patients with epilepsy had a liability to mental disease. If it occurred early in life, it was nearly always caused by a mental defect. Coming on later, the trend was toward gradual impairment of mental faculties and loss of memory. The striking features in sane epileptics were irritability and impulsiveness, which could lead to frequent acts of violence.[73] Numerous specific therapies were employed in the treatment of epilepsy, the most popular in the early nineteenth century being mistletoe, silver nitrate, and ammoniate of copper.[74] However, none proved to be able to prevent fits or reduce their frequency. The first drug to achieve this effect was potassium bromide, first reported in 1857, having been tried as a result of a chance association. Subsequent reports over the next three decades confirmed that it had virtually superseded all other drugs in the treatment of epilepsy, though it did have severe side effects consisting of physical weakness, mental dullness, and skin rashes, known as bromism.[75] The next development in drug therapy, the introduction of phenobarbitone, did not take place until 1912.

Experiencing Epileptic Seizures

Restraint was often justified for epileptic patients to prevent them sustaining injury during a seizure. However, those with less frequent or predictable fitting and not thought to require restraining were also at considerable risk. In Wolverhampton in 1859, Edmund Howell sustained a severe injury to his nose when he fell at the onset of a seizure and the commissioner in lunacy recommended the use of low reclining chairs. Fifteen years later, one epileptic patient was confined to bed after fracturing an ankle by banging it on the bathroom floor during a fit.[76] To prevent injury at night, the commissioner suggested in 1873 that low bedsteads with padded headboards be used for the "worst of epileptics" and all eighteen epileptic women and the twenty-five men were sleeping in them four years later.[77] However, these beds were not in use in Birmingham infirmary fifteen years later, although an attendant was present throughout the night to provide surveillance.[78] Maria Morton received immediate attention from the nurse when she started to fit, but this did not prevent the sixty-year-old epileptic from dying from regurgitation of food.[79] Inmates were also at risk of being accidentally injured during a fit by a fellow patient. When James Bentham sustained a fit in Birmingham workhouse in 1846, he made contact with William Williams, dragging him to the ground and breaking his leg.[80]

The risk of epileptic patients injuring themselves would depend on how frequently fits occurred, and prior to the introduction of effective drugs, accounts of the frequency of fits occurring on the wards indicate that it must have been a daily occurrence. During a visit by a commissioner in lunacy to Wolverhampton workhouse in the late 1860s, several of the thirty epileptic patients were lying on the floor fitting.[81] Downes Ireland, aged thirty-two, had been admitted in January 1870 to Birmingham workhouse and transferred to the asylum on two occasions, returning back to the workhouse for the second time in December. He was having fits about once per month, was ill tempered, used bad language, but had no delusions. Although fit to be discharged from the workhouse, he was unable to get work. Eli Ensor, a twenty-eight-year-old woman, was admitted in November 1867, was subject to fits about every seven days, was sometimes morose, but appeared contented. Elizabeth McGuire's fits had occurred every seven to ten days since her admission in November 1870 and, although the thirty-two-year-old was sometimes noisy, she could not be regarded as dangerous. Adam Simpson, workhouse medical officer, did not consider that any of them needed to be moved to a lunatic asylum.[82] Dr. Cornelius Suckling, visiting physician to Birmingham workhouse, provided details of the number of fits occurring per week among the thirty-three to thirty-nine men in the epileptic wards over nine weeks in 1889 (table 3.6). They ranged between 89 and 168, with a mean value of 138 and a median of 149. In addition, one man suffered 150 fits in week eight.[83]

Improving Standards of Living for Epileptics

The management of epileptic and insane patients changed at the beginning of the twentieth century and behavioral difficulties were seen as less problematic. In the case of epileptics, the availability of drug therapy with the ability

Table 3.6. Average weekly number of fits over nine weeks in the male epileptic wards in 1889

Week	Number of patients	Number of fits
1	36	168
2	37	157
3	37	129
4	37	97
5	38	89
6	33	127
7	36	149
8	39	307
9	39	167

Source: BCL, Infirmary Management Committee, GP/B/2/4/4/1, February 11, 1889.

to modify and control the frequency of fits may have played a large part in this. For instance, Annie Evans, an epileptic in Wolverhampton workhouse, was allowed out of bed from time to time to sit in a chair by the fireside.[84] In Birmingham epileptic patients were engaged in boot making, tailoring, and basketmaking before the turn of the century.[85] The state of accommodation in the epileptic wards in Birmingham was praised as very favorable at the start of the twentieth century. A dining hall and recreation room had been erected in the male epileptic block and there were greater facilities for outdoor exercise.[86] The majority of inmates could by this time spend their time in useful employment, with some women working in the laundry and men in the garden.[87] The nurses gave concerts for the patients every two weeks. Three years later, Mrs. George Allbright treated the epileptic women to a drive followed by a tea, despite the medical officers' concern that the vehicles used were unsafe for these patients. Despite this, outings such as this became a regular feature for both men and women over the following decade, and by 1906, took place three or four times per year.[88] However, outings were not without hazard. Miss Palmer, superintendent of the female insane ward in Wolverhampton workhouse, had taken twenty-one of her patients out for exercise onto Penn common in 1880 and failed to count them on the return. As a result, Emma Barker and Ann Kendrick had wandered away and were reported missing. Only Barker was found on Cannock Chase and taken to Stafford Asylum, but nothing was heard of Kendrick.[89]

Lunatics retained in workhouses were not legally required to be certified until 1889, but this was followed by an act five years later disallowing certification of inmates suffering only from "epilepsy pure and simple." However, this caused a problem in Wolverhampton workhouse with their placement within the workhouse's classification system. They were not thought suitable for either the able-bodied or the ordinary sick wards due to the lack of supervision. The commissioner in lunacy agreed they could still reside in the insane wards provided they were "not kept against their will." At that time, there were four females and six males who were not certified.[90] At the end of the century, there were twelve sane epileptic patients admitted to a workhouse from Wolverhampton County Borough and 118 from Birmingham County Borough. In Wolverhampton at that time, 13 percent of patients in the insane wards were sane epileptics.[91] However, the definition of sanity merely meant that the individual could not be certified as a lunatic under the conditions of the act. It did not mean that they were free from any degree of mental disability and many were considered to have minds that were "feeble" or exhibited minor mental defect, but had the ability to respond to advice.[92] No doubt this close relationship between sane epileptics and mental disability led the commissioner in lunacy to allow them to reside in the insane wards in Wolverhampton.

Another improvement in the management of epileptics toward the end of the nineteenth century was the establishment of dedicated institutions or epileptic colonies. The secretary of the West Midlands Poor Law Conference wrote to Wolverhampton guardians in 1897 regarding the erection of an institution for the "care and treatment of epileptic and weak minded persons." There had been moves by several unions in the locality to collaborate in providing suitable accommodation. Although the guardians approved of this development, they did not agree to join the scheme until fifteen years later.[93] Following the presentation of a paper at the West Midlands Poor Law Conference in 1901 advocating the establishment of "industrial colonies" under medical supervision, a joint committee between Aston and King's Norton unions and Birmingham parish was set up in 1904 in order to erect a building as an epileptic colony at Monyhull estate in the south of the city.[94] Birmingham guardians approved the project on the grounds that the "advantages of separate institutions [were] well known." In the colony, patients could be "of some useful service" such as working on the land and rearing poultry, instead of "sitting in the wards looking at each other and waiting for the fits to come."

Each board of guardians assessed their inmates for suitability on the basis of whether the medical officer felt they might improve with treatment in the colony (table 3.7) plus those who were not certified as insane and would appreciate the new surroundings, but would probably not improve (table 3.8). Feebleminded people were assessed on whether or not they might improve and if not, whether they would also appreciate being in the colony

Table 3.7. Epileptics who might improve

	Aston	Birmingham	King's Norton	Total
Men over 45 years	–	6	–	6
Men aged 16–45 years	2	20	3	25
Women over 45 years	2	10	2	14
Women aged 16–45 years	4	13	4	21
Children under 16 years	1	1	3	5
Total	9	50	12	71

Source: BCL, BBG, GP/B/1/2/73, May 18, 1904.

Table 3.8. Epileptics not classed as insane and capable of appreciating such a home

	Aston	Birmingham	King's Norton	Total
Men over 45 years	1	18	1	20
Men aged 16–45 years	2	4	–	6
Women over 45 years	4	18	3	25
Women aged 16–45 years	6	10	2	18
Children under 16 years	–	–	1	1
Total	13	50	7	70

Source: BCL, BBG, GP/B/1/2/73, May 18, 1904.

Table 3.9. Feeble-minded persons

	Aston	Birmingham	King's Norton	Total
Those who might improve:				
Adults	12	26	31	69
Children	3	21	12	36
Those who probably will not improve:				
Adults	27	105	11	143
Children	–	7	3	10

Source: BCL, BBG, GP/B/1/2/73, May 18, 1904.

(table 3.9).[95] Out of a total of 5,644 inmates in the three workhouses, 399 (7 percent) were identified as suitable to move to a colony. The joint committee decided to exclude children and adults over forty-five years old from the number of those who would benefit from transfer and so built a home to accommodate 200 inmates with 40 places allocated to Aston Union, 104 to Birmingham parish, and 34 to King's Norton. After the initial transfer from the workhouses, patients would be admitted directly to the colony. Because of a delay in the progress of the scheme, inmates were not transferred until 1908.[96] Of the 159 colonists resident at the end of the first year, 81 were classed as epileptic and 78 as feebleminded.[97] The only other poor law colony in existence at that time was Langho Colony, set up by Chorlton and Manchester Board of Guardians. Although this development had been approved by the Local Government Board in 1897, it took almost ten years to open.[98] The Monyhull Colony was established while the Royal Commission on the Care and Control of the Feebleminded was gathering evidence and members of the commission were impressed by the scheme, hailed as a "bold venture." As a result, Monyhull Colony acted as a pioneer in the care of people with what is now called learning difficulties and was copied by authorities all over the country.[99]

Venereal Disease

Venereal disease was the term in common use in the nineteenth century to cover a host of sexually transmitted diseases, the major ones being syphilis (or "Great Pox") and gonorrhea. However, Kevin Siena has cautioned against assuming that those diseases were precisely the same as the ones that are known by the same names at the present time.[100] Workhouse inmates suffering from venereal disease posed a different management problem partly because of their uncooperative behavior, but more so on account of the perceived need to keep them separate from other workhouse inmates due to the disease's association with prostitution and immorality. Segregation had less to do with their behavior after admission and more with the condemnation of how they had behaved beforehand. The immoral associations surrounding venereal disease was no doubt the reason for the House Committee in Wolverhampton debating in 1902 the advisability of probationer nurses being involved in the venereal wards, despite being under the supervision of charge nurses. The committee concluded that attendance on these wards was a necessary part of their training to become a "fully informed nurse." However, at the board meeting, Reverend Johnson had an amendment accepted that they should not do so within three months of their appointment.[101]

However, venereal patients could pose difficulties for workhouse staff. In April 1842 the master of Wolverhampton workhouse called the guardians' attention to the case of Mary Spruce, a fifty-nine-year-old married woman, admitted "very badly diseased" with venereal disease and that of Priscilla Hodgkins, a young woman of nineteen years, who had died from the disease in the same week. Both had become infected at The Pheasant public house, where Spruce had worked apparently as a servant, but in reality she was a prostitute. The following year, the master also sought the guardians' advice as to "the proper mode" of punishing the behavior of two other inmates who were prostitutes. May Perry and Fanny Porter had scaled the walls one Saturday evening to go into town. When they returned during the night, they were unable to gain access to their ward and so walked around in the yard till morning. Unfortunately, the guardians' response to the master is not recorded. Nor was it only the women who misbehaved. Thomas Nokes, admitted with venereal disease, absconded with the workhouse's clothes along with a female inmate who had previously applied to the guardians for clothes for the purpose of going into service. Toward the end of 1844, two more prostitutes in the venereal ward, Ellen Wells and Ann Ashley, absconded on a Wednesday evening, once again in the union's clothing. They had been apprehended and were due to appear before the magistrate the following afternoon, no doubt to be charged with stealing the workhouse clothes.[102] No further reports of misbehavior were reported in Wolverhampton workhouse thereafter and the only incident in Birmingham will be discussed later in the chapter.

Syphilis first appeared in Europe in Italy at the close of the fifteenth century and rapidly spread as an epidemic, thereafter remaining endemic throughout the continent. The disease goes through three distinct phases after an incubation period varying from ten days to ten weeks. It first presents as a local infection, with a painless genital ulcer, or chancre, which heals. Secondary syphilis develops six to eight weeks later with fever, a rash of variable character, though usually maculopapular. Mouth ulcers may be present, as well as condylomata, which are warty lesions on the perineum. There follows a latent period of many years before late symptoms become manifest, with abscesses, destruction of the bones and face, as well as cardiovascular and neurological defects. The disease can be transmitted to the fetus from an infected mother, resulting in deformities in the child, such as the diagnostic "peg-shaped" teeth, blindness, and deafness.[103] Advances in etiology and diagnosis did not take place until early in the twentieth century, with the isolation of the causative bacterium, called *Trepenonema pallidum* since 1906. The same year a diagnostic blood test, the Wassermann reaction, was developed, based on detecting antibodies to the bacterium. The test proves positive between five and eight weeks after infection has been contracted.[104] In 1914, Wolverhampton guardians agreed to make the test available at a cost of fifteen shillings per case, so that the medical officer could make an accurate return of the number of syphilitic patients in the workhouse for the Royal Commission on Venereal Diseases.[105] However, in the commission's report, Wolverhampton declared that the test was not used in the workhouse. It was used occasionally in two out of forty-seven provincial workhouses and regularly in only eight, one of which was Birmingham, where the test was carried out by the guardians' own pathologist.[106]

Gonorrhea is a bacterial infection that results in urethritis with a urethral discharge in the male and cervicitis, vaginal discharge, and urethritis in the female. In both, a systemic reaction may occur with arthritis and a vasculitic rash. It was not clearly differentiated from syphilis until 1837 and the causative organism, *Neisseria gonorrhoea* (also known as the gonococcus), was identified in 1879. The major complications are urethral stricture in men and infertility in women due to infection ascending to the uterus and ovaries. The main form of local treatment was the instillation of antiseptic solutions of silver salts into the male urethra and the vagina in women, but oral therapy with copaiba was thought useful in men.[107]

Segregating Venereal Patients

The poor law medical service was responsible, by default, for the management of the majority of patients with venereal disease. Those suspected of suffering this condition were frequently denied admission to voluntary hospitals, often on moral grounds, although the South Staffordshire General Hospital at Wolverhampton was an exception. In general, hospital facilities for patients suffering from venereal disease were inadequate. For example, London hospitals in 1856 had only 297 dedicated beds for a population of almost 2.5 million and 53 of those beds were in the London Lock Hospital, the only institution in the country devoted to venereal patients at that time.[108] The situation in the rest of the country was no different and half a century later, little had changed. Dr. R. W. Johnstone was "struck by the paucity of indoor accommodation provided for venereal disease in the infective stages" when visiting 30 general hospitals for his report to the Local Government Board. None of the hospitals reserved beds for such cases and hospital committees did not encourage their admission.[109] Specialist hospitals, often called Lock or Skin Hospitals, were not established outside London until the later part of the century; for instance, the Skin Hospital in Birmingham (founded in 1881) first took inpatients in 1886 and then only twelve.[110] A quarter of a century later, the number of beds had not quite doubled. Although no tickets were required for admission, few women presented themselves for treatment and prostitutes rarely did so.[111] Siena found it difficult to estimate the general prevalence of sufferers of venereal disease in eighteenth-century workhouse infirmaries in London, as their proportion varied over time. For instance, in St. Margaret's parish workhouse in London, there were around 4 percent in 1733, but 12 percent the following year.[112]

The majority of workhouses had dedicated "venereal" or "lock" wards. In 1844 Birmingham provided just four beds for men, but thirty-six for women with venereal disease. This difference was maintained throughout the next two decades, although the number of beds had increased to twenty for men and sixty for women in 1856 and to one ward of ten beds for men and three wards with a total of thirty-one beds for women in the mid-1860s when Wolverhampton provided one ward of five beds for men and three wards, each with five beds, for women.[113] However, Birmingham's provision became equalized in the early 1870s with around thirty beds for each sex, although there were only twenty-four men in their ward for thirty-one, but three more women than the number of beds in the female ward.[114] During the first week in January 1876, there were fifty-five patients with venereal disease in the Birmingham wards, comprising 6 percent of all sick patients, and eight (5 percent) in Wolverhampton, compared with an average of 2 percent in English workhouses.[115] At times, there were no venereal patients in Wolverhampton and only twenty-six beds were allocated for "syphilitic and skin" patients in the infirmary in the new workhouse in 1903.[116] By 1914 only four of forty-seven provincial unions did not provide dedicated wards for either sex, while one had beds only for men and four only for women.[117] The occupancy in these wards did vary considerably over time. On one day in December 1869, there were only two venereal patients in Wolverhampton workhouse, but fifty in Birmingham, comprising 7 percent of sick inmates, well above the national average of 2 percent. This was still the case six years later.[118] The latter survey details the individual diseases suffered by inmates and the number who died as a result of them (table 3.10). Many of those deaths may well have occurred at an early age. For instance, of the six inmates in Wolverhampton workhouse who died of venereal disease in 1840, Thomas Roberts was twenty-one years old, the four women were aged between seventeen and twenty-seven years, and the youngest, Maria Lee, had been born just five weeks before her death, having contracted the disease from her mother.[119]

Dedicated wards were one means of separating venereal patients from other sick inmates, no doubt on the grounds of the immoral connotations of the disease. However, other ways had to be devised at times to ensure complete segregation, particularly at times when the workhouse wards were overcrowded. Birmingham guardians set up a committee in 1856 to consider the best means of separating women with venereal disease from other inmates when well enough to be moved off the venereal wards into the main body of the workhouse. However, the committee's report was not recorded, although it was accepted by the board.[120] This issue arose again twenty-four years later when it was thought that some women who did not have the disease had been placed in the venereal ward. The medical officer examined the six women in question, who were the ones with young babies, confirming the diagnosis. He suggested that the "worst and most infectious cases" be accommodated in a building detached from the main workhouse. Those next in severity should be in the upper story of a building that housed a convalescent ward. In addition, a receiving ward should be made available for pregnant women who might be infected before transfer to an appropriate ward. Thus, his classification entailed a probationary (receiving) ward, a ward for "what may be termed the better class of cases," and a ward for "the worst cases."[121] When the new detached infirmary was due to open in 1889, patients suffering from venereal disease were not considered appropriate for transfer and the wards remained in the workhouse.[122] After the formation of the combined Birmingham Union in 1914, the female venereal patients were transferred to wards in the infirmary. The men were to be accommodated in a new block, consisting of two wards of thirteen beds each, and all venereal men from within the new union would be treated there. At that time, there were thirty-two men and twenty-eight women with gonorrhea and forty-one men and fifty-three women with syphilis in the workhouse.[123] This arrangement was not unusual as venereal wards in the majority of unions were in the workhouse rather than the infirmary and separating the sexes between the two institutions was not uncommon. Also, it was usual to choose the wards in the worst condition for venereal patients. Some unions attempted to separate "the more advanced female patients" from those less infected. Women were sometimes not allowed to exercise in the open air and men not allowed to leave their ward.[124] Thus, even at the beginning of the twentieth century, patients with venereal disease in poor law institutions were suffering discrimination.

The segregation of venereal patients from other workhouse inmates had the added advantage of preventing spread of disease. However, the risk of becoming infected came not just from patients. An outbreak of ophthalmia occurred in Birmingham in November 1875, starting in the schools and spreading to adults, but with no fresh cases after June 1876. Ophthalmia was due to an infection causing inflammation of the conjunctiva, which could

Table 3.10. General and venereal patients in workhouses during the first week of June 1876 and the number of deaths during 1875

	Birmingham	Wolverhampton	England and Wales
Number of inmates on medical relief books	861	287	44,735
Number of cases of gonorrhea	19	–	121
Number of cases of primary syphilis	17	10	226
Number of cases of secondary syphilis	19	2	413
Number of cases of unspecified venereal disease	–	6	195
Total deaths from all causes	512	176	28,574
Deaths due to syphilis	7	2	184
Deaths due to gonorrhea	–	–	4

Source: HCPP, 1877 (260), *Returns of General Diseases and of Venereal diseases*, 10–11, 17.

lead to blindness. In the nineteenth century, the most common infecting agent in children was the gonococcus. The medical officer, Adam Simpson, traced a total of 195 cases in the following locations: infants' school, 97; girls' school, 22; nursery school, 26; lying-in ward, 5; bad head ward, 4; sewing room, 3; oakum room, 1; fever ward, 2, plus 35 patients had been admitted to the house with the disease. Simpson had initially put the cause down to measles in the schools, but had found that a pauper acting as an undernurse in the infants' school for five weeks was suffering from gonorrhea. Subsequently, two other pauper undernurses were also diagnosed with gonorrhea and removed from duty in the school. In addition, a patient had been admitted from the infants' school to the female venereal wards in February 1876. He felt unable at that point to "positively assert this as the cause but it is suspicious," the locations where the disease occurred tending "to prove my suspicions." He treated those infected by attending to general overcrowding, bad ventilation, provision for open-air exercise, lack of cleanliness, and diet.[125]

Treatment of Syphilis

The mainstay of treatment from the sixteenth century onward was mercury, either ingested as a pill or applied locally as an ointment, although they were not curative. One of the most popular forms was the blue pill, which also contained confection of roses and powdered licorice. However, as the massive doses prescribed were not always effective and produced side effects, a nonmercurial plan of treatment, known as the "simple plan" and based on the antiphlogistic regimen and local bloodletting, came into favor in the early nineteenth century.[126] Langston Parker, a surgeon at Queen's Hospital, Birmingham, and an expert on venereal disease, recommended that treatment with mercury be withheld in primary syphilis until the patient had been prepared for it by means of the simple method. However, he preferred to start it immediately for secondary manifestations.[127] The most important of the many alternative forms of treatment that were tried was iodide of potassium, introduced in 1836, but it became restricted to the treatment of tertiary disease. Powerful caustics such as nitric acid were used to treat sores and other local manifestations.[128] Although both mercury and iodine are treponemacidal, it is likely that they were only suppressive of clinical symptoms rather than curative.[129] In 1910, Paul Ehrlich, a German medical scientist, developed salvarsan, an arsenical compound as an effective curative treatment, although it was subsequently amended to neo-salvarsan because of toxic side effects of the earlier preparation. It had to be administered with caution by intravenous injection and a number of injections were required until evidence of healing of lesions took place.[130]

Mercury was used to treat syphilis in both Birmingham and Wolverhampton workhouses. The medical officer of the latter visited the female venereal wards twice weekly in 1856 and prescribed a "white medicine," which he denied was "salts and magnesia" on the grounds that they were "inappropriate to the disease."[131] Birmingham's workhouse medical officer, John Wilmshurst, expressed the view at that time that venereal patients were "neglected in many Unions and the surgeon never examined them" and they were "simply dosed with salt and senna and discharged cured." This followed the guardians becoming concerned about the large increase in syphilitic cases and whether it was due to more liberal treatment being extended to "that unfortunate class." Wilmshurst claimed to provide superior treatment compared to that in other workhouses and felt it was not surprising that they came "where they can get some specific medical treatment in wards set apart for the cure of these complaints."[132] He attributed his treatment to attracting an increased number of venereal patients to the workhouse and his view was given some support by the following statement provided for the guardians by workhouse inmate Emma Rose, aged twenty-three years:

I belong to Kidderminster—I have been in the workhouse there about three months and suffered from venereal disease all the time I was in that workhouse. I was in bed all the time—I often asked the Medical Attendant for Medicine but during the last 2 months, I could not obtain any. Mrs Priddy, the Nurse of the Sick Wards examined me one morning in the early part of last week and said I was worse than when I went into the workhouse and was in a very bad state indeed. She said that if I came to the Birmingham Workhouse, I should be sure to get cured and she advised me to come to the Birmingham Workhouse. I arrived in Birmingham last Thursday evening . . . and on Friday morning I (in company with Emma Bayliss) went to the parish offices to ask for a Note of Admission into the workhouse. (BCL, BBG GP/2/1/20, November 18, 1857)

An inquiry by the guardians to Kidderminster Union elicited a denial by Mrs. Priddy that she had said Rose would be treated better in Birmingham. She attributed the comment to Elizabeth Edwards, an inmate at Kidderminster suffering from venereal disease, claiming Edwards had said "she had had more good done to her in six weeks" in the Birmingham workhouse than in two years in Kidderminster. The medical officer there reported that Emma Rose was treated with nitrate of silver almost daily for the removal of condylomata, having refused to have "the better and quicker remedy, nitric acid."[133]

In 1867, Wolverhampton guardians accepted that there would be "those who have come to be cured of venereal disease" and inquired of the Poor Law Board whether they could have the power to retain patients in the workhouse for a certain period after they were deemed cured.[134] However, they did not record the reply. The power of compulsory detention in the workhouse was again raised in 1913 by Dr. Johnstone, but the unanimous opinion was that it would deter patients from coming for treatment. He raised the question because of the considerable difficulty in retaining patients for treatment in the institution until the most infective stage had passed. In over half the workhouses he visited, the doctors and officials confessed to extreme difficulty in retaining venereal patients for a sufficient time for treatment and had acquiesced in "their coming and going as they pleased."[135] It seems that little had changed in over fifty years since Emma Rose exhibited the same behavior when she was in Kidderminster workhouse.

Despite the possible difficulty with compliance with treatment, Birmingham guardians, toward the end of the century, hoped to transfer venereal patients to the Lock Hospital on a payment-per-patient basis. Their number had diminished, totaling three males and seven females in September 1892. However, this did not prove possible due to the pressure of work at the hospital and the limited number of twelve beds.[136] In 1912, the guardians arranged that venereal patients could be transferred temporarily to the Skin and Lock Hospital for treatment with salvarsan for a course of therapy of up to ten days' duration. They agreed to a fee of twenty-one shillings for one week or part of one week, plus the cost of the drugs. In the following three months, Mary Whitehouse, Margaret Timmins, George Thomas, and John Whitcombe all received salvarsan injections. Timmins returned to the workhouse much improved, but returned to the Lock Hospital for a second course of treatment, as did George Thomas.[137] The guardians' preference to refer these workhouse inmates to the specialist hospital for treatment, rather than arrange it at their own infirmary, was in line with the national trend to use specialist institutions.[138] In the report of the Royal Commission on Venereal Diseases, the medical officer for Wolverhampton declared that salvarsan had been used in only a few cases, although around seventy-seven venereal patients had been admitted in the previous twelve months. However, he did not identify where the treatment had been carried out.

Punishment or Treatment?

Mechanical restraint and seclusion were employed not only to control behavioral disorder in mentally ill patients, but generally to punish any form of bad behavior or dissent by any of the inmates. Their use could also have had a deterrent effect on those inmates who witnessed others being restrained. Another method found to be useful as an effective punishment was the cold shower or a "forcible plunge into a cold bath." Both warm and cold baths had originally been thought to have therapeutic properties and continued in use on that basis. As a result, the use of baths as treatment and as punishment inevitably became intermingled.[139] The fact that the medical officer was seen to have a disciplinary as well as a medical role within the workhouse makes the distinction between treatment and punishment indistinguishable.[140] In general, methods of workhouse punishment and medical ideas on treatment of pauper lunatics was a controversial area throughout the nineteenth century.[141]

One of the complaints against the Wolverhampton medical officer, George Cooper, in 1851 (referred to in chapter 4) was that he had confined William Newell in the lunatic wards in the workhouse for three days as punishment. John Bytheway, eighty-six years old and partially blind, also complained of being punished in 1873 because he had written a letter of complaint to the Local Government Board regarding his treatment when he was admitted severely ill three years before. He maintained that the medical officer had certified him as a lunatic as soon as his letter was forwarded to Wolverhampton Board. He wrote again to the central authority requesting that a commissioner in lunacy reassess his mental state.[142] Wolverhampton guardians made the distinction between treatment and punishment in 1902, when William Lewis complained that the medical officer had sent him to the "syphilitic ward" after he had been "misbehaving himself" and causing annoyance to other patients, although he was not suffering from venereal disease. The infirmary had been full and only one patient in the ward had been suffering from venereal disease. The guardians accepted that the medical officer had the authority to send patients to any ward he deemed best for medical treatment, but informed him that it was improper to do so as punishment.[143]

A more detailed examination of the question came about during a Local Government Board inquiry into the practice of Adam Simpson, workhouse medical officer in Birmingham, with regard to Ellen Peters and Mary Jane Skett. The conduct of Ellen Peters, a patient in the venereal ward, was strange and she had been removed to the imbecile wards and put in the padded room by order of Charles Mitchell, assistant workhouse medical officer. She had a shower bath administered as a punishment for "exposing her person" and a blister carried out by Nurse Burns on the instructions of one of the other assistant medical officers.[144] Later, she tried to cut her throat and broke windows with a poker, for which she was taken before the magistrates and jailed. Skett, an imbecile, had been resident in the workhouse for three years and had had four shower baths and two episodes of blistering that she declared had been carried out as a punishment. The chairman of the committee that carried out an inquiry into the matter expressed the view the use of padded rooms, blisters, and shower baths were cruelties rather than punishments. However, it was pointed out to him that these were medical treatments. Indeed, physical forms of therapy, such as blistering and bloodletting, were frequently employed in the treatment of mentally ill patients at that time. Simpson did not clarify the position directly himself, leaving the committee to conclude that his orders had been meant as punishment. The guardian requested a Local Government Board inquiry, following which he was censured for committing a grave error of judgment in secluding a sane inmate in the padded room. Simpson's actions were defended by Joseph Rogers, president of the Poor Law Medical Officers' Association and a leading reformer of the poor law medical service, who had personally encountered "malingering and deception" among workhouse inmates on a daily basis. For those who tried to gain sympathy for "their imaginary sufferings," he considered mustard poultices, blisters, the galvanic battery, or the shower bath the "most fitting treatment." He pointed out that such "heroic treatment" was also used in voluntary hospitals on the suspicion of malingering.[145]

This real-life story exemplifies the difficulties for medical staff in controlling the behavior of patients in workhouses, both in those with and without mental health issues. Other institutions could choose their patient clientele, whereas the workhouse could not refuse admission to those who were destitute. The possibility of discharge was always open to hospitals and asylums, with the workhouse available if no other avenues of removal were possible. We need to see the struggle to provide care within this context. The architecture of workhouses was not a suitable one in which to provide accommodation for the mentally ill. It was severely criticized at times by the commissioners in lunacy, but neglect and maltreatment of lunatics was found to be endemic in all the various types of institutions they visited in the early to mid-nineteenth century.[146] Conditions in the new county asylums were an improvement and unions did seek to move as many lunatics as possible out of the workhouse as soon as one became available in the locality. Thereafter, transfer between the two institutions became problematic. This study does not support the view that the major reason for so few workhouse lunatics being admitted to asylums was the guardians' reluctance on the grounds of parsimony. Rather it appears multifactorial and those whom the medical officers recommended did get transferred to asylums. It is easy to be critical of the standard of care and accommodation afforded to what were seen as undesirable inmates, often being allocated the worst-kept wards and often within the main part of the workhouse rather than the infirmary. However, we must remember that to the present day, mental health services in Britain have suffered from chronic underinvestment even after the National Health Service was in place.[147] The result has been insufficient and less satisfactory accommodation for patients with mental illness compared with services for patients with physical health problems and inadequate levels of both medical and nursing staff. It is to the doctors who worked in the poor law medical service that we turn our attention in the next chapter.

Chapter Four

Day-to-Day Doctoring

Under the Old Poor Law, parishes paid for medical attendance on a fee-for-service basis, but by the early nineteenth century, many found it more convenient to contract with a medical practitioner based on an annual salary.[1] The latter arrangement was cemented after the Poor Law Amendment Act (1834) when the Poor Law Commissioners authorized boards of guardians to appoint medical officers for the provision of outdoor medical relief and for the attendance on sick inmates in workhouses. Consequently, guardians treated medical officers on the same basis as other officers or servants employed by them. For instance, William Sturrock, workhouse medical officer in Birmingham in 1900, complained that he was allowed only three weeks' annual leave, whereas other first-class officers had four. He claimed that this "seems like a slur on Medicine that its representative should be ranked with subordinate officers."[2] Immediately after the New Poor Law, guardians appointed the doctors by utilizing the tendering process, usually choosing the lowest submitted. This arrangement was abolished after the General Medical Order of 1847 required a salary decided by the guardians to be stated at the time the post was advertised. Medical officers were usually appointed on an annual basis, despite the order directing that tenure should be permanent. It also required them to be qualified as surgeons and apothecaries.[3] This was modified by an order in 1859 to require qualifications to practice medicine and surgery in England and Wales, thereby ensuring that poor law medical officers were better qualified than practitioners in private practice. However, the dual requirement could be circumvented if a doctor lived outside the district of his responsibility. Although salaries were set by guardians prior to appointment, they remained very low, varied greatly, and were a cause of frequent complaint.[4] Despite this, medical officers were the one common denominator within a patchwork of welfare practices and fundamental to medical welfare.[5]

This chapter will consider the conditions under which the workhouse medical officers of Birmingham and Wolverhampton labored and will provide an estimate of their workload. The questions it attempts to answer include to what extent the New Poor Law influenced the institutional medical care of paupers and how the development of infirmaries affected medical staffing. A comparison between the arrangements in Birmingham and Wolverhampton has allowed exploration of possible differences in the performance of resident and nonresident medical officers. For instance, was the greater continuity of medical care that occurred with the appointment of nonresident staff a positive advantage? How they came into conflict with guardians and other poor law officers over patient care and why medical officers were at times exonerated while others were charged with medical negligence will be explored. To what extent did the imposition of charges reflect the approach of medical officers to their patients? The chapter will commence with details of the medical officers, followed by an analysis of their conditions of employment and the number of patients they cared for. It will question whether the medical officers' workload compromised their management of patients.

Appointment and Duties of the Workhouse Medical Officer

The duties of the medical officer were prescribed in Article 78 of workhouse regulations in the Second Annual Report of the Poor Law Commissioners in 1836. These required him to attend at times stated by the guardians and in emergencies at the request of the master; to visit the sick as their condition necessitated; to examine all lunatics; to give directions for inmates' diets; to provide and dispense all medicines; to keep a register of morbidity and mortality; and to provide the guardians with regular reports on the inmates treated. He was required to inform the guardians of defects in sanitation, ventilation and heating, and the conduct of the nursing staff. All admissions to the workhouse were to be examined by him and classified into the appropriate group. In particular, he had the task of separating the "able-bodied," who could be assigned work, from the "non-able-bodied." This and his duty to decide the fitness of inmates for punishment meant that he was seen as much a part of the disciplinary system as the provider of medical care.[6] In 1847, the task of vaccinating all children entering the workhouse was added to his list of duties. According to Kim Price, his workload must have been immense, making it almost impossible for him to carry out his duties conscientiously. As he was able to appoint an assistant without medical qualifications, it was often left to that individual to attend to those in the workhouse, while the medical officer devoted his time to his private patients.[7] This was possible as the most usual arrangement for medical care for inmates of the workhouse was for guardians to engage a private practitioner, whose contract may have included duties as a district medical officer in addition. Jeanne Brand is of the opinion that the regulations were so general that they allowed not only considerable variation in performance but "outright abuse."[8]

Less frequent practice was the appointment of a full-time doctor specifically for the workhouse, sometimes with the requirement to reside within it. His workload was considerably greater than those of resident medical officers in voluntary hospitals. For instance, *The Lancet* commented in 1867 that Bethnal Green workhouse had only one officer for 600 patients, while a similar-sized voluntary hospital in London would have had fifteen doctors. Full-time employment within workhouses was a controversial issue, opposed by *The Lancet* and Dr. Edward Smith, medical officer to the Poor Law Board. Joseph Rogers, a reformer and workhouse medical officer in the 1860s, was instrumental in getting the requirement for the infirmaries in London to have resident surgeons supervised by visiting physicians included in the Metropolitan Poor Act of 1867.[9] Over the following four years, those who were resident increased in the capital from three out of a total of twelve to seven of thirteen.[10] By the early 1880s, a majority of metropolitan medical officers served full-time and no longer carried out private practice.[11] In the provinces, they were most likely to be appointed in large urban workhouses, such as Liverpool, Nottingham, Manchester, and Birmingham (see table 4.1).[12] Although full-time contracts became more usual from the 1870s, 93 percent of the 625 unions in England and Wales still had no resident medical officer in 1900. Birmingham was unusual in appointing a resident surgeon to the workhouse as early as 1823, but was not unique for a provincial workhouse as Nottingham had one from 1822.[13]

Legacy of the Old Poor Law

After 1834, there was a marked reduction in the number of medical officers' posts in the new unions. In seven examples given by Irvine Loudon, the extent of the removal of medical men ranged from 50 percent to 81 percent.[14] Birmingham, at the time of the New Poor Law, employed six surgeons who received thirty pounds per annum, were each allocated to a district, with responsibility for attending patients in their homes and at the town dispensary. They all had duties in the Town Infirmary, where the medical staffing also consisted of one resident house surgeon and apothecary, plus two assistant apothecaries. The surgeon was paid an annual salary of seventy pounds and received free accommodation and board. His duties, prescribed

Table 4.1. Resident workhouse medical officers in Birmingham workhouse, 1830–1914

Name	Time in office	Annual salary	Reason for termination
Joseph Pedley	March 1830–March 1837	£50–£70	Died
A. H. Nourse	March 1837–July 1839	£70	Resigned; private practice
Charles Smith	July 1839–March 1850	£70	Reorganization of medical officers
John Humphrey	March 1850–April 1855	£150–£175	Appointed to civil hospital
William Fernie	May 1855–April 1857	£150	Resigned
John Wilmshurst	May 1857–May 1858	£150	Resigned
John Redfern Davies	June 1858–October 1861	£150–£200	Resigned at request of guardians
Edmund Robinson	October 1861–January 1869	£200–£350	Appointed public vaccinator
Edmund Whitcombe	February 1869–July 1870	£200	Appointed to Borough Lunatic Asylum
Adam Simpson	August 1870–August 1886	£200–£350	Removed from office by Local Government Board
Charles Mitchell	August 1886–January 1890	£207	Resigned
Edmund Corder	February 1890–April 1890	£150–£200	Resigned
Ebenezer Teichelmann	April 1890–September 1891	£150–£200	Resigned
George Ferraby	October 1891–October 1894	£150	Appointed district medical officer
George Barber	November 1894–May 1895	£150	Resigned
Alexander McDougall	May 1895–March 1899	£150–£200	Appointed district medical officer
William Sturrock	May 1899–September 1914	£150–£200	Granted leave to take up active service

Source: BCL, BBG, GP/B/2/1/3–67, March 1830 to September 1899; Advisory Sub Committee, GP/B/2/8/2/1, September 23, 1914.

prior to the New Poor Law, included visiting each ward twice daily and providing a list of necessary drugs, plus responsibility for cleanliness and "good
order" of the sick wards and "superintendence" of the nurses. The assistants
were nonresident and had an annual salary of fifty pounds; their duties were
not stated, but would have included dispensing drugs. The inpatient workload of all the medical officers from April to June 1834 consisted of between
116 and 123 patients, while that for the surgeons also included 2,722 seen
in the dispensary, 1,385 seen at home, and 108 midwifery cases, which they
monitored in association with the poor law midwives.[15] By comparison, the
medical officer of Nottingham Union in July 1837 was responsible for 58

patients in the union hospital, 47 in the workhouse, and 351 outpatients, with the help of only a dispenser in the institutions.[16] In Birmingham ten years later, it was decided to separate the indoor and outdoor medical relief, as the house surgeon was being "called out of the workhouse" frequently, and six additional surgeons were appointed for district work only. It was planned to reduce the existing surgeons (who were to work in the infirmary only) to four as vacancies arose, with a reduced salary of ten pounds per annum. At that time, the number of patients in the infirmary had increased to around 150, while that of dispensary patients had fallen by half. Rather than a reduction, more surgeons were appointed, so that by March 1847, sixteen were in post, with annual salaries of between ten pounds and twenty pounds.[17]

As Birmingham parish had been established by an individual act of Parliament, the guardians could resist aligning with the regulations of the New Poor Law for many years. However, the increasing influence of the central authority, exerted through the Poor Law Board inspectors, resulted in a radical reorganization of medical staffing in 1849, with a substantial reduction in the number of medical officers. The number of sick in the infirmary (160) had not shown an increase in the years before this, but the new workhouse was in the planning stage with a proposed infirmary of just over 300 beds.[18] Inpatients were to be cared for by only one resident surgeon at an enhanced annual salary of £150, plus "lodgings, coals and candle." His duties would be governed by the workhouse regulations laid down by the Poor Law Board, and the guardians would continue to cover the cost of drugs. The salary may have been improved in the hope of obtaining a more experienced practitioner or it may have reflected the anticipated increase in workload. The surgeons were reduced to six, with responsibility for only outdoor medical relief, at an annual salary of £150, which was to include the cost of all "drugs, medicines and surgical appliances." Notice was given to the assistant apothecaries and surgeons that their services would not be required after Lady Day in 1850.[19] Charles Smith, house surgeon, did not apply for the redesigned post, although the fact that he was then sixty-six years old may have influenced his decision. Fifteen candidates applied and John Humphrey was elected. Five of the preexisting surgeons were appointed to the six new district medical officer posts, out of a total of forty-six applications.[20] The workhouse medical officer was no longer supported by more senior colleagues, although the guardians allowed him to request a second medical opinion from physicians and surgeons in the town, who were paid a fee for their services. Despite the increasing medical role of Birmingham infirmary, the central authority had succeeded in reducing medical staffing and thereby the quality of patient care.

Meeting an Increasing Workload in the New Infirmary

John Humphrey transferred to the new workhouse when it opened in March 1852. From then until 1914, fourteen medical officers held the office of resident surgeon, serving for periods varying from one month to sixteen years with an average just over four-and-a-half years (table 3.1). With only four spending more than five years in office, there was little continuity of medical care, which varied according to the practices of individual officers.[21] This is similar to the situation at the town's General Hospital where the resident medical officers between 1857 and 1875 had an average length of service of approximately three years. However, continuity was provided by eight honorary physicians and surgeons, whose periods in office ranged from eight to thirty-seven years.[22] A similar situation was not initiated at the workhouse until 1882, when a visiting physician was appointed, followed by a visiting surgeon five years later. The stimulus for these appointments was a visit, at the request of the guardians, by two Local Government Board inspectors, one of which was Dr. Frederic Mouat, MD. They suggested that two nonresident medical officers should be appointed to provide adequate medical cover.[23] The guardians' reaction was to send a deputation to assess the medical administration of the workhouse at Liverpool, which housed around 3,000 inmates, compared with about 2,500 in Birmingham. Both the medical and surgical officers in Liverpool were nonresident, visited the workhouse daily, and supervised the three assistants. The Liverpool guardians allowed the nonresident officers to have private practices in order to attract high-quality candidates and by so doing could manage with fewer medical staff.[24] Comparing the cost of the medical departments at the two workhouses, Birmingham appears generous in its payment to medical staff since it was very unusual for poor law medical salaries to rise above £250 per annum (table 4.2).[25] Birmingham guardians decided to appoint only one visiting physician, Dr. Cornelius Suckling, who already held an appointment as honorary physician to the Queen's Hospital and became professor of medicine at Mason's College, the precursor to the University of Birmingham.[26] Five years later, Dr. George Jordan Lloyd was appointed visiting surgeon at the workhouse at the same annual salary of £150.[27] At the time of his appointment to the workhouse, Lloyd was honorary surgeon at the Queen's Hospital and later became professor of surgery at the University of Birmingham. In making these appointments, the guardians were emulating the staffing arrangements at the voluntary hospitals. The workhouse medical officers continued to be employed on a full-time basis, were required to be resident, and were not permitted to practice privately. Starting salaries rose from £150 per

Table 4.2. Annual cost of medical administration in Liverpool and Birmingham workhouses in 1882

Liverpool		Birmingham	
Medical officer	£150	Medical officer	£350
Surgical officer	£150	Assistant MO	£200
3 Assistant MOs	£240	Assistant MO	£150
Dispenser	£80	Dispenser	£130
Assistant dispenser	£78	Assistant dispenser	£18
Total annual cost	£698	Total annual cost	£848

Source: BCL, HSC, GP/B/2/3/3/8, July 4, 1882.

annum, plus board, lodgings, and a personal servant, to £200 per annum in 1861, but returned to the previous level in 1890 after the new infirmary opened (table 4.1).[28]

Workhouse medical officers during these decades resigned for a variety of reasons. For example, in 1855, John Humphrey took up an appointment at a new civil hospital near Constantinople.[29] Barber left because of ill health, and Fernie resigned due to the heavy workload. A few were appointed to public posts locally, for instance as public vaccinator in 1869 and two as district medical officers in the 1890s. Edmund Whitcombe received his medical education at Sydenham College in Birmingham and was appointed to the workhouse the year after becoming MRCS.[30] He resigned eighteen months later to take up the post of assistant medical superintendent at the Borough Lunatic Asylum and was appointed to a chair of mental diseases at the University of Birmingham in the late 1880s (table 3.1).[31] Charles Mitchell left to set up a private practice and Ebeneezer Teichelmann to return to his native Australia. William Sturrock was called up for active service in 1914, having joined the Territorial Army six years before.[32] In general, there were few workhouse medical officers in Birmingham who left public service and were appointed to positions at local voluntary hospitals, one exception being Redfern Davies, who was honorary surgeon to Birmingham Children's Hospital three years after resigning from the workhouse. As those acting as resident surgeons in workhouses were at an early stage in their careers, poor law records rarely contain detailed information about their practices after resignation. However, part-time workhouse medical officers could hold honorary appointments at voluntary hospitals in addition to their poor law duties, for instance, Dr. L. M. Guilding at Battle workhouse was also assistant surgeon at the Royal Berkshire Hospital.[33]

Humphrey's workload increased when around 250 children were transferred from the Infant Poor Asylum to the new workhouse a few months after it opened in 1852 and his salary was increased by twenty-five pounds.[34] Within a few months, he was complaining of an "extensive increase in duties," having attended 1,048 patients over the past year, with 706 coming under his care in the last six months. He felt in need of help as "the continuous strain presses hard on physical and mental energy when only a single acting individual."[35] He requested help in the form of an articled pupil, as was allowed to the district medical officers. The guardians agreed, but the Poor Law Board refused because it would have permitted someone to be resident in the workhouse and not be directly responsible to the guardians through the master.[36] Two years later, he again appealed for help:

> The continued and regular increase in the number of sick persons admitted into Birmingham Workhouse renders it absolutely necessary to apply to you for some assistance. Since the commencement of this year I have admitted into the Infirmary 448 patients, making with 273 persons in the sick wards on the 1st of January, a total of 721. Besides the patients in the Infirmary, I have a large number to attend to in the Workhouse and my duties . . . become so great as at times completely exhaust me. The daily average of patients in the Infirmary is 318 and this number prevents me from giving that attention to some of them, which their cases require. (BCL, BBG, GP/B/2/1/15, February 28, 1855)

Although a nonresident dispenser was appointed at an annual salary of seventy-five pounds, John Humphrey resigned a few months later to take up an appointment at a new civil hospital near Constantinople.[37]

The following year the guardians decided to compare the workhouse's staffing levels and salaries with those in England and Wales built for the accommodation of 1,000 inmates or more. Returns were received from eleven unions. The workhouses of Liverpool, Manchester, and Marylebone Street in London with over 2,000 inmates employed four, two, and two medical officers and assistants respectively, while the others employed only one (table 4.3). Salaries ranged from £70 to £250 per annum, but most were between £100 and £150.[38] As Birmingham's salary was compatible with the other unions, the guardians took no action on the basis of the returns.

Humphrey's successor in 1855 was William Fernie, but he resigned within two years because he felt unable to "continue the necessary performance of my unremitting duties [sic] with no reasonable opportunity for recreation of body or relaxation of mind." In his testimonial, the guardians accepted that his duties were "onerous" because of the crowded state of the workhouse, but took no action to rectify matters and merely advertised for a replacement. One of the two candidates selected for interview for the vacant post was

Table 4.3. Number of medical officers with remuneration, in workhouses in England built to accommodate 1,000 inmates or more, 1856

Union or parish	Number of inmates	Number of medical officers	Annual salaries	Extra remuneration
Birmingham	1,663	1	£150	Board
City of London	1,016	1	£175	Rations
Clifton	1,186	1	£70	–
Greenwich	1,044	1	£175	–
Lambeth	1,100	1	£250	Board, rations
Liverpool	2,345	4	£100, £100, £80, £80	Rations for two juniors
Manchester	2,000	2	£130, £85	–
Marylebone Street	2,000	2	£150, £80	Rations
Nottingham	1,150	2	£120, £120	–
Portsea Island	1,150	1	£150	–

Source: BCL, Returns, GP/B/18/2/1, October 15, 1856.

assistant surgeon at St. Pancras workhouse, but he withdrew his candidacy when he discovered the extent of the duties at Birmingham.[39] The successful candidate was John Wilmshurst, who was resident surgeon at Birmingham Lying-in Hospital, but when his request in the first year of his tenure for additional help was turned down, he resigned three months later. The reason the guardians gave for their refusal was that other large workhouses in England, such as City of London, Clifton, Greenwich, and Lambeth, had only one medical officer, although Manchester, St. Marylebone, and Nottingham had two.[40]

In 1864, Edmund Robinson, after two years in post, reported that his workload had significantly increased, so that he was occupied all day and part of the night with his workhouse duties.[41] His request for an increase in salary, rather than for assistance, was granted, raising his remuneration from £200 to £250 per annum. In Edward Smith's report on provincial workhouse infirmaries two years later, Robinson is recorded as being satisfied with his workload and did not need assistance, in spite of having to care for between 600 and 700 sick inmates. Interestingly, his salary had by then been increased to £350 annually and this level would not have been possible with additional medical personnel.[42] Commenting on Smith's report, *The Lancet* praised Birmingham workhouse as one of the best managed in the provinces, but found it hard to believe "that the whole of these 600 sick are properly attended to, even granting the chronic nature of a large number of the cases."[43] The employment of only one medical officer was also severely criticized in 1865 by a local doctor, who found it unbelievable that "a rich and progressive town like Birmingham" would permit "an infirmary containing 599 beds to be officered by one medical man."[44] In early 1874, *The Lancet* once again criticized Birmingham guardians for employing only one resident surgeon, suggesting "the medical supervision of the infirmary, with its 958 patients, must be merely nominal."[45] A few months later, following a Local Government Board inspector's criticism of the adequacy of the staffing of the medical department, the guardians eventually agreed to the appointment of an assistant medical officer at an annual salary of £100.[46] However, Cuthbert Fitzsimmon was not appointed until June 1876, but both he and his successor, Aird Jolly, remained in post for less than a year. Charles Mitchell followed them in 1877 and eleven years later he was promoted to workhouse medical officer.[47]

A subcommittee was set up in October 1877, at the instigation of the central authority, to consider medical and nursing arrangements in the workhouse. The medical officer, Adam Simpson, considered that he had had no particular difficulty in performing his duties before an assistant was appointed, but admitted there was more work with the patients than he could perform, although he had given them satisfactory attention. He had needed to work hard, but had "broke down" on occasions, so that it was not the patients who had suffered, "rather it was himself." Simpson estimated that three surgeons were needed to provide sufficient care for the number of patients, which he put at 900 to 1,000. The two assistants would share the work between them and visit their patients daily; he would provide supervision and be available for consultation over difficult cases. Charles Mitchell, assistant medical officer, agreed that patients did not suffer, but they were liable to be overlooked and with more time, could be more carefully examined. Mitchell spent from 9:00 a.m. to 12:00 p.m. daily going around the wards and seeing people in the body of the house, and saw admissions in the afternoon. He was called up at night about twice per week.[48] The subcommittee recommended the appointment of a third surgeon to improve the medical care of patients. When Suckling was appointed visiting physician in 1882, he took charge of the medical wards, leaving Simpson to cover the surgical wards. The assistants were divided between the medical and surgical departments, and when Jordan Lloyd took up office as visiting surgeon five years later, he became responsible for the surgical wards of the infirmary. The central authority had finally recognized the need for adequate medical staffing in workhouses. The guardians on the subcommittee in 1877 were impressed by the large number of acutely ill patients, which had turned the workhouse into "a large Hospital containing cases of so many various kinds of disease."[49] In doing so, they were recognizing in their own institution the national trend toward the increasing involvement of workhouses in medical care and this development will be explored in the next section.

Developing the Infirmary into a General Hospital

After the new Birmingham infirmary opened in 1889 on a separate site adjacent to the workhouse, the medical staffing began to align with that of the voluntary hospitals. The two assistant medical officers in the workhouse were transferred as resident surgeons and Charles Mitchell, who had been acting as workhouse medical officer, was appointed to the post on a substantive basis. The visiting physician and surgeon had their duties apportioned between the two institutions, with the majority of their time spent at the new infirmary. An editorial in *The Lancet* was once again extremely concerned that the medical staffing was inadequate, stating:

> The 1,700 beds will . . . be occupied by sick persons requiring active medical supervision and treatment. For this number of persons there is to be a medical staff consisting of a visiting physician and a visiting surgeon, and two resident assistant medical officers . . . there is to be no medical superintendent. We have no hesitation in saying that it is impossible the sick can be properly cared for under these circumstances. The varying wants of sick people needing personal attention requires a detailed supervision, of which there can be none in the Birmingham Infirmary. (Anonymous, "Editorial," 1244–45)

In a letter of reply the following week, Cornelius Suckling, visiting physician, defended the staffing arrangement by pointing out there would also be two qualified resident clinical clerks, so giving a complement of six doctors and that many patients suffered chronic ailments, not requiring frequent examination. Throughout the previous six years, Suckling had paid a daily visit, usually lasting two hours, during which he examined "every fresh case" on the medical side, commenced treatment, and saw any case with which the resident officers required help. He claimed that in his time at the workhouse, more clinical reports had been published in the medical journals and more cases shown at medical societies from the infirmary than any other in the country, proving that the "cases there are gone into properly."[50] His account was challenged by an anonymous workhouse medical officer, who doubted that Suckling's stated workload could be completed in two hours.[51] Three years after the infirmary opened, improved arrangements for medical

Table 4.4. Visiting surgeon and physicians to Birmingham infirmary, 1882–1913

	Name	Time in office	Annual salary	Reason for termination
Surgeon:	George Jordan Lloyd	January 1887–April 1913	£150–£200	Died
Physicians:	Cornelius Suckling	November 1882–January 1892	£150–£200	Resigned due to pressure of private practice
	Alfred Carter	April 1892–April 1898	£100	Resigned
	John Barrett	April 1892–January 1893	£100	Resigned as he had insufficient practical experience
	Sydney Short	April 1892–June 1913	£100	Post abolished
	Otto Kauffman	April 1893–June 1913	£100	Post abolished
	Thomas Wilson	May 1898–March 1903	£100	Resigned
	Ross Jordan	April 1903–June 1913	£100	Post abolished

Source: BCL, BBG, GP/B/2/1/50–82, 1887–1913.

staffing were introduced, with the appointment of two additional visiting physicians (table 4.4). Each of the physicians and the surgeon was allotted one of the resident medical officers, who rotated every six months.[52] The resident surgeon held office for short periods of time, sometimes being succeeded by one of the clinical clerks. In the early 1900s, the tenure of the posts was fixed at one year, but with renewal possible.[53] The majority of the visiting physicians were of high professional standing in the town, with honorary posts at the voluntary hospitals. Otto Kauffman, for example, became professor of medicine at the University of Birmingham, after visiting posts at the infirmary were abolished in 1913.[54] At this time, Frederick Ellis, FRCS, MD, was appointed medical superintendent at an annual salary of £750, to increase incrementally to £1,000.[55]

After the new infirmary opened in 1889, the medical officer at the workhouse, Charles Mitchell, continued to have a heavy workload, as not all patients had been moved to the new institution. Initially, he had the support of the visiting physician and surgeon, who had a minor portion of their duties allocated to the workhouse. The visiting physician's input lapsed when Suckling resigned, but was restored two years later with the appointment of the senior physician at the infirmary, Alfred Carter, at an annual salary of twenty-five pounds. However, when four years later he had not completed the required reports for almost a year and did not have evidence to prove his attendance at the workhouse, he was asked to resign.[56] No subsequent appointments appear to have been made. The workhouse medical officer spent a considerable amount of his time seeing patients in the venereal and bedridden wards. He spent two-and-a-half hours each morning examining tramps and outpatients and visited the receiving wards five times each day between 12:00 p.m. and 10:00 p.m. He admitted thirty to forty inmates daily, with each one taking up to fifteen minutes, so that he could be busy until 11:00 p.m.[57] In addition, he had to assess all potential admissions to the infirmary at the workhouse. Likewise, all patients were discharged from the infirmary to the workhouse before being allowed home. In 1880, the board of guardians had decided that it was not desirable for patients to be admitted directly to the infirmary and this policy had the Local Government Board's approval.[58] This was partially relaxed when it was agreed in 1900 that cases sent in by ambulance could be sent directly to the infirmary, but only when the workhouse medical officer was on leave.[59] When a young woman admitted to the infirmary in 1903 refused to stay, the medical officer suggested she should be discharged directly through the infirmary gate. However, the guardians reemphasized their previous stance that all patients must be transferred to the workhouse before taking their final discharge.[60] By this time, the majority of unions had accepted that the principle of deterrence no longer applied to sick paupers.

Having only one resident medical attendant in the workhouse returned the institution to the inadequate level of medical staffing of the 1870s. Difficulties in medical attendance arose when he was on afternoon and occasional leave. The resident infirmary medical officers were required to perform his duties at these times, but it was often difficult to obtain their assistance. Delays occurred because of the time they took to arrive at the workhouse, after being called to see new admissions or sick inmates in the wards. This often arose because they were busy with duties in the wards or accompanying the visiting physicians. Eventually, in 1903, the Infirmary House Subcommittee recommended that all cases sent to the workhouse by the district medical officers, as well as ambulance cases, should be received directly at the new infirmary lodge during these periods of leave.[61] However, that did not solve the problem of attendance to sick patients arriving at the workhouse on their own initiative. On one occasion in January 1904, a man in pain arrived at the workhouse at 3:40 p.m., forty minutes after the workhouse surgeon had left, and the infirmary medical officer had not turned up to see him by 6:00 p.m., when a further telephone message was sent. After several more telephone calls, Dr. Cooper eventually arrived at 7:40 p.m., but the patient had not waited, returning the next day to be admitted to the infirmary.[62] A further incident occurred three years later, also involving

Dr. Cooper. Night Nurse Crocker had telephoned him at 9:00 p.m. to see Thomas Jeffrey with a "very bad ulcerated leg" in the probationary ward. He arrived an hour later, was annoyed at being called, made a cursory examination of the wound, and ordered the patient to the tramp ward without prescribing a dressing.[63] These were not the only problems resulting from the workhouse medical officer being sole resident in the workhouse, available both day and night. For instance, on one occasion in 1901, William Sturrock apologized for the four-hour delay in attending a patient, Edward Porter. Sturrock had been called out of bed three times during the night, then taken a "sedative draught to obtain sleep." After Nurse Brisbane called him at 6:30 a.m. to see Porter, he had gone off to sleep again and the nurse did not call a second time.[64] At that time, the 959 non-able-bodied and 575 able-bodied but temporarily disabled inmates present in the workhouse were likely to impose a heavy workload on one solitary surgeon.[65] Difficulties in the provision of adequate medical care due to large numbers of patients also occurred in Wolverhampton workhouse.

Part-time Medical Attendance in Wolverhampton Workhouse

The advantage of appointing workhouse medical officers on a nonresident, part-time basis and allowing them to practice privately in addition was that they were more likely to stay in post for many years, providing greater continuity of medical care. This was the arrangement in the first Wolverhampton workhouse, providing a contrast to that in Birmingham, but was more in keeping with most moderately sized workhouses in England. The first two medical officers also acted as district officers, but after 1852, district work was separated from that in the workhouse (table 4.5). All surgeons' posts were advertised for tender in 1839, and Charles Hodgkin was appointed to the workhouse at twenty-five pounds per annum.[66] Following readvertisement two years later, George Cooper took over the workhouse and Charles Hodgkin one of the districts.[67] Thereafter, the medical officers for the workhouse remained in post for many years (just over thirteen years on average), usually until they died or were asked to resign by the guardians. Only Richard Nugent resigned voluntarily, presumably to take up another appointment, as he had requested a testimonial three weeks before his resignation.[68] Wolverhampton medical officers rarely requested assistance when their workload increased, preferring to ask for an increase in salary, which would presumably help them to appoint assistants. George Cooper requested a bonus because of the influx of patients suffering from fever that had broken out in some lodging houses, but was rejected even though the guardians accepted that his duties had been onerous during the crisis. Their reason was that it was a contingency to which all contracts were liable. Mr. Perks, one of the guardians, was particularly unsympathetic, stating that "when the medical officer took his situation, he took it as a man took his wife, for better or worse."[69] When Nugent's salary was increased within a year of his appointment, it was on condition that he promptly attended every case of midwifery to which he was summoned, and the nurse was directed to call him as soon as any difficulty was suspected.[70] Henry Gibbons's salary was increased in 1866 to enable him to take on an assistant to carry out the dispensing. He supported his case by pointing out that the workhouse infirmary had 300 beds and the annual number of cases was 1,706. Whereas, at the local voluntary hospital, there were only 100 beds, with 750 cases in the year, and the patients were cared for by eight "medical men" and two pupils.[71] Eight years later, the guardians agreed to pay the salary of a dispenser (twenty pounds per annum) without altering Gibbons's salary.[72] At the beginning of the twentieth century, a Local Government Board inspector questioned whether the medical officer's two hours in the workhouse daily were sufficient to provide satisfactory care and suggested that a resident officer should be appointed. A motion to the board of guardians to do so was defeated, but it was agreed to appoint a dispenser at a salary of £130 per annum.[73] Agreement on the appointment of a resident surgeon was not reached until prior to the opening of the new workhouse in 1903. Surprisingly, considering the proposed increase in infirmary accommodation from 230 to 360 beds, Thomas Galbraith requested the decision be rescinded and the current arrangement remain in place, with himself as sole doctor.[74] The guardians decided to proceed with the appointment and George Anderson commenced in January 1904 with an annual salary of £130. His duties included examining all tramps daily, dispensing on Sundays and at other times in the absence of the dispenser, administering anesthetics, and lecturing to and instructing probationer nurses. Among the eleven applications for the post, two were female, but they were summarily rejected.[75] Anderson remained in post for eight years and was replaced by William Coghill, who left to take up a post in Coventry after three years.

Some poor law historians have been critical of part-time poor law medical officers for their lack of attendance on sick paupers and for leaving this task to their unqualified assistants.[76] However, both Brand and Hodgkinson point out that it is not possible to assess their efficiency with any degree of accuracy as the complaints of the sick poor were rarely recorded.[77] The Wolverhampton guardians, in a special meeting in 1890, included in the

Table 4.5. Workhouse medical officers in Wolverhampton workhouse, 1839–1914

Name	Time in office	Annual salary	Reason for termination
Charles Hodgkins	March 1839–March 1841	£40	Retendering process
George Cooper	March 1841–September 1852	£40–£80	Requested to resign
Richard Nugent	October 1852–December 1859	£80–£130	Resigned
Henry Gibbons	December 1859–April 1882	£130–£180	Died
Edward Watts	April 1882–August 1894	£130–£180	Died
Thomas Galbraith	September 1894	£175–£200	In post in 1914

Source. WALS, WDG, PU/WOL/A/2–25, 1839–1914.

regulations for the medical officer that he must attend at least once daily. Four years later, they required that he should arrive no later than 10:30 a.m. every morning.[78] However, when the occasion demanded it, officers could spend long periods in the workhouse. George Cooper was in attendance from 5:00 a.m. one morning in June 1845 to attend a woman with a difficult and protracted labor and he stayed till she had given birth at 12:00 p.m. On an earlier occasion, the labor of "E.D." was also protracted and the master reported that the safety of the mother and child was due to Cooper's skill and the "great attention" he gave to the delivery.[79] Despite this dedication, the infrequency of his attendance at the workhouse became a source of conflict between Cooper and the guardians eight years later. Because of discrepancies between the entries in the medical report book and porter's book relating to his times of attendance, he was reprimanded after being found guilty of "gross carelessness in bookkeeping" and inflating the amount of time he spent in the institution. However, the board did so reluctantly because of his previous good service.[80] Around this time, the Poor Law Board had informed the guardians that Cooper was entitled to hold his appointment on a permanent basis.[81] However, the guardians wished him to forgo the permanency by resigning in the following March and recorded his verbal agreement in the board minutes. Cooper maintained that he was opposed to resigning as he approved of the Poor Law Board's ruling on the permanency of medical appointments and he had merely agreed to respond in writing to the guardians' formal request for his resignation.[82] Subsequently, further charges of failing to enter details of patients with infectious diseases in the medical relief book were laid, with the implication of medical negligence.[83] However, it is likely the guardians were looking for a way to terminate his contract, as he had not complied with their request for his resignation.

Conflict between the Guardians and the Medical Officers

Disputes between medical officers and guardians over conditions of employ-ment and the state of the workhouse were numerous, with guardians fre-quently ignoring their requests for treatment and improvement to workhouse conditions. Power struggles between medical officers and guardians or other workhouse officials often resulted in charges of neglect. The medical ethos of striving to cure patients was at variance with the principle of less eligibility, which prevailed in keeping the standard of medical welfare low. An extensive study of the employment, disciplining, and dismissing of workhouse medical officers after the New Poor Law demonstrated that most charges for negli-gence arose out of the issues of attendance and record keeping; the former being one of the most common causes of dissatisfaction with general prac-titioner services in the 1970s.[84] Extremely low salaries, the conflict between poor law doctors' private and public duties, and their immense workload were instrumental in making it virtually impossible to attend to all ill inmates promptly. However, there have been few studies of this aspect of their work. Reforming doctors were at greater risk of being charged, but almost 40 percent of medical officers in workhouses were disciplined throughout the nineteenth century. The tightening of the rules of employment in 1871 was a major factor in the increased number of charges of malpractice and the crusade against outdoor relief was a "barely concealed attempt to set poor law medical officers up as the nation's 'fall-guy.'"[85] Although unable to carry out their contractual obligations, they were held responsible for negligent conditions that were beyond their control to alter.[86] Guardians could cre-ate "groundless charges" to rid themselves of troublesome surgeons and, as a result, doctors bore the brunt of the failings in the poor law medical ser-vice.[87] Before considering the events in Birmingham and Wolverhampton, it is necessary to have an understanding of the context in which charges arose. In the nineteenth century, a doctor's practice was judged on the basis of what "an ordinary man" would consider reasonable, rather than by standards set by the medical profession.[88] Medical officers were viewed as providing a ser-vice similar to any business, and failure to carry it out efficiently was regarded as negligence. This differs from the twentieth-century concept of negligence, which is failure to practice acceptable standards of clinical care.

The frequency of visits to the workhouse was a common cause of con-flict between guardians and medical officers in Wolverhampton. The report of the inquiry into the charges of negligence against Cooper in December 1851, referred to earlier, was generally favorable to him, but he was severely reprimanded by the guardians. The seven charges mostly reflected his nonattendance and poor bookkeeping. First, he had neglected to see Ellen Dunnock, a sick child, who had died twelve hours after admission to the workhouse in the early evening. He had confined William Newell in the lunatic wards for three days as punishment, but omitted his name from the list of patients in those wards. For sixty-nine hours from one Saturday, he had been absent without leave and failed to provide a deputy, and in that time Thomas Franks, nine years old, was admitted badly burnt. Franks did not receive medical attention for twenty-six hours, only being seen one hour before he died. Cooper had not attended to Lydia Gidderidge during her fifty-eight-day stay in the workhouse and omitted her name from the medical relief book. He had failed to record many of the episodes of illness among the children. Thomas Day, a lunatic, had been confined to bed by means of straps for several days, but Cooper had not recorded it, nor reported it to the guardians, who had recently expressed their disapproval of such treatment. The way he treated individual inmates was the subject of only one charge, in which he was accused of acting "contrary to decency." He had allowed between twenty and thirty boys and girls, of around ten years old, to be in a "state of nudity" in one room together, while they were being treated for skin disease. Similarly, two adult males suffering from venereal disease were left naked in a ward with other inmates present.[89] The Poor Law Board's inquiry blamed these instances on the breakdown in the proper classification in the workhouse and so the treatment of the inmates was not directly attributable to Cooper. Nevertheless, the board censured him for not bringing the guardians' attention to the lack of classification.[90] In doing so, the board was giving higher priority to the administration of the workhouse than to the personal dignity of its inmates. The guardians had hoped that the central authority's warning would secure for the inmates "that amount of professional attention" that they wished. However, within a few months, errors in bookkeeping and complaints by inmates regarding Cooper's treatment continued. Following a further inquiry by Andrew Doyle, Poor Law Board inspector, Cooper was requested to resign in the "interests of the Union."[91] Dr. Mannix, one of the guardians, was of the opinion that Cooper had initially been "an active and efficient officer," but had later "relaxed" for reasons he could not fathom.[92] One likely reason could have been a burgeoning private practice, since tension between public and private responsibilities often resulted in difficulty attending the workhouse.[93]

Cooper's successor, Richard Nugent, was investigated for poor attendance at the workhouse within a few years of his appointment. He had recorded in the medical relief book in 1855 that he had visited every patient daily, whereas he was accused of failing to see Josiah Tomkinson, aged seven years, despite being requested to do so on two occasions. When he did see him, eight days before the boy died, he diagnosed skin disease, but entered "scrofula, rickets and spinal" on the death certificate. The guardians admonished Nugent, but they agreed to his request not to inform the Poor Law Board after he had given them an explanation of his conduct. One month later, he was reappointed as medical officer with 57 percent of the guardians' votes in an election involving three other candidates.[94] However, within a few weeks, inmate Benjamin Lane complained of not receiving treatment from Nugent, whose explanation on this occasion was judged unsatisfactory. The Poor Law Board members were notified and they subsequently issued Nugent with a censure, pointing out the importance of listening to the complaints of sick inmates with patience.[95] Three months later, Nugent's conduct in the management of Mary Shaw was also called into question. She had developed severe abdominal pain, which worsened the same evening, so she requested Nugent be called to see her. He attended between 8:00 p.m. and 9:00 p.m., but threw off her bedclothes in what the nurse described was "an indecent manner" and examined her very roughly. He was obviously in a "very bad temper" and used threatening language when Mary complained of headache. Nugent admitted to the guardians that he was annoyed at being called out by the matron, as she had no authority to do so, and to "a simple case" of abdominal pain. When requested to apologize for the language he had used, Nugent denied that he had been abusive, but was prepared to make an apology if the board were of the opinion that he said what the inmate and nurse had reported. The board stopped short of dismissing him, instead issuing a final warning.[96] No further disagreements over Nugent's attendances occurred for three years, but at that time the guardians had a return prepared detailing his conduct over two years. Nugent or his deputy had attended the workhouse for 539 days (74 percent) in the period, although the chairman of the guardians pointed out that they had often visited when there were no patients needing attention. The average length of visits was sixty-two minutes, but could be as short as five to twenty minutes, even when there were 200 sick inmates in the workhouse. Discussion of the report was postponed, but there is no record that it subsequently took place before Nugent resigned the following year to take up another appointment.[97] By comparison, the medical officer for Nottingham workhouse spent on average two-and-a-half hours on his daily visits in 1866, with an average of 300 patients under his care.[98]

His successor, Henry Gibbons, was in post for over twenty-two years, and the only complaint regarding his conduct took place two years after his first leave of absence due to ill health in 1870. However, he had previously been reported by the Local Government Board to the guardians for failing to enter the dates of an order for medical extras in the medical relief book.[99] In April 1877, Patrick Reddington, an inmate of the workhouse, complained to the board about his treatment on admission, but the guardians subsequently found "no cause for complaint" against Gibbons.[100] Two years later, he was again off work, but this time for around six months, prompting the guardians to consider whether to grant continuing leave. However, one of them commented that sick inmates were "perfectly satisfied" with the attention Gibbons gave them and he was able to resume his duties shortly thereafter. When he died suddenly in April 1882, approximately fifty years of age, the guardians' response suggested admiration.[101] While deputizing for Gibbons in August 1881, Edward Watts was exonerated by the guardians after a complaint from Mrs. Blower regarding her treatment in the workhouse.[102] After Gibbons's death, he was elected as medical officer on the casting vote of the chairman of the board, defeating four other candidates. A further complaint, in 1890, of neglecting William Thomas, a patient in the infirmary, also found that Watts was not to blame.[103] However, after sustaining an accident a few months later, lapses in his performance started to arise. In May the following year, the board's auditor reported errors of omission and accuracy in the medical relief book, all of which were accepted by Watts and he was cautioned to be more careful in his record keeping. The following month, Watts failed to visit the workhouse for three days, following which the master requested the medical officer's deputy to attend. Watts's reason for his nonattendance was that he had been taken ill with influenza, but it is obvious he had failed to inform his deputy. Although the guardians were dissatisfied with his attendances over the previous three months, no action was taken against Watts after an exchange of letters between the guardians, Watts, and the central authority.[104] A more serious charge of neglect of duty on the part of Watts related to the treatment of Joseph Freeman, an inmate who died on June 8, 1894, and the guardians requested an inquiry by the Local Government Board. Watts saw Freeman on admission, two days before his death, suffering from abdominal pain and allocated him to the old men's ward. However, the nurse later had Freeman transferred to the infirmary as his condition had deteriorated. Watts visited the workhouse the next day, but did not see Freeman, although he discussed his condition with the nurse. At the request of one of the guardians, who was medically qualified, Watts went to see Freeman and instigated treatment. Watts was also questioned as to why he had not attended a case of "Acute Scorbutis" in the same ward when attending Freeman. He replied that he did not think it necessary. The master reported that the medical officer was often in "a muddled state" when visiting the workhouse.[105] Watts died before the Local Government Board's inquiry into his conduct over Freeman could be completed. It is clear that both Watts's and Gibbons's performance of their duties deteriorated when they suffered ill health, but they strove to continue at work. Price found that almost one quarter of poor law medical officers died in office due to many carrying on into old age, when they were more likely to make mistakes.[106]

This did not apply in Gibbons's case and was unlikely to have applied in Watts's case, as the majority of Wolverhampton's medical officers were appointed in their twenties. One exception was Thomas Galbraith, who was in his early thirties when he succeeded Watts. He was still in office in 1914 and until that time, the only serious complaint against him arose once more because of illness. He needed reminding of the times he was required at the workhouse because of late and irregular attendance in his early years of appointment. It was also impressed upon him that his "first and principal duties" were to the inmates of the workhouse. Two years later, he was again requested to be more punctual as his later arrival at the institution disrupted the serving of meals.[107] Early in the twentieth century, a tramp, William Buck, complained that the medical officer had not seen him, although he had requested a visit on his arrival at the workhouse late one evening. Galbraith was unwell at this time and his deputy, Dr. Carter, had left the workhouse before Buck arrived, although he had returned in the late evening to visit patients in the infirmary. He did not see Buck, as the nurse informed him that everyone in the tramp wards would be in bed and no one needed to be seen urgently. Carter did not visit the following day (Monday), as he assumed Galbraith would be fit for work and Buck left the workhouse early the following morning. He turned up at Walsall workhouse a day later and was diagnosed as having severe smallpox. The Walsall officials accused the Wolverhampton guardians of "grave dereliction of duty." When questioned, Galbraith stated he had set out for work on the Monday, but returned home, as he felt his physical strength was insufficient to continue and arranged a locum from London. His sister had telephoned the workhouse to explain the arrangements, and had spoken to the superintendent nurse, who unfortunately did not inform the master. Galbraith regretted that his illness had been the primary cause of the "neglect in his duties," but felt he had done his best in difficult circumstances. Nevertheless, the board instructed Galbraith that, in future, he must ensure the master is made aware directly of the arrangements in place if he is unable to attend.[108]

Over the period of this study, Reading Union workhouse employed three medical officers on a part-time basis similar to Wolverhampton, but there are no recorded incidents of nonattendance or charges of neglect of duty.[109]

Similarly, no charges were brought against the workhouse medical officers for Nottingham Union. They were employed on a full-time basis and not allowed to practice privately, but also had district duties. Although they were designated as resident, they were required only to live as close to the workhouse as possible.[110] Leicester Union workhouse medical officers had contracts similar to Wolverhampton, and while two remained in post for around ten years, one did so for thirty-four years. John Moore, appointed in 1857, suffered ill health toward the end of his ten-year appointment. When he failed to reduce a fracture of an inmate's leg, which developed gangrene and resulted in her death, he was asked to resign. The longest-serving surgeon, Clement Bryan, was a lax record keeper, which resulted in him being questioned several times, but no charges against his conduct in other matters were ever brought, and no complaints by patients about their treatment were recorded.[111]

By requiring medical officers to be resident in the workhouse, it might be assumed that Birmingham guardians had insured that attendance on patients would not be an issue. However, the officers were not required to be present at all times, although their movement in and out of the workhouse was recorded in the porter's book. As a result, one surgeon, Redfern Davies (in post 1858–61) was required to resign because of insufficient time in the institution. He first came into conflict with the guardians over his attempts to carry out major operations in the workhouse, rather than transfer patients to the local voluntary hospitals, as preferred by the guardians. He defended his views vigorously at first, but eventually apologized and accepted that he could operate in the workhouse only in cases of urgency and when the patient was unfit to be transferred.[112] Davies was an enthusiastic and ambitious surgeon, who published reports of his practice in the medical press. The son of a local physician and Birmingham's first coroner, Birt Davies, he had extensive local medical connections. After he had sustained an accident in December 1860, he thanked the guardians for allowing him leave to recover as he felt "I should have broken my heart" if not permitted to return to work.[113] Around this time, it came to light that Davies had been absent from the workhouse on numerous occasions, although he had been accustomed to do so prior to his accident. He had been leaving the workhouse daily, usually for about five or six hours for health reasons and stated his intention to continue to do so.[114] Although he initially declined to resign when requested by the guardians, he eventually agreed after they requested an inquiry by the Local Government Board and he accepted that his absences were more numerous than he had thought, due to "want of memory."[115] It is possible that he did so to pursue medical interests elsewhere.

The only other Birmingham medical officer to face charges of negligence was Adam Simpson, LRCS, Ed. He was born in County Tyrone in Ireland in 1836 or 1837 and remained single. After he left the service of Birmingham workhouse, he lived in nearby Gillott Road with his unmarried sister.[116] He was appointed as medical officer to the workhouse in August 1870, but the records for that period of the Visiting and General Purposes Committee, which recommended his appointment to the board, are missing from the archives. He suffered at least four episodes of ill health in his first five years in office, one of which was described by the master as a "serious illness."[117] When he unsuccessfully applied for the post of surgeon to West Riding Prison in 1875, the guardians' testimonial stated he had given them "utmost satisfaction" in the performance of his duties.[118] He was the sole medical officer in the workhouse until the appointment of an assistant in 1876 and an additional one two years later. With the appointment of a visiting physician in 1882, Simpson's duties were limited to the surgical side of the infirmary.

The first Local Government Board inquiry into his conduct took place sixteen months after the first assistant had been in post and it centered on whether the deaths of Henry Binks and a man named Washbrook were due to medical neglect. Simpson had admitted Binks to the infirmary in the mid-afternoon after diagnosing bronchitis, but did not consider his condition needed urgent further attention. In the ward Binks was given milk, beef tea, and a dose of the cough mixture kept on the ward when he became breathless. When Simpson saw him again at 8:00 p.m., he had deteriorated and was prescribed brandy and a linseed poultice for his chest. The coroner accepted the cause of death as bronchitis, but the jury at the inquest were of the opinion that Binks should have received earlier attendance. Simpson disagreed that this would have affected the outcome.[119] After the Local Government Board requested the guardians to obtain his resignation, Simpson placed the matter before the board of guardians, remarking on the kindness and courtesy he had "invariably received at [their] hands" over the previous seven years. The guardians considered he had not given "all attention" required to Binks, but there was no direct evidence to "inculpate" him in the Washbrook case. They concluded that censure was sufficient and gained the central authority's consent to retain him in office. In deciding Simpson's future, the guardians undoubtedly took into consideration the remarks by the Local Government Board that he had under his care more patients than he could properly attend to, even in the most cursory manner and that he was uniformly kind to his patients.[120] This incident led the guardians to set up an inquiry into the deficiency in medical and nursing staff in the infirmary and to the subsequent appointment of the second assistant medical officer. Four years later, Simpson was charged with using medical treatment as a punishment for patients by confining Ellen Peters, of reputed sound mind, in the padded room. There were also allegations by Nurse Burns that blisters and shower baths were being used to punish Peters and Mary Jane Skett. Again, the guardians referred the matter to the Local Government Board as Simpson no longer retained their confidence, but the central authority merely censured him.[121] This incident led to the appointment of the visiting physician the following year. In December 1884, Simpson was called before the guardians for using "improper language" to a nurse in one of the wards, which he explained was done in "moments of irritation." He was found to have interfered with the "perfect harmony" required for the efficient running of the infirmary and requested to refrain from such language in future.[122] At this time, there were around 1,200 patients in the infirmary, cared for by three resident officers and one visiting physician.

The final inquiry arose after an outbreak of puerperal fever in the lying-in wards in April 1885. Elizabeth Wood, aged thirty-one years, was admitted on November 12 to the lying-in wards, which at the time were in the girls' school. Later that day, she was delivered of twin boys by Nurse Rebecca Williams after a labor lasting three hours and ten minutes (appendix D). She had a two-year history of pulmonary tuberculosis. Her temperature was higher than normal on admission, but increased markedly after four days and remained at this level until her death on December 6.[123] Simpson was of the opinion that she was not suffering from puerperal fever, although the two assistant medical officers were not in agreement.[124] He requested a second opinion from Dr. Edward Malins, obstetric physician at the General Hospital and vice-president of the Obstetric Society of London, who confirmed the diagnosis of "puerperal septicaemia," whose origin was intrinsic to the patient, but which was communicable to other lying-in patients.[125] When the lying-in wards were moved to the girls' school, the members of the Infirmary Sub-committee were concerned that no one involved in the wards up to that date should have any further attendance on lying-in patients. This included Simpson and they resolved that Henry Cook, one of the assistants, should have sole charge of these wards. Simpson was informed of this on his return from a four-day stay in Ireland on November 3. However, he continued to examine patients in the lying-in wards, including Elizabeth Wood, and perform deliveries until Malins confirmed Wood's diagnosis.[126]

The guardians referred the matter of Simpson's conduct to the Local Government Board with a request that the inquiry would be limited to whether he had disobeyed orders.[127] At the inquiry, Mr. Price, chairman of the Infirmary Sub-committee, stated that he had informed Cook on October 30 that he was in "sole charge" of the lying-in wards and, three days later, told Simpson of Cook's position and that the guardians wished to release him (Simpson) from attending cases in the girls' school. Both Cook and Simpson denied that Price had said Cook was to have "sole and entire" charge. In addition, Simpson denied that Price had forbade him to enter the wards, and pointed out that he had not received any written confirmation of such an order. While the members of the inquiry, J. J. Henley and Dr. F. Mouat, criticized the guardians for not making the order explicit and for failing to ensure all officers concerned were aware of it, they took the view that "in charge" implied complete professional control as the only medical officer. They concluded that Simpson had disobeyed an important order and failed to justify his disobedience; the guardians were justified in their opinion that he had forfeited their confidence; and the Birmingham board should request his resignation.[128] However, he refused to resign, protesting to the central authority that there was no evidence that Price had informed him not to attend the lying-in wards. He received support for his retention from the Medical Defence Union, local newspapers, and some of the Birmingham guardians. At a special meeting of the Birmingham board on June 15, there were sufficient guardians present who wished Simpson to be removed from office to confirm his dismissal, despite strong support from some of the others.[129] The previous inquiries into Simpson's conduct were taken into consideration by the Local Government Board in refusing to alter its decision.[130] In light of Simpson's continued refusal to resign, the board declared him "unfit for the office of Medical Officer" and ordered him to cease to perform the duties of the office. He left the workhouse on September 3, 1886.[131]

It is obvious from the records that Simpson engendered strong feelings both toward and against him among the guardians and other officers, creating tension within working relationships in the workhouse. The matron, in 1877, was overheard to say he was not fit to be medical officer and, if he had been in Liverpool, would have been quickly dismissed. However, she and her husband, the master, were under investigation at that time and resigned before it could be concluded.[132] Kim Price claims that, as a council member of the Poor Law Medical Officers' Association, Simpson was a reforming poor law surgeon, but there is no evidence for this in the local records, in which he appears to have carried out his duties as required and no more. Likewise, Price's opinion that he repeatedly asked for more staff is not borne out in the guardians' minute books, in which there is not one instance of him complaining of overwork.[133] Although he did admit to finding the work stressful, he denied that he found it particularly difficult to perform his duties before the first assistant was appointed. In addition, he did not concur with the guardian who suggested that patients had suffered as a result of his workload.[134] He ought to have been aware of the possibility of the transmission of puerperal infection and sought clarification of his position, when, as he claimed, he was not given precise verbal instructions. In not doing so, perhaps he was the architect of his own downfall. It is also interesting to note that his professional conduct seems to have been less satisfactory after he had medical help, rather than during the period when he was on his own and suffered ill health. Nor was he in the vanguard of nursing reform. When the guardians asked his opinion on the appointment of a trained nursing superintendent, he replied that a professional nurse was not necessary, only "a clever woman."[135]

Patient Care

This chapter has drawn out the characters of previously unknown workhouse medical officers who struggled day after day to provide care to sick inmates in as humane a way as possible. Those in Birmingham and Wolverhampton carried a heavy workload that increased as the nineteenth century progressed. Although this caused some to resign or to request medical help, others merely used it as a tool to increase their salaries. By doing so, part-time medical officers could employ their own assistants, but it is surprising that some full-time officers were content with extra payment only. An example is Edmund Robinson in Birmingham, who denied he needed assistance, despite the presence of between 600 and 700 sick inmates on his wards. He subsequently became one of the most highly paid poor law medical officers (table 4.1).[136] There is a marked difference between the employment of resident surgeons in Birmingham, supported at times by visiting medical personnel, and the single part-time doctor in Wolverhampton. Part-time officers offered more continuity of care as they served for longer periods, but difficulties could arise if they suffered poor health or as they aged. As Birmingham's resident officers could spend most of the day and evening on the wards and be called during the night at times, it is difficult to imagine that Wolverhampton's officers could be providing adequate care with a visit of a few hours each day, even with a smaller number of sick inmates since understaffing can result in a failure to provide basic care.[137] Birmingham's medical staffing levels were exemplary in the early years of the New Poor Law, but as the central authority imposed its rules governing medical duties, the reduction to one resident medical officer was highly unsatisfactory. The change to the medical arrangements resulted in the surgeons losing the right to admit urgent cases directly to the infirmary without the permission of the guardians or an overseer and so imposed more completely the principle of less eligibility. To give some credit to the Local Government Board, it was at their insistence that the number of medical officers was subsequently increased. One result of the new infirmary being separately managed from the workhouse was that medical cover in the latter was again reduced to one lone officer, with subsequent difficulty in providing twenty-four-hour medical attention for patients.

One issue that resulted from the heavy workload of the medical officers in the workhouse is conflict between them and the guardians, which led to charges of medical negligence. According to welfare historians John Stewart and Steven King, the poor working relationships in many unions between guardians and medical officers was unlikely to lead to effective or conscientious medical care.[138] Examination of Simpson's dismissal brings to the fore the role that poor communication played, both between doctors and patients and medical officers and guardians. The lack of satisfactory communication is a factor that continues to be one of the most important in current medical complaints made by patients against doctors.[139] In Linda Mulcahy's study of patients' complaints in the late 1990s, the lowest incidence was in those medical specialties in which the patient was least empowered and of low social status.[140] As the main objective of the New Poor Law was the disempowerment of indoor paupers, it might be expected that they would not feel able to question a doctor's practice. However, inmates in both locations felt sufficiently empowered to complain about the treatment they received. On at least one occasion, it concerned the medical officer's unsympathetic attitude during examination (by Mary Shaw in Wolverhampton in 1855), the second most common type of complaint in Mulcahy's study.[141] The majority of the other charges related to nonattendance at the workhouse, but were not exclusive to nonresident officers. Although part-time officers in Wolverhampton were particularly guilty of this offense, it was associated with ill health on more than one occasion and the two workhouse medical officers who died in office were middle-aged. A low salary may have played a part in the frequency of attendance in the case of Cooper, but the others were paid an amount that was in the top 10 percent of the salary range throughout the nineteenth century. The majority of charges took place before the onset of the crusade against outdoor relief and so is at variance with the national picture.[142] Medical officers were often exonerated or merely cautioned when charges were related to subjecting patients to degrading or unsatisfactory treatment, as in the matter of Cooper's handling of children in Wolverhampton, whereas failure to cooperate with the guardians' wishes or keep accurate records were taken more seriously. Reporting deficiencies in the workhouse premises or inadequacies in the nursing staff could bring them into conflict with the guardians, but failure to do so could lead to a charge of breach of contract. Crowther has commented that guardians were prepared to defend a medical officer, whatever the charge, if they were subservient to the guardians' standards.[143] Whether subservience to the guardians had an influence on the medical treatment that medical officers prescribed for sick inmates will be discussed in the next chapter.

Chapter Five

Medical Therapies

The nature of medical care in workhouses and of the clinical treatment inmates received after the New Poor Law is not well understood. Neither is it certain how representative it was of nineteenth-century therapeutics.[1] This chapter analyzes the therapies that medical officers utilized in the management of patients in Birmingham and Wolverhampton workhouses and attempts to reconstruct the treatments they prescribed. Because workhouse medical officers were often required by boards of guardians to pay for the drugs they used from their salaries, historians have accused them of withholding effective treatment. Joseph Rogers recounts that, when he was appointed medical officer to Westminster workhouse in 1872, the retiring physician expressed pride in the fact that the only medicine he gave inmates was peppermint water.[2] Was this true of other workhouses, or just an unrepresentative anecdote? At the beginning of the nineteenth century, medical treatment was much as it had been for many centuries, with the emphasis on depletive therapies, and it was not until the end of the century that the production of effective treatments in the form of the first vaccines for infectious diseases took place.[3] However, from the perspective of twenty-first-century pharmacology, the only really effective drugs were opium and aperients, and the only one that could cure disease was, arguably, quinine for malaria. One advance in therapeutic technique was Edinburgh physician Alexander Wood's introduction of the hypodermic syringe for subcutaneous administration of drugs in 1855.[4] Despite the lack of apparent ineffectiveness in the drug armamentarium, medical historians agree that nineteenth-century medical therapeutics worked in the context of the culture of the time and that patients had visible evidence of the effectiveness of the regimens employed.[5]

Four approaches will be used to uncover therapeutic practice in the workhouses. First, therapies, such as natural and physical medical treatments, the use of food and alcohol as treatment for disease, and the drugs prescribed, will be described. Alcohol was an important and widely used therapy in the nineteenth century, but its prescription in workhouse infirmaries has not previously been investigated. An alternative approach to aid the understanding of therapeutic practice will investigate the management of specific conditions, such as respiratory disease and skin conditions. Third, the management of individual patients and their perspective on the treatment they received will be addressed through the complaints they made to the guardians. Finally, how sanatorium methods of management for tuberculosis were implemented in workhouses will be described. The chapter will also address the question of the extent to which guardians limited the treatments that inmates could receive and to what extent they overruled medical officers' prescriptions and advice.

Therapeutic Principles

Before considering individual treatments, it is necessary to understand the principles on which they were prescribed. The antiphlogistic, depletive regimen of the eighteenth century remained the mainstay of medical treatment at the beginning of the nineteenth. Bloodletting, purgation, a debilitating diet, sedating drugs, and bed rest were employed to relax the state of excitement that disease was thought to induce in the body. However, by the middle of the eighteenth century, a stimulant regimen was also used when the physician considered the illness was producing a debilitating state in the patient, rather than an excitatory one. A major proponent of this system was the Edinburgh physician, John Brown (1735–88), who postulated that all diseases were due to an excess or deficiency of natural energy or "excitability."[6] He called the condition with excess *sthenia*, while deficiency resulted in asthenic disease. He did not believe in the healing power of nature to overcome disease, but considered all maladies required a stimulant. Sthenic conditions required antiphlogistic regimens of bloodletting, purging, cold applications, and physical rest, which were all weak stimulants to reduce excessive excitement. Strong stimulants were required to increase deficient excitement in asthenic conditions and these included wine or spirits, gentle exercise, increased mental activity, and the drugs opium, camphor, musk, and ether. The choice of stimulant for any individual patient depended on the speed of action and level of stimulation required. Brunonian therapeutics was not taken up enthusiastically in Britain because judging the degree of bodily excitability and distinguishing asthenia from sthenia was problematic. Nevertheless, the importance of his theory lay in providing an alternative form of therapy to the exhausting eighteenth-century medical treatments of purging and diuresis.[7] The other components of the stimulant regimen were a fuller diet containing meat, hot baths rather than cold, exercise, alcohol, and tonics. However, whichever regimen was chosen depended on the physician's judgment as to the effect of the disease on the patient. On some occasions, an initial depletive regimen would be replaced by a more stimulating one as the patient's condition improved.[8]

Natural and Physical Therapies

Medical practitioners employed therapies utilizing the natural environment to aid the body's natural healing process or to combat the spread of disease as understood at the time. One of the more important environmental measures in institutions was efficient ventilation, and the duties of the workhouse medical officer included advising on the adequacy of ventilation and sanitary arrangements. The miasma theory of disease, dating back to around the sixth century, postulates that disease could arise spontaneously in rotting matter, human waste, and stagnant water and spread in the emanations given off into the atmosphere from these sources.[9] Many physicians continued to cling tenaciously to this mode of disease transmission late in the nineteenth century. It followed that to combat cross-infection in hospitals and infirmaries, adequate ventilation was required and the pavilion system of building these institutions was devised to ensure this. Although wards with windows placed opposite each other were first suggested in *An Essay on Parish Workhouses* in 1867 by Edmund Gillingwater, it was not adopted generally until the Poor Law Board issued a circular a century later stating that all new infirmaries must adopt the pavilion principles.[10] These involved long wards with opposing windows, built in separate blocks. A few years before this circular, Edmund Robinson, medical officer in Birmingham workhouse, suggested that new infectious disease wards should be built with the windows unrestricted by other buildings, so as to enable as much fresh air as possible.[11] Both the new Birmingham infirmary in 1889 and the second Wolverhampton Union workhouse in 1903 were erected according to the pavilion plan.

Robinson, like many of his contemporaries, held a strong belief in the curative power of fresh air: "Pure air is the very life and blood, so to speak, of the sick and without it, the most consummate skill in medical or surgical treatment is of little or no avail."[12] However, twenty years before, Charles Smith, the house surgeon at the infirmary, cautioned against the excessive use of fresh air in the sick wards in the winter as the patients suffered mainly from "pulmonary, bronchial, rheumatic affections." He pointed out that the result would be an exacerbation of pain in those with rheumatism and coughing and dyspnea in those with lung conditions. He emphasized that these patients were susceptible to sudden changes of temperature, which could worsen their condition.[13] The therapeutic benefit of fresh air was one of the basic principles behind open-air treatment for tuberculosis and we will return to this issue later in the chapter.[14] In the first decade of the twentieth century, Arthur Foxwell, physician at the Queen's Hospital, introduced an open-air ward on the top floor of the building to be used for the treatment of nontubercular patients.[15]

The medicinal use of water dates back as far as ancient Greece, when water was thought to both stimulate and tranquilize the nervous system and its healing properties could restore harmony to bodily humors.[16] The therapeutic benefit of cold baths were promoted in England by Sir John Floyer, an eminent physician from Lichfield, in his 1702 treatise on the use of hot and cold baths.[17] In the early nineteenth century, Vincenz Priessnitz, an Austrian layman, developed a new system of treatment, of which the main tenets were that disease resulted from the body's attempts to expel foreign matter and only cold water, used internally and externally, could separate and remove it. His water cure became extremely popular and was brought to England in 1842 by Dr. James Wilson.[18] However, therapeutic bathing had been in use in hospitals prior to that time; for instance, just over 115 patients in the Royal Infirmary of Edinburgh received some form of bathing as part of their treatment in the last quarter of the eighteenth century. The hospital provided separate hot and cold baths for patients' use only, although they could also use portable tubs in the wards. Baths were thought to exert a tonic effect on the nervous system, to be useful in skin conditions, and the relaxing effect of a warm bath for fifteen to twenty minutes was used to help patients with chronic rheumatism and postparalytic muscular contractions.[19] Vapor baths were in use in Birmingham Skin Hospital to treat a variety of dermatological diseases in 1882.[20] Richard Nugent, medical officer at Wolverhampton workhouse, prescribed three warm baths per week for children with skin diseases in 1858. Four boys and thirty girls over the age of two years were suffering from "impetigo," which he put down to poor personal cleanliness and inadequate ventilation in the building.[21] More than three decades later, Edward Watts, the workhouse medical officer at the time, was using large quantities of mineral water in the treatment of patients. One of the guardians, Dr. Totherill, a hospital physician, considered it an ineffective therapy, but could not persuade Watts to discontinue its use. Totherill accepted that Watts had the authority to order it and the guardians were powerless to overrule him.[22] One medical officer in Birmingham workhouse also used Buxton water to treat a patient in 1855 with good effect.[23] The Victorian period witnessed a profusion of spas and mineral water hospitals, which specialized in the treatment of chronic rheumatic diseases.[24] Birmingham guardians utilized such facilities for Thomas Regan, a young inmate suffering from chronic gout, by arranging his attendance at Droitwich Salt Baths in 1883.[25]

While water was thought to strengthen the body, bloodletting weakened the body as it effected a cure.[26] The rationale behind its use was based on the causation of diseases by the imbalance of humors. At the time of the Roman Empire, Galen of Pergamon had postulated that certain diseases, such as fevers, resulted in a buildup of blood or "plethora" and could be corrected by bloodletting. Despite advances in the understanding of human physiology from the seventeenth century onward, it remained the mainstay of the antiphlogistic regimen. In the late eighteenth century, 25 percent of patients in the Royal Infirmary of Edinburgh were subjected to one or other forms of bleeding, despite a degree of popularity for John Brown's stimulant treatment.[27] In the early nineteenth century, the medical system proposed by François-Joseph-Victor Broussais, renowned as the leader of Paris medicine at the time and acclaimed as the inventor of "physiological medicine," resulted in a resurgence in the use of therapeutic bleeding.[28] He considered that all diseases were due to overstimulation of bodily function, resulting in local inflammation, most frequently in the stomach, but which could spread throughout the body. Thus, the appropriate treatment for all diseases was an antiphlogistic regimen of a debilitating diet and bloodletting by means of locally applied leeches.[29] The practice of removing blood from the body declined substantially after the "blood-letting controversy" in Edinburgh in 1857, in which John Bennett, professor of the institutes of medicine, challenged the principles behind the bleeding of patients.[30] For instance, all methods were reduced from 35 percent of patients in Massachusetts General Hospital in the 1830s to only 1 percent in the 1880s.[31] However, its value as treatment continued to be accepted theoretically.

The most common method of general bloodletting was by venesection, the opening of a vein using a lancet. It produced a reduction in pulse rate, a decrease in body temperature, and a feeling of relaxation, considered necessary in sthenic conditions. If local extraction of blood was required, for instance from an inflamed joint or around the eyes in ophthalmia, leeches were used. Leeches had been in use in medical practice in ancient Greece and the species preferred for this purpose was named *Hirudo medicinalis* by Linnaeus in 1758. It took from thirty to sixty minutes for the worm to extract sufficient blood to drop off the skin, but bleeding can continue from the site for up to one hour because the leech produces an anticoagulant transmitted to the host via its mouth.[32] Leech therapy gained great popularity in the early nineteenth century, as Broussais promoted it as his preferred method of bloodletting. However, its use continued unabated after Broussais's theories were discredited.[33] Local bloodletting could also be carried out by cupping, using vessels attached to the skin to induce a partial vacuum, and by blistering or applying plasters containing irritative substances to the skin. There is no record of venesection being used in either Birmingham or Wolverhampton workhouse, but Birmingham guardians spent between eleven pounds and twenty-four pounds per quarter on the purchase of leeches between 1847 and 1849.[34] At that time, Mary Hill was employed in the workhouse as the "Leech Woman in Surgery" and earlier in the decade, two male inmates were paid one shilling each per week as "leech bleeder[s]."[35] The guardians agreed that leeches could be supplied from the infirmary to treat the sick poor at home on the instruction of the district surgeons.[36] In 1868, Edmund Robinson, medical officer in Birmingham workhouse, requested leave to have treatment for inflammation of his eyes by the production of blisters.[37]

The other common physical therapy was carried out using static electricity. The greater understanding of the principles of electricity in the early eighteenth century led to its promotion as a medical treatment. Within two decades, it had become "the fashionable wonder of mid-Georgian England."[38] Machines generating static electricity, such as the Leyden jar, were developed and used to deliver both a generalized electrical stimulation to the body and localized "shocks" to specific areas. Around 5 percent of patients in the Royal Infirmary of Edinburgh in the late eighteenth century received electrical therapy, mainly for paralysis and rheumatism.[39] An electrical machine was one of the first pieces of medical equipment purchased at the Birmingham General Hospital after it opened in 1779.[40] Electrotherapeutics became more widely used from the 1830s, reached its height of popularity in the 1890s, but fell into relative disuse from the 1910s.[41] Local application of an electric current through a particular part of the body was preferred, avoiding the occurrence of an electric shock or the production of pain.[42] Electrical therapy was used to treat a variety of chronic diseases, but more specifically neurological conditions such as paralysis and chorea.[43] Because it was thought also to influence internal organs, it was preferred instead of surgery for gynecological conditions.[44] The electric current applied to the patient could be generated by an induction coil (faradic electricity) or by a battery (galvanic electricity). An "Electro Galvanic Battery" was purchased by Birmingham guardians in 1850 for use by the medical officer, John Humphrey. In his successful request for the purchase of an additional battery for the machine, he praised the "beneficial effect" it had on patients.[45] Thirty years later, a further "Faradic" battery was ordered and the "Voltaic" battery repaired.[46]

Nutrition

Diet was considered important in the therapeutic regimen because of its ability to provide a stimulus to the human system and had been promoted by Galen to this end.[47] Foodstuffs were central to premodern therapeutics and, although the rise of pharmaceuticals may have blurred the connection between food and health, food as a therapeutic tool flourished well into the nineteenth and early twentieth centuries. Yet its contribution to health has been relatively neglected within the social history of medicine. No doubt, this is why food has been labeled "The Forgotten Medicine."[48] Different types of diet were prescribed for specific indications and medical institutions incorporated them into their official regulations. The aim was to manage a patient's diet in order to allow the healing process to proceed unhindered. In the 1860s, German chemist Justus von Liebig, who had a seminal influence on nineteenth-century chemistry by applying it to the functioning of living organisms, put forward his principles of nutritional physiology.[49] He divided food into those components, such as protein, that were converted into organized tissue and those, such as carbohydrate and fat, that were oxidized to assist respiration and provide heat.[50] He postulated that a "vital force" caused the decomposition of food and its assimilation into the tissues of the body and also provided resistance to destructive influences. He explained the cause of diseases as an inability of the "vital force" to neutralize all disturbing factors. Oxygen was the principal factor causing diseases because of its ability to destroy living tissue, but certain foods could minimize tissue breakdown.[51]

Doctors in institutions organized a series of dietaries for different conditions: regular, full, low, fever, ordinary sick. A low debilitating diet was an essential ingredient for the antiphlogistic or sedative regimen. It was lacking in animal food products other than milk, given in small quantities, and prescribed for all inflammatory conditions.[52] As the century progressed and the theories of disease altered, so the therapeutic manipulation of the diet led to the increasing use of stimulant regimens, similar to those proposed by John Brown almost a century before. John Warner has shown that the low diet declined in use, from 16 percent of patients at Massachusetts General Hospital in the 1830s to 2 percent in the 1870s. Prescription of a high diet underwent the reverse process, from nil in the earlier period to 20 percent in the later one.[53] The main ingredients in the strengthening diet were beef, mutton, or chicken as meat was considered a powerful stimulant.[54]

Dr. Edward Smith, medical officer of the Poor Law Board, reported on "Dietaries for the Inmates of Workhouses" in 1866, with recommended dietaries for different classes of inmates. However, these did not include guidance for sick inmates as their diet was under the control of the medical officers, who adapted them to the individual needs of each patient. He did note the variability in the ordering of medical extras, from a wide variety in some workhouses to almost nothing in others. Arrangements for set dietaries for the sick, which could be adjusted as necessary, were advised for the convenience of food preparation; and he gave examples of such diets in use in the sixty-eight workhouses he had surveyed. The main constituents of the "Full Diet" for sick inmates were bread, butter, and tea for breakfast and supper; meat, potatoes, and bread at dinner. Named dietaries included low, extra, milk, special, liquid, convalescent, while some unions labeled them only by numbers. The majority of unions provided three or four sick diets, although each diet was also available with a lower quantity of food for women. Fifteen unions had no set dietaries, leaving the medical officer to order individual diets, and of those unions that did have them, 74 percent provided specific fever diets.[55] The sick dietaries in Cardiff workhouse in the 1880s similarly relied mainly on bread, cooked meat, potatoes, and soup. The fever diet, consisting of eight ounces of bread and two and one-eighth pints of milk with beef tea when required, was prescribed to all acute cases as well as to patients with fever.[56] The "Full Sick" dietary in Birmingham workhouse in the early years after the New Poor Law contained bread, milk pottage, cooked meat, potatoes, soup, cheese, and suet puddings. For those who could not manage the quantity involved in the full diet, there was the "Half Sick" diet, which was smaller in quantity, with similar ingredients except for the meat, which was unsalted.[57] Birmingham guardians sought permission from the Local Government Board in 1886 as their medical officers wished to make a fish diet available for patients. This was made up of ten ounces of bread daily, with a half pint of milk for breakfast, eight ounces of boiled fish and half a pound of potatoes for dinner, and one pint of gruel for supper. Presumably, the intention was to use it to treat certain conditions, as Dr. Suckling was of the opinion that there were about twenty-five patients under his care in the infirmary who would benefit from it. The Local Government Board pointed out that "dietaries" for sick inmates were at the sole discretion of the medical officers and did not require the board's approval.[58] When it issued new regulations for dietaries for different classes of inmate at the beginning of the twentieth century, infirm men and women were included, with reduced amounts for those could not take the full ration.[59] However, no recommendation was made for inmates with an acute illness. Consequently, minutes of the guardians in Wolverhampton and Birmingham contain little information on the diets prescribed for sick inmates. The nutritional content of these diets may not have been entirely adequate, however, as an outbreak of scurvy occurred in the mental wards of Wolverhampton workhouse in January 1908.[60]

Medicinal Use of Alcohol

Alcohol, especially in the form of wine, was an important therapeutic agent in the treatment of the sick, used externally as an antiseptic on wounds and burns, internally before and after surgery as an analgesic and sedative, and medically as an appetite stimulant and diuretic.[61] The prescription of wine reached its greatest medical popularity during a period from the seventeenth to nineteenth centuries, but its use declined in the late nineteenth century following doubts about its efficacy and the appearance of new pharmacological agents.[62] The system of medicine proposed by John Brown in the seventeenth century and its corollary, Brunonian therapeutics, provided a rational basis for the prescription of alcohol and led to its more widespread use. According to W. F. Bynum, alcoholic beverages along with opium were Brown's favored remedies for asthenic conditions.[63] Alcohol was a popular remedy among Brown's colleagues, and his esteemed mentor, William Cullen, prescribed beer liberally in fever cases.[64] The increasing cost of the consumption of alcoholic-containing drinks in the 1790s forced the Royal Infirmary of Edinburgh to tighten its procedures for their prescription by requiring the physicians to record them each day.[65]

By the middle of the nineteenth century, "alcoholic therapeutics" had gained a prominent position in British medical practice, replacing the use of bloodletting and purgatives. In the words of Warner, "the brandy bottle replaced the lancet."[66] Samuel Wilks, physician at Guy's Hospital, suggested "the most important question in therapeutics at the present day is the value of alcohol in disease."[67] Physicians did not doubt that alcohol was an effective therapeutic agent, and used it as the stimulant of choice. Scientific validity of its mode of action was based on the theory of Liebig that alcohol had a greater capacity to become oxidized in the bloodstream than food and so was more efficient in preventing tissue breakdown. Robert Todd, a physician at King's College London, used this concept to justify the medicinal use of alcohol. He believed that all diseases resulted in the depression of vital power and disintegration of tissue, secondary to inflammation, and alcohol could protect healthy tissue from being broken down.[68] For Todd's theory to hold, alcohol had to be completely metabolized within the body, but the experiments by Ludgar Lallemand and colleagues in the late 1850s appeared to contradict this mode of metabolism. Attention now turned to the effect of alcohol on the body's temperature. Rather than raise body temperature by the production of heat as had previously been postulated, it was observed that ingested alcohol could have the opposite effect in a healthy individual. This led to its widespread use in high dosage in the treatment of fevers, and by the early 1870s it had become the mainstay of treatment for typhus and typhoid.[69] The use of large doses of alcoholic stimulants in febrile illness was challenged by William Gairdner, professor of the practice of medicine at the University of Glasgow. In 1864, he reported a reduced mortality in typhus patients treated without alcohol and concluded that its use poisoned, rather than supported, the body.[70] Despite this, alcohol continued to be prescribed widely as a therapeutic agent until the 1920s.[71] By the late nineteenth century, the majority of doctors were recognizing the harmful effects of alcohol on the body, particularly cirrhosis of the liver, and were aware of the condition of alcoholism. This recognition and the influence of the growing impact of the temperance movement led to more moderate doses being used.[72] Teetotalers strongly attacked the theories of alcohol's medicinal qualities and were supported by a few medical men, such as Benjamin Ward Richardson, who later became a physician at the London Temperance Hospital.[73] Some influence on medical practice was achieved as practitioners subsequently limited their prescribing of alcohol, although this occurred in the context of a reduction in the general consumption of spirits of 80 percent and of beer of 38 percent between 1831 and 1931.[74]

Workhouse inmates were supplied with alcoholic beverages for a variety of reasons. Beer was provided in the dietary for able-bodied inmates in some workhouses, more often in the early years of the New Poor Law. For instance, the ordinary dietary in Birmingham in 1834 included beer at dinner on five days each week and, four years later, it was increased to one pint of beer every day for both men and women. However, paupers in the infirmary were restricted to one-half pint daily, but, six years later, beer had been withdrawn from those on the "half sick" diet.[75] Patients in West Ham Union Infirmary were also given beer at dinner and supper, with those on the full diet allowed one-and-a-half pints and on the half diet one pint, but patients on the low and fever diets were not permitted alcohol.[76] Voluntary hospital patients were also allowed regular alcoholic beverages; for instance, in the Royal Infirmary of

Edinburgh in the eighteenth century, a "house" beer of low alcoholic content of 1.2 percent was served during breakfast and supper.[77] Alcoholic beverages were frequently provided to inmates who carried out tasks within workhouses, including the pauper nurses. Edward Smith, in his report on Metropolitan Workhouses in 1866, noted that paupers in many workhouses were given a daily allowance of either one pint or one-and-a-half pints of strong porter, plus one or more glasses of gin for carrying out disagreeable work.[78]

Medical officers could prescribe alcohol on an individual basis, as part of "medical extras" paid for by the guardians, for both pauper nurses and patients. As the majority of their contracts stipulated that they were required to pay for the drugs they prescribed, guardians were suspicious that medical extras were frequently substituted for drugs in order to avoid this expense. Both they and the central authority strove continually to control the cost of alcohol consumption in workhouses, but this proved difficult due to alcohol's status as a medicine, although this was challenged in the latter part of the nineteenth century. Jonathan Reinarz and Rebecca Wynter assert that a decline in the prescription of alcohol in institutions had more to do with cost than a change in prevailing theories. They give as an example the marked difference at the General Hospital in Birmingham between 1865–67 and 1881–84, where the consumption rate of wine reduced from 0.09 to 0.02 bottles, spirits from 0.07 to 0.03 bottles, beer from 0.55 to 0.01 quarts, and ale from 0.58 to 0.09 quarts.[79] A similar situation with increasing costs leading to restrictions in the prescription of wine and beer at the Royal Infirmary of Edinburgh in the 1790s has already been mentioned.[80] At the time when alcoholic beverages were more freely prescribed at the General Hospital, Edward Smith considered that the quantities of "spirituous liquors" ordered in provincial workhouses and the length of time during which they are ordered are "sufficiently astonishing, and will, I do not doubt, ultimately engage the attention of the Poor Law Board."[81] This issue was the only one he had encountered where there was widespread disagreement between the views of guardians and those of the medical officers. Smith's assumption proved correct and the first of a number of returns relating to the consumption of alcoholic beverages by paupers was issued in 1872.

Historians' criticism that workhouse medical officers ordered extras, including alcohol, to avoid the cost to themselves of prescribing drugs did not apply in Birmingham as the guardians continued to meet the cost of drugs ordered in the workhouse after 1834, as they had previously. Wolverhampton guardians did not agree to pay for medicines until 1874, but before this time, there had been no concerns raised in Wolverhampton over the cost of extras, despite the consumption of alcoholic beverages rising significantly between

Table 5.1. Inmates, patients, and alcohol consumption in Wolverhampton workhouse, 1842–46

	1842	1843	1844	1845	1846
Mean no. of inmates	442	478	419	374	–
Mean no. of patients	40	69	69	63	–
Ale (pints)	5,321	7,057	9,489	10,536	11,497
Wine (pints)	163	244	166	413	446
Brandy (pints)	1.5	10.5	5	8.5	9
Gin (pints)	173	307	457	685	823

Source: *Wolverhampton Chronicle*, December 2, 1846; WALS, Master's Journal, PU/WOL/U/2, April 16, 1842, to August 16, 1845.

1842 and 1846, while the number of inmates stayed the same (table 5.1).[82] Although the number of patients increased in 1843, it remained static thereafter and the increased consumption most likely reflected increased prescription and possibly the opening of fever wards. Wolverhampton guardians discussed the cost of alcohol consumption in 1867, as it had risen eightfold compared to a few years earlier. For the quarter year ending 1866, they had spent nearly eighty-five pounds at a cost of two shillings and three pence per inmate, while Birmingham spent above £134 at only one shilling and three pence per head. The matter was raised by Mr. Barker, who was denounced as a teetotaler by the other guardians, one of whom, Mr. Willcock, was proud that the medical officers gave the sick poor those stimulants he considered necessary, as he felt they did more good than all the medicines that were prescribed.[83]

The amount spent on wines and spirits to treat sick inmates in Birmingham workhouse increased from a weekly average of approximately forty-three pounds for the year 1832–33 to nearly eighty pounds for 1842–43, but declined to annual costs of just under fifty-seven pounds in 1849 and nearly thirty-nine pounds in 1871. Over the same period, the number of patients rose from 122 to around 700.[84] The guardians did not raise the issue of cost at that time and the mostly likely reason for the reduction in the prescription of alcohol was a change in medical practice. Nevertheless, when the guardians were presented in 1876 with details of alcoholic "liquors" prescribed over the previous five years, they instructed the medical officer to revise the list of inmates for whom it was allowed with a view to reducing consumption. This was despite considering the return as satisfactory.[85] At this time, Birmingham was already frugal in the amount of alcohol consumed in its institution, compared with Wolverhampton workhouse and the national average (table 5.2). This is reaffirmed by the cost per

Table 5.2. Quantity and cost of alcohol consumption in Wolverhampton, Birmingham, and all English and Welsh workhouses, 1871–92

Place and year	Quantity in pints			Cost in £s			No. of inmates	Cost per inmate in £s
	Ale	Wine	Spirits	Ale	Wine	Spirits		
Birmingham								
1871	30,440	479	303	130	19	30	1,761	0.10
1881	7,656	302	1,264	36	11	131	2,119	0.08
1892	6,258	151	1,735	32	19	186	2,263	0.10
Wolverhampton								
1871	28,870	1,180	1,208	210	65	101	716	0.53
1881	28,584	447	1,037	183	29	104	972	0.33
1892	22,960	280	1,242	143	18	138	845	0.35
England and Wales								
1871	8,675,337	168,700	232,711	48,362	11,231	22,962	140,000	0.60
1881	6,541,128	114,497	183,233	33,839	7,148	19,316	170,566	0.35
1892	3,643,504	38,597	124,367	16,951	4,256	14,428	182,000	0.20

Sources: HCPP, 1872 (391), *Paupers (Consumption of Liquors)*, 22–25, 36; 1883 (108), *Workhouses (Consumption of Spirits, &c.)*, 4, 14–15; 1895 (44), *Workhouses (Consumption of Spirits)*, 4, 25; Census data for 1871; Williams, *From Pauperism to Poverty*, 159.

patient, which is available for 1871 only. Birmingham spent four shillings and five pence per patient, while Wolverhampton was more spendthrift at over one pound, although this was two-thirds less than the national average, despite the workhouse medical officer having to meet the cost of the drugs he prescribed.[86]

A national return on alcohol consumption in workhouses for 1881 was brought to the attention of Wolverhampton guardians. Birmingham had spent less, but could obtain ale and brandy at a lower cost and port wine at half the price per gallon.[87] When a further return from the Local Government Board was considered at the request of the chairman of the Workhouse Drink Reform League in 1888, the cost of consumption of wine and spirits had dropped to eight pounds and forty-two pounds respectively and the cost per inmate had fallen to three shillings and five pence and to eight shillings and seven pence per patient. Out of the 423 patients in the infirmary, only 14 had been prescribed alcohol, but it was also being given to inmates employed in disagreeable work, including those caring for epileptic patients. Without their help, eight extra nurses would have been required, costing an estimated £400 annually. The guardians were encouraged that the cost per inmate was lower than the average for urban unions and made no changes to existing arrangements.[88]

Table 5.3. Cost of consumption of wines and spirits in Wolverhampton workhouse, for the years ending Lady Day, 1900–1906

	1900	1901	1902	1906
Wine	£8	£12	£14	£16
Spirits:				
Brandy	£56	£67	£66	£31
Whiskey	–	–	–	£33
Gin	–	–	–	£1
Total for spirits	£56	£67	£66	£65

Source: WALS, WBG, PU/WOL/A/32, April 6, 1906.

Birmingham guardians were also concerned in the early 1880s that medical extras had become excessive and sought advice from the central authority. Their inspector, Dr. Mouat, reiterated that one of the principles of the poor law in treating the sick, namely "that they should be denied nothing that was essential to their health . . . but must not have luxuries or what they would not have in their own station in life." He was, thus, applying the principle of less eligibility to sick inmates, but if alcohol was an essential treatment, those who were destitute would qualify for it whether at home or in the workhouse, and those who were poor could receive it in voluntary hospitals. He appears to have been using poor law principles to limit consumption, as he went on to say that the effect of alcohol could be obtained by prescribed medicines, such as beef tea and Liebig's Extract. Despite this, medical extras increased the following year by 21 pints of brandy, as well as by 188 quarts of milk and 134 eggs, although the number of patients fell by 110.[89] Table 5.3 shows that ale and wine were ordered less over the twenty years, but that the amount of spirits rose. Overall, the cost per inmate stayed constant, although the proportion of sick inmates must have increased in that period. In the separate infirmary in 1892, the cost of alcohol per patient was three shillings and seven pence, only slightly less than in 1871 and about half the cost per patient of seven shillings and five pence of fifty years earlier.[90] Thus, Birmingham's resident surgeons were sparing in their use of alcoholic beverages, possibly because they did not pay for prescribed drugs, but another factor may have been that the temperance movement was strong in Birmingham.[91] For example, Joseph Chamberlain introduced schemes for municipalizing the drinks trade in the town in the second half of the nineteenth century.[92] At the end of the century, the amount of beef, eggs, milk, tapioca, poultry, port wine, and brandy had increased in the infirmary despite the same average number of patients, but the volume of whiskey consumed had decreased.[93]

In the last decade of the century, Wolverhampton guardians considered the latest parliamentary return on the consumption of alcoholic liquors in workhouses.[94] One guardian expressed the view that it was much greater in Wolverhampton than the majority of other workhouses and showed no sign of decreasing if the current medical officer remained in post. However, rather than calling for his resignation, the guardians decided to call his attention to the desirability of reducing it, as the amount prescribed to the sick was in excess of other workhouses. They also prohibited the issue of alcohol to inmates not requiring it for medical reasons.[95] Table 5.2 suggests that Wolverhampton was above the national average for consumption per inmate, but that it had not changed from ten years before, whereas there had been a decline across the country. The following year, the auditor's report alleged misconduct on the medical officer's behalf in the prescription of "intoxicating liquors" in the workhouse. Edward Watts denied the accuracy of the charges and gave an explanation of his practice of ordering stimulants in a written response, which the guardians accepted as a satisfactory answer.[96] Early in the twentieth century, the expenditure on spirits for the infirmary in the new workhouse was again under scrutiny. The additional bed capacity may have led to greater consumption, but as table 5.3 shows, the cost had increased before the move into the new institution in 1903, following which a greater range of spirits were provided.[97]

Although Wolverhampton guardians were concerned over expenditure on alcohol, they also expressed a desire to obtain a good-quality product. In 1899, they expressed a wish to pay twenty-five shillings per gallon for port wine, but on being told by the clerk that this was not economic, they reduced the amount to fifteen shillings.[98] However, three years later, they raised this to eighteen shillings and decided that brandy should be three-star in quality.[99] The alcoholic strength of sherry was confirmed to be satisfactory for its use in making white wine whey, administered to patients suffering from diarrhea. The other ingredients of this concoction were milk and boiling water and it was also used in the treatment of fevers.[100] Thus, there was conflict between the guardians' continual attempts to control the cost of alcohol consumption and their desire to ensure that what was available was of sufficient quality to be an effective remedy.

The use of alcohol by workhouse medical officers for its perceived therapeutic benefits varied considerably between workhouses throughout the country. For example, Edward Davies, medical officer in Wrexham workhouse, abandoned the use of alcoholic drinks in the treatment of disease in 1873. Cases of erysipelas, typhoid fever, and pneumonia were managed with "medicinal stimulants and nutritious diet," such as milk, eggs, and beef tea.

The mortality rate in the workhouse fell from forty-one for the three years before his prohibition to thirty-six for the same period afterwards.[101] On the other hand, Alfred Sheen, medical officer at Cardiff workhouse and senior surgeon at Glamorgan and Monmouthshire infirmary, although cautioning against the liberal use of stimulants, advised that they should be ordered with the same care as was taken with the prescription of medicines and recommended the same approach as with patients in an "ordinary hospital." He was against complete nonuse because "Cases of sickness occur where it would be a gross dereliction of professional duty, if not an act of culpable negligence . . . to withhold stimulants."[102] His expenditure at Cardiff workhouse on alcohol was modest at ten shillings and seven pence per patient in 1871 and at similar levels per inmate in 1881 and 1892 (nine and eight pence respectively) as Birmingham.[103] The medicinal use of alcohol continued to remain a controversial topic among the medical profession throughout the nineteenth century.

Drug Therapy

Treatment in the nineteenth century was essentially symptomatic and most drugs were herbal products or mineral preparations. The choice of treatment regimen did not depend on the diagnosis or nature of the illness, as there were only two specific therapies, quinine for intermittent fever and mercury for syphilis.[104] The major component of the depletive regimen was cathartic drugs, which purged the patient, but were also thought to have a systemic stimulant effect. Although aloes, rhubarb, and senna were used, the most popular purgative was calomel (mercurous chloride). However, it produced severe side effects, with excessive salivation, inflammation, and bleeding of the gums, loosening of the teeth, profuse sweating, and, in more severe poisoning, loss of teeth and necrosis of the mandible.[105] Emetics, anodynes (analgesics), hypnotics, and diaphoretics (drugs increasing perspiration) were included in the depletive regimen. Stimulant drugs consisted mainly of bitters and tonics to increase the general strength of the body and promote appetite and diuretics to promote the excretion of urine. The most popular stimulant was Peruvian bark containing quinine, but iron compounds were also used. Arsenicals, most commonly in the form of Fowler's solution, were thought to be useful for numerous conditions and regarded as a "multipotent drug."[106]

Wolverhampton board of guardians became concerned in 1855 at the method employed in dispensing medicines in the workhouse. The nurse whom the medical officer had instructed in the preparation of pills of calomel passed the task onto one of the older female inmates. As a result, the pills were given to patients without the required amount of mercury being weighed. Calomel was used to treat fevers and, for cholera, was given as a "blue pill with soap." The other drugs in general use in the workhouse were described by the medical officer, Richard Nugent. The "Universal Assafoetida Pill" was given to old women and "asthmaticals." It contained gum resin that was considered to be an antispasmodic and expectorant, useful for treating cough in older people. The others included *Pil Hydrarg*, which contained only mercury dissolved in nitric acid, and *Pil Saponis cum Opio*, the soap considered beneficial for digestive disorders. However, the most frequently used medicine was "Salts and Magnesia," which may have been a term used for *Magnesii Sulphas*, or magnesium sulfate, used as an antacid.[107] Because of the disquiet regarding the system of dispensing, Nugent was requested to change the practice. The guardians deferred discussion on the issue of whether all medicines should be purchased by them, so that the medical officer continued to pay the cost of drugs he prescribed.[108] In 1866 he estimated this as £50 per annum out of his salary of £130 and considered the guardians should have covered the cost of the castor oil and quinine required by patients.[109] However, the guardians did not decide to pay for medicines until ten years later, at which time they also appointed Samuel Richards as workhouse dispenser.[110] Eleven years later, they became concerned at the rising cost of the drugs bill and took steps to limit the amount of any drug dispensed to no more than that indicated on the prescription and to move to a common form of the main drugs used as agreed by the workhouse and district medical officers.[111]

Prior to the passing of the Poor Law Amendment Act (1834), Birmingham guardians employed two resident dispensing apothecaries in addition to the house surgeon.[112] Because of the increasing influence of the Poor Law Board, the guardians relieved the dispensers of their duties in 1850, in spite of the number of sick inmates increasing from an average of 135 in 1834 to 233 in October 1847.[113] The increased workload of the medical officer eight years later, with an average of 318 patients in the infirmary, made it necessary to reemploy a nonresident dispenser.[114] Concern arose over the increase in the expenditure on drugs by over £217 in the six months from September 1886 to March 1887 compared to the equivalent period the previous year. The dispenser reported that prescriptions had increased by 120 daily between the two periods and a greater variety of drugs were used instead of "stock" items. The purchase of iodoform, which was expensive, had cost around forty pounds and the use of another expensive drug, iodide of potassium, had increased threefold. The Infirmary Committee considered the additional outlay was justified as the number of sick inmates discharged from the infirmary to the workhouse or their homes had increased from 1,856 in the earlier period to 1,947 in the later one and deaths in the infirmary had decreased from 630 to 557. The committee concluded that "we can confidently assert that the Sick Inmates are made most comfortable, that their lives are prolonged, and that they are fully treated up to the scientific attainments of the present day."[115]

When the infirmary moved to its new building in 1889, a temporary part-time dispenser was employed for the workhouse only, although the guardians considered doing without one. Ebenezer Teichelmann, workhouse medical officer, estimated that the thirty prescriptions he wrote daily for the treatment of workhouse inmates would take two hours to dispense and recommended the dispenser be continued for three hours each day. The large number of prescriptions was necessary as the majority of the ninety-eight patients in the convalescent and new chronic wards were on medication.[116] In the new infirmary, it was decided to keep a stock of drugs in locked cupboards in the wards, but to have them sent to the dispensary for checking monthly (appendix C). They consisted mainly of purgatives, laxatives, expectorants, astringents, analgesics, tonics, and stimulants, as well as ointments for local application. The following year, the ward list also contained morphine, cocaine, and ether. Senior nurses were now allowed to give hypodermic injections in the presence of the surgeon.[117] In order to gain a better understanding of how these drugs were employed in the workhouse, we will now consider how specific disease states were treated.

"The Itch"

Itch was an ambiguous condition of the skin, which covered a variety of dermatological diseases. Despite its omnipresence in poor law institutions and its links to immorality and poverty, few historical studies have been undertaken since the first half of the twentieth century.[118] Although the itch was associated with venereal disease and leprosy, a common but not universal cause was scabies caused by the mite *Sarcoptes scabiei*, which burrows into the epidermis where the female lays her eggs, usually in the hands of those infected. Intense itching follows with a rash, which spreads up the arms. The disease is transmitted by direct skin contact and was accepted as contagious by the nineteenth century. The mite was identified in the mid-seventeenth century, but was not accepted as the cause of the disease until 200 years later because doctors found it difficult to comprehend how a localized infestation could result in widespread pathology and the mites were considered second-ary to the infection.[119]

Many workhouses had dedicated wards for sufferers, for instance, in the mid-1860s, 52 percent of forty-eight provincial workhouses had itch wards or cutaneous wards. However, they were often in detached buildings, such as an outhouse, and were dirty and repellent, partly due to "a sense of disgust" at the nature of the condition.[120] For example, the two rooms used for the "cure of the itch" in Birmingham workhouse in 1842 were described as in a filthy and disgusting state and alternative rooms were found.[121] Around the same time, patients with itch in Wolverhampton workhouse were being placed in the same ward as venereal patients.[122] The itch was very prevalent in workhouses, which led to it being perceived as a disease of the "immoral" poor. Two years later, the workhouse had been free of the disease for some years and the guardians praised "the diligent and successful service" of the medical officer.[123] The Lancet investigation into the state of workhouse infirmaries reported that the 100 or so boys appeared generally healthy, but personally dirty. Three were under treatment in the infirmary, although 3 others that the investigators examined showed evidence of the disease. The report concluded that itch was rarely absent from the school and to eradicate it completely, the schoolmaster and the boys must all be treated together and the wards cleansed from top to bottom.[124] Two years later on one day in December, there were 14 cases of itch on the medical officer's books out of a total for England and Wales of 653.[125] Although there were none in Birmingham at that time, large numbers (between 1 percent and 2 percent of inmates) were admitted over a two-year period at the end of the following decade (appendix A). Thereafter, although the absolute numbers increased in the early twentieth century, inmates with itch constituted only 1 percent of patients.[126]

A severe outbreak of skin disease occurred among the children in Wolverhampton workhouse in the autumn of 1858, with 53 out of about 130 affected at its peak. The medical officer stated the cause as their debili-tated constitution and treated them with a full diet plus a small quantity of ale or beer after dinner. The guardians expressed surprise at giving alco-hol to children and one of them thought it "a great evil" and would induce them to become drunkards in the future. The medical officer explained that his prescription was a tonic regimen that had been successful in other institutions. By the following February, the number had reduced to 13.[127] However, a further outbreak took place 21 years later, affecting 22 children, resulting from the admission of infected patients.[128] Children appear to have been particularly susceptible. When Mary Kitson and her 5 children were transferred to Walsall workhouse from Wolverhampton in 1893, they were noted to be suffering from the itch and the heads of 2 of the children were in a "filthy condition."[129]

The traditional treatment was with sulfur, which was made into an ointment by mixing it with butter or hog's lard and had an offensive odor.[130] It was applied to the whole body, except the face, and was reapplied over several days. It contaminated bedding and prevented patients from dressing. In 1857, John Wilmshurst, medical officer at Birmingham workhouse, requested permission to use a new method imported from Belgium, using a solution of sulfur and lime. This required only one application to achieve a cure and he pointed out it would allow more rapid discharge of patients and create more space in the infirmary for urgent cases. Wilmshurst introduced this treatment to Birmingham ten years before it became standard treatment in other workhouses and this is one example of the introduction of innovative treatment by a doctor in a workhouse.[131]

Respiratory Disease

The invention of the stethoscope in the early 1800s by René Laennec, one of the greatest physicians of the French school, permitted him to identify normal from abnormal breath sounds and, as a result, to differentiate a variety of pulmonary diseases.[132] Respiratory disease was one of the most common reasons for admission to hospital, accounting for 11 percent of admissions to the Royal Infirmary of Edinburgh in the late eighteenth century.[133] The mortality attributed to bronchitis, pneumonia, and influenza increased in the second half of the nineteenth century, but declined sharply thereafter.[134] In December 1869, 8 percent of patients in workhouses in England and Wales were suffering from a nontuberculous respiratory illness. However, in Birmingham they constituted 39 percent of patients, and in Wolverhampton 27 percent, reflecting the industrial nature of those towns.[135] Respiratory diseases other than tuberculosis accounted for between 18 percent and 22 percent of deaths in Birmingham Borough in the 1880s.[136]

Cornelius Suckling, physician at the Queen's Hospital, Birmingham, and visiting physician at Birmingham workhouse, published an account in September 1884 of his treatment of lobar pneumonia in 100 workhouse inmates over the previous 16 months. The disease is the most common bacterial cause of community-acquired pneumonia, affects only one lobe of the lungs, and is known now to be caused by *Streptococcus pneumoniae*. The overall mortality was 43 percent, rising with the increasing age of the patients.

Patients he treated for pneumonia at the voluntary hospital were fitter premorbidity and had better outcomes than those at the workhouse. He pursued a stimulant plan of treatment in most of these cases, starting with cinchona and ammonia, and was convinced he had saved several lives by "free stimulation" with alcohol. Quinine and occasionally a cold pack were used to treat a raised temperature. Pain was alleviated by "morphia injections," hot poultices, and a few leeches. He believed bloodletting to be dangerous in most cases of pneumonia and, on the only occasion he used it, the patient, who had marked cyanosis, had died. In four cases he had seen early after the onset of the illness, he believed that he had aborted the disease by one dose of ten grains of quinine.[137] Early in the twentieth century, pneumonia was one of the most common causes of death in Birmingham infirmary, declining from 14 percent (55 patients) in the first six months of 1905 to 6 percent (31) for the same period three years later. The guardians credited the decrease in morbidity to the change in the treatment of pneumonia that had taken place over those years, but, unfortunately, did not elucidate what that alteration had been.[138]

Dr Suckling's usual treatment for cough in patients with chronic bronchitis and emphysema, and chronic phthisis was a mixture of ammonia and senega.[139] He added a few grains of iodide of potassium if expectoration was difficult and a small quantity of lobelia if dyspnea was marked. Most patients were also given cod-liver oil, as he considered it one of the most useful drugs in these conditions. Of 100 cases he treated in the winter of 1885, 28 were discharged well, with the chest examination being clear, and 68 discharged relieved. After reports of the benefit of pure terebene for winter cough, he gave it a trial in a further 100 patients, giving five drops orally every four hours initially and increasing the dose to ten drops, whereas his previous mode of administration had been to let patients inhale it.[140] Oral administration resulted in 72 percent of patients with chronic bronchitis and 67 percent of the 6 cases of chronic phthisis being relieved, although the beneficial effect was mainly on their breathing as many requested an antitussive in addition. Suckling concluded that oral terebene was very effective in relieving the dyspnea of chronic bronchitis.[141]

Tuberculosis

Pulmonary tuberculosis became a major public health concern in the nineteenth century, exacerbated by the rapid population expansion in towns with overcrowded housing conditions. Mortality, though high, declined throughout the century, although the reasons for this has been a matter of considerable debate. Raised standards of living, better nutrition, sanitary improvements, legislation to control the disease, and greater institutionalization have all been proposed as factors. However, the argument is far from being settled in favor of any one cause.[142] The medical officer of the Local Government Board in his report for 1905–6 dismissed the proposition of Dr. Arthur Newsholme that segregation of tubercular patients in workhouse infirmaries had played a dominant role in the decline. He did so on the grounds that the infectivity of tuberculosis was not sufficiently high to be influenced by isolation, when more highly infectious diseases had not been controlled in this way. In addition, he felt the average length of stay of tubercular patients in workhouses was too short to prevent the spread of the infection; for instance in Birmingham in 1897, it was only seventy-four days.[143] Newsholme's view gains support from the historian L. G. Wilson, who argued that the influence of segregation was sufficient to be the decisive factor. He made the point that by 1905, workhouse infirmaries were being used very extensively for tubercular patients in England and Wales.[144] Throughout the nineteenth century, there was no change in the medical approach to tuberculosis, nor was there any treatment available that could account for the decline.[145] Deaths from pulmonary tuberculosis declined steadily throughout the second half of the nineteenth century and the annual death rate in England and Wales decreased by 71 percent between 1840 and 1905 (table 5.4). The national rate for other forms of tuberculosis also fell, but only by 21 percent between 1858 and 1900.[146] All types of the disease accounted for 13 percent of all deaths during the period, but for 33 percent of those aged between fifteen and thirty-four years, making it primarily a disease of young adulthood.[147] The mortality rate was greater in females until the mid-1860s, when it changed to become more predominant among males.[148] Tuberculosis was more prevalent in urban areas, such as Birmingham, where the death rate was higher than the national average and the decrease between 1870 and 1910 was 5 percent lower than the country as a whole (tables 5.4 and 5.5). The Black Country also suffered high mortality from the disease. It dominated the causes of death among all sections of society and killed more people than any other disease throughout the Victorian era.[149] Despite the mortality decline, tuberculosis was the most common cause of death after heart disease at the end of the nineteenth century.[150]

Tuberculosis has a long history dating back 20,000 to 35,000 years and evidence of its presence has been found in skeletons in ancient Egypt.[151] Yet, attempts to control the spread of the disease and improve the condition of sufferers did not occur until the late nineteenth century. A major reason

Table 5.4. Annual number of deaths and annual death rates from phthisis in England and Wales, 1840–1905

Year	Total deaths	Death rate per 10,000
1840	59,923	38.9
1850	46,614	26.2
1860	51,024	25.5
1870	54,231	24.1
1880	48,201	18.6
1890	48,366	16.8
1900	42,987	13.3
1905	38,950	11.4

Source: HCPP, 1907 [Cd. 3657], *Thirty-Fifth Annual Report of the Local Government Board*, 36.

Table 5.5. Cause-specific death rates for phthisis, Birmingham registration district, 1871–1910

Decade	Total deaths	Death rate per 10,000
1871–80	5,913	24.8
1881–90	5,232	21.5
1891–1900	4,887	19.9
1901–10	3,036	12.9

Source: Woods, "Mortality and Sanitary Conditions," 180.

why it was not seen as a public health issue earlier was the belief that it was an inherited condition arising spontaneously within the body of susceptible individuals, possibly as a result of "bad living."[152] Although Robert Koch identified a bacterium as the cause of the disease in 1882 and established it as contagious, medical opinion in Britain was slow to change. The majority of doctors combined the new bacteriological findings with the old idea of hereditary susceptibility. As the infective nature of tuberculosis gained greater acceptance, attempts by medical officers of health to institute specific preventive measures yielded success toward the end of the century, although compulsory notification of the respiratory form was not achieved until 1912.[153]

Small nodules in the lungs filled with caseous material, called tubercles, had been identified in the seventeenth century, but it took another 100 years for them to be recognized as pathognomonic of pulmonary tuberculosis, known at the time as phthisis by doctors and consumption by the general public. These three terms are similar and will be used to mean the same disease, bearing in mind the difficulties over accurate diagnosis in the nineteenth century.[154] Tuberculosis is spread by airborne droplets from the sputum of infected humans or bacilli in milk from infected cattle. It can affect many organs throughout the body other than the lungs, most commonly the skin, causing lupus vulgaris, and the lymph nodes, known as scrofula. Only about one in ten of those infected develop the pulmonary form, which results in cough, low-grade fever, hemoptysis, night sweats, and general wasting, giving it the name White Death.[155] It killed 80 percent of sufferers within 5 to 15 years.[156]

Open-Air Treatment

Treatment in the early nineteenth century was palliative, focusing on the most distressing symptoms of cough, night sweats, and diarrhea. Later, but prior to Koch's discovery of the tubercle bacillus, therapy strove to concentrate the body's ability to overcome the disease through rest, to improve nutrition by a suitable diet, and to strengthen the lungs by moving the patient to purer atmospheric conditions. Cod-liver oil and bathing were also popular remedies. In the 1880s, the inhalation of antiseptics, such as creosote, came into vogue. In 1890, Koch introduced tuberculin, an extract from culture plates of the bacillus, as a specific treatment, but it was soon dismissed as ineffective.[157] Nevertheless, Birmingham guardians acceded to the visiting physician's request to order "50 marks worth" of Dr. Koch's lymph from Berlin.[158] Climatic treatment became the gold standard, aiming to place the patient in the environment most likely to limit progression of the disease. It was often combined with exercise to promote full ventilation of the lungs.[159] This developed later into "open-air treatment," in which the location became less important than spending as much time outdoors as possible, as outdoor air would contain less bacteria than indoor.[160] The essential factors in open-air treatment were described by a sanatorium physician in 1909 as "air, rest, feeding and supervision," plus "time."[161] Open-air treatment, which was developed in Germany in the 1860s and introduced into Britain thirty years later, became an established part of the therapeutic regimen in sanatoria. Although isolation of infected individuals was a significant part of their role, these institutions were promoted as providing a cure through a therapeutic regime of diet, exercise, strict monitoring of temperature and weight, as well as exposure to fresh air, either in huts on the sanatorium grounds or in wards with the windows wide open.[162] Because of the stress on the curative role of sanatoria, admission was not granted to patients with advanced diseases, who frequently ended their lives in poor law infirmaries.[163] Consumptives were also excluded from admission to voluntary hospitals for similar reasons. Specialized facilities were very inadequate, with only 14 sanatoria and 1,000 beds in Britain by 1910.[164] As a result, many poor law infirmaries included sanatorium wards; 12 in London provided open-air treatment and a sanatorium ward was in place in Sheffield around 1904. Purpose-built poor law sanatoria were established in Liverpool in 1902 and Bradford in 1903.[165] Reading Union did not establish dedicated facilities until 1912, providing 1 ward with 4 beds for women and 1 for men with 8 beds.[166]

From the early 1850s to 1890, the number of patients suffering from consumption in Birmingham workhouse was usually in single figures and constituted between 3 percent and 5 percent of sick inmates (appendix B).[167] When Edward Smith visited on November 12, 1866, there was a designated ward for consumptive cases, containing 19 beds out of a total of 630 in the infirmary.[168] In a national report four years later, there were 26 patients in the infirmary categorized under the "Phthisis and Tuberculosis" heading, constituting 3.7 percent of patients under the care of the medical officer, 1 percent greater than the national average. However, there were no patients with phthisis or consumption in Wolverhampton workhouse in that year.[169] Around 80 patients with consumption were present in Birmingham infirmary when the guardians decided to provide a dedicated ward for open-air treatment in the early twentieth century, prompted by moves nationally to take measures to manage tuberculosis.[170] Dr. Short, one of the visiting physicians, cautioned against having all phthisis patients together because of cross-infection between patients. Many of the patients were, he considered, in Class I in the last stages of the disease. Those in Class II also suffered from bronchitis and because of this were not suitable for open-air treatment. He estimated that there were no more than 6 cases of those in the early stages (Class III) who had been in the infirmary in the year and only they would benefit. However, he was not in favor of open-air treatment being carried out on the infirmary grounds because of the cold and windy atmosphere to which the patients would be exposed and he cautioned that treatment for less than six months would be useless. Dr. Kauffman agreed with him, except that he thought it worthwhile trying it at the infirmary and that Class II would benefit. The third visiting physician concurred with Dr. Kauffman, but added that patients would need to agree to undergo treatment for a minimum period of six months. The committee agreed to go ahead with special provision for a few patients, but also to transfer some to a sanatorium. Three sufferers who showed willingness to stay for at least three months were transferred to the Midland Open-Air Sanatorium at Belbroughton at a cost of

Table 5.6. Phthisis patients in the "phthisis hospital" in Birmingham workhouse on September 16, 1904

Name	Age	Time since admission (weeks)	Progress
W. Hexley	49	60	Improved; signs of active disease decreased
James Bunn	40	59	Slight improvement
Harry Overton	37	34	Improved; signs of active disease modified
Robert Jones	47	36	Some improvement; signs persist but modified
Charles Sampson	45	13	Doing well; signs of disease much diminished

Source: BCL, IHSC, GP/B/2/4/5/3, September 26, 1904.

one pound, eleven shillings, and six pence each per week, as there was no sanatorium provision in Birmingham at that time.[171] The phthisis hospital in Birmingham infirmary, which cost £444, was operational by the beginning of July 1903, all 6 beds being occupied by men, each having a separate room.[172] From that date to September 26, the next year, there had been 15 admissions and 10 discharges; details of the 5 remaining patients are contained in table 5.6. The ages of 9 of those discharged ranged from 19 to 58 years, with a mean of 41. Four were discharged at their own request, 3 as they had not improved, and 3 described as "unfit," presumably meaning not suitable for treatment. In the following six months, 18 men were admitted, 14 discharged, leaving 4 remaining in the ward. Dr. Kauffman reported that patients with relatively advanced disease did badly, while those with bronchitis and suspected phthisis were apparently cured. Overall, "hopeful" cases showed marked retardation of disease after three months, with the greatest improvement in the early period of stay.[173]

The number of admissions of patients with phthisis decreased from 297 in 1904 to 177 in 1905 and 156 in 1906.[174] On May 21, 1906, there were 85 men and 10 women in the infirmary at different stages of the illness. Two women and 14 men were in the early stage, 3 women and 33 men in the active middle stage, and 4 women and 15 men in the active advanced stage. One woman and 23 men had the chronic stage of the disease and the medical officer recommended separate accommodation for them to prevent spread of infection.[175] The reduction in admissions resulted in no patients being transferred to the phthisis block in the three months to January 1908. Two patients in the block had developed renal inflammation; 1 had died and the other had been transferred to a ward in the infirmary. As a result, the guardians debated the benefit of continuing with the arrangement. Dr. Jordan, who had taken over the care of patients in the block, advanced two reasons why it had not been as successful as expected. First, the quality of the atmosphere was too impure because of many surrounding factories, which also restricted the amount of sunshine.[176] In saying this, he was attributing the therapeutic benefit to the inspired air, a belief supported by Flurin Condrau, who asserts that the prime ingredient of institutional therapy was "fresh air." However, Michael Worboys disagrees, claiming that it was not pure air that was the therapeutic agent, but the regime in the sanatoria.[177] This accords with Dr. Jordan's second reason for failure of the phthisis block, namely the lack of supervision of patients due to its distance from the main building. He added that on one occasion, one of the medical staff paid a surprise visit to the block and found that the inmates had closed all the windows and doors, which, he claimed, would delay their progress by two months.[178] The inmates' actions support Condrau's assertions that patients are not merely objects of institutional therapy and that an institution exists independently of its inmates.[179] Dr. Jordan suspected that tuberculosis sufferers would not present for admission to the infirmary at an early enough stage of the disease to be suitable for open-air therapy since they would prefer to continue working as long as possible. He concluded that patients would gain more benefit in dedicated wards within the infirmary. The decision was taken to close the block accordingly, no doubt aided by the fact that the efficacy of sanatorium treatment was beginning to be questioned at that time.[180]

The workhouse medical officer at Wolverhampton also introduced open-air treatment. Early in the twentieth century, the guardians requested the architect to determine how the buildings proposed for the new workhouse could be adapted to provide "outdoor treatment of phthisical cases."[181] However, no dedicated facilities are included in the plan of the hospital dated 1902.[182] After the new workhouse had been operational for one year, the medical officer suggested converting a window into a doorway in the surgical ward, which contained patients suffering from tuberculosis of bones in the leg and spine. This would prevent them from being carried out through a corridor and airing court and instead give direct access to the outside of the ward. He stressed that open-air treatment was necessary for these patients. It took the guardians almost two years to seek the approval by the Local Government Board for the alteration, and a further year for the board's inspector to visit to give his approval. Three years later, the guardians agreed to widen a door so that patients could be moved out of the ward in their beds.[183] In the meantime, the guardians approved the purchase of six coats to enable phthisical men to get out in the open air as much as possible.[184] They also inquired of the medical officer whether phthisical patients could be put to work on the land and were advised that outdoor employment would be very beneficial in certain cases.[185] They were also concerned regarding tubercular patients "expectorating on the floors" because of the danger to other patients and threatened any doing so with prosecution for disobeying rules.[186] Birmingham guardians also considered the provision of "receptacles for the spittle of phthisis patients" and the best way of disposing of it safely.[187]

In the year ending Michaelmas 1908, there had been 346 admissions due to tuberculosis into Birmingham infirmary, with 69 admitted more than once. Of the 277 patients admitted, 201 were men, 62 women, plus 5 boys and 3 girls under 15 years of age. Only 6 women were admitted for a second time, but of 40 men who took their own discharge, as they wished to resume work to provide for their families, 25 were admitted for a second time, 9 for a third time, 5 for a fourth time, and one had 6 admissions.[188] Over the next few years, the number of admissions remained constant, except for the third quarter of 1911, and the number of phthisis patients present in the infirmary (table 5.7) was similar to that at the turn of the century (80) and in 1906 (85 men and 10 women).[189] The high mortality rate reflects the severity of the disease in patients admitted who were frequently in the terminal stages, but compares favorably with an estimated mortality rate of around 20 percent at the City of London Hospital for Chest Diseases in the 1880s.[190] When Edinburgh City Hospital opened in 1906, the death rate of the first 104 admissions was as high as 46 percent because many of the patients were in the later stages of the disease. Of the 48 who died, 11 did so within 10 days of admission.[191] Phthisis was responsible for the largest number of deaths in Birmingham infirmary in the years 1905 to 1908 inclusive, causing 16 percent of the 1,707 who died. It was the most common reason for admission in the year ending May 31, 1910, affecting 246 patients and accounting for 7 percent of the 3,338 admitted.[192] This is in stark contrast to Smith's estimate, based on extrapolating data from Liverpool, that 60 percent of admissions to workhouse infirmaries in England and Wales were of consumptive patients.[193]

An alternative to open-air treatment that became popular in Britain in the early twentieth century was a model of occupational therapy or graduated labor. It was pioneered by Marcus Paterson, medical superintendent at the Brompton Hospital Sanatorium at Frimley in Surrey. Patients started with walking and after they were able to do ten miles, carried baskets, which

Table 5.7. Tuberculosis patients in Birmingham infirmary for specific time periods, 1909–11

Time period	Present on first day of period	Admitted	Discharged	Transferred to workhouse	Died	Mortality rate
1st quarter of 1909	73	64	35	2	20	15%
2nd quarter of 1909	80	67	53		35	24%
1st quarter of 1910	72	78	32		37	25%
2nd quarter of 1910	81	66	45		35	24%
1st quarter of 1911	74	80	64		31	20%
2nd quarter of 1911	79	80	79		25	16%
3rd quarter of 1911	55	118	70		29	17%
Year: 1909	73	333	197		119	29%
Year: 1910	72	282	128	12	140	40%

Source: BCL, WIMC, GP/B/2/4/4/5–6, 1909–11.

gradually were made heavier, and finally they progressed to digging.[194] Paterson claimed that it prepared patients for an immediate return to work on discharge. This was one of the reasons given by Thomas Galbraith, workhouse medical officer at Wolverhampton, for implementing a similar scheme of graduated exercise for men in 1913. However, four years before he had agreed with the guardians that "work on the land" would be beneficial for some patients. The exercise program started with walking for half a mile daily after their temperature had returned to normal on bed rest. After they could manage six miles daily, graduated labor was begun. This consisted of very light work, such as carrying a basket, weeding, potting, watering plants, and was increased to heavier carrying, planting out, or cutting vegetables after about one week. Further stages included sweeping paths, cutting edges, hoeing; then light digging, mowing grass; and finally digging, trenching, or sawing until they were fit to resume their previous occupations. Galbraith estimated this would take fourteen to seventeen weeks and that fifteen male patients in the workhouse would benefit from the scheme. Its other advantage would be overcoming the demoralizing effects of long periods of mental and physical inactivity. The guardians agreed to proceed and delegated the newly appointed male charge nurse to provide close supervision of the men who would be taking part. They decided not to erect dedicated buildings for the men to sleep at night, but chose to add balconies to the existing wards. Once again, they made alterations to the doorway in the male surgical ward to enable patients to be taken out into the open air in their beds. Galbraith did not think that there were a sufficient number of female patients to justify instituting the same arrangements. It was agreed that the ward in which they resided should be portioned so that their part could be provided with as much ventilation as possible.[195] Strict adherence to the exercise program was considered necessary for success. The medical officer in Reading Union workhouse found it difficult to persuade patients to remain for the full course of treatment, as the regulations for phthisical patients were so detailed and tedious. However, patients were notified that the program would be of "no use to them" if they did not "co-operate heartily . . . in every detail of the routine" by "cheerfully acquiescing in every direction given to them." They were also informed that the average length of stay was three months, which was similar to the time that tubercular patients were required to commit to treatment in Birmingham infirmary.[196]

Although it has been acknowledged that poor law infirmaries provided the larger share of accommodation for patients with tuberculosis, they have not been given credit for instituting current methods of treatment. Both Birmingham and Wolverhampton guardians began taking steps to provide dedicated accommodation and access to fresh air for patients early in the twentieth century, whereas many urban workhouses had not done so by the end of that decade.[197] Following this, they adopted the regime carried out in sanatoria, which has been described as being "the bedrock of treatment" for nearly 100 years.[198] That it did not succeed in Birmingham may have been because the environmental conditions were not conducive. Within the historiography of tuberculosis, the poor law sanatorium set up at Heswall at the start of the twentieth century gets a brief mention.[199] The intention was to provide treatment for those at an early stage to return them to employment. However, it had the disadvantage that all patients had to be admitted via the workhouse. As happened in Birmingham, patients were reluctant to enter the workhouse until they were in the later, nonambulant stages and Heswall became "a staging post of the dying."[200] Perhaps it was because poor law infirmaries were seen to cater mainly for tuberculosis patients who were terminal that they have received so little attention from historians. The initiative in instigating current methods of treatment for patients was taken by the medical officers in both workhouses.

Patient Management and Mismanagement

A greater understanding of how treatments were utilized can be gleaned from consideration of the management of individual patients. Workhouse inmates had high expectations of treatment from their medical attendants and would readily complain to the guardians if they were not satisfied. Benjamin Lane, an inmate of Wolverhampton workhouse in April 1855, had initially been suffering from "white swelling" of the knee, for which he was prescribed a flannel to wrap round the joint.[201] Later, he developed a pain in his side and diarrhea, for which he was given a mustard plaster and he subsequently recovered. However, he complained that it took three requests to the medical officer, Richard Nugent, before he received treatment for his bowel complaint.[202] Joseph Freeman had also been complaining of abdominal pain on admission in June 1894 and explained that it was four days since he had had a bowel movement. The medical officer gave him a "draught to relieve pain." He was transferred from the old men's ward to the infirmary as the doses of laxatives and castor oil were unsuccessful and his condition had deteriorated. An injection of an analgesic and oral lime water and brandy produced a little improvement, but he died the next day.[203]

Patients were also critical of the type of treatment prescribed for them. William Stanley and John Dyer criticized Nugent's practice of using the same medicine for between twenty and thirty different cases in Wolverhampton infirmary. They considered that not everyone's sickness was alike and that therapy should have been prescribed according to individual complaints and constitution. Nugent dismissed their criticism by claiming that "this class of case" would never be satisfied whatever treatment was used.[204] An anonymous letter to the *Birmingham Journal* in 1857 complained that Birmingham guardians did not believe in any medicines more expensive than "epsom salts," and restricted the surgeon's use of drugs. The accusations, which had been made by Daniel Smith, who had been an able-bodied inmate, were denied by the medical officer, who stated that he treated inmates with the same drugs and stimulants as he would use for private patients.[205] However, there were few complaints over eighty years and the most likely explanation is that patients usually received the attention they expected.

Inmates were also at risk of inadvertently being given the wrong medication, although only one incident has been recorded in the minutes of both boards of guardians. In 1898, probationer Nurse Stockwin in Birmingham workhouse infirmary admitted that she gave two patients a dose of lead lotion instead of ward mixture. She called promptly for medical attention and both patients recovered without incident. Both medicines were contained in identical bottles, although that containing lead lotion had the word "poison" on it. It was usually kept in the poison cupboard, but had been lying out on the ward as it had been in use. The nurse was reprimanded for carelessness and the guardians took steps to provide distinctive bottles in future for poisons.[206] The lotion in question was likely to have been lead acetate, also known as sugar of lead, which was used as an astringent.

Therapeutic Practice

In 1887, Birmingham guardians considered that the medical treatment of patients in the workhouse was in accord with current scientific knowledge.[207] This chapter has provided evidence to support this claim. The volume of medical prescriptions ordered by the medical officers at both workhouses required the services of a dispenser over most of the study period. There is a tendency among medical historians to decry nineteenth-century drug therapy as dubious because little of it was deemed curative. To do so is to deny the palliative aspects of treatment as well as the placebo response. It has been postulated that placebos may have a pathophysiological response on the body.[208] Even today's highly effective drugs do not always benefit patients to the same extent and the doctor's attitude during a consultation can make the difference in a patient's response to the prescription. According to medical historian John Harley Warner, nineteenth-century medicine did work, but not when judged by the criteria of twentieth-century pharmacology.[209] The drug therapy used in the workhouse was similar to that prescribed in voluntary hospitals and in private practice. The point here is that workhouse patients were not deprived of treatments in common use at the time because of funding constrictions by either the guardians or the doctors. Some medical officers introduced therapies that were innovative, for instance, John Wilmshurst's treatment for scabies and Suckling's use of oral terebene for chronic bronchitis; or treated workhouse inmates more rigorously than patients in the voluntary hospital, as in the management of pneumonia. Medical officers in both workhouses introduced open-air therapy for tubercular patients, a treatment regimen that had recently become popular in Britain's sanatoria. Redfern Davies attempted to introduce new surgical techniques and groundbreaking surgery into Birmingham workhouse, with some success in spite of the guardians' objections. However, much of this innovative medical practice in Birmingham comes to light only because the medical practitioners were motivated to publish their practice to improve their standing in a competitive medical market. The presence in the town of a medical school further encouraged publication in the medical press to enhance a practitioner's standing. The fact that the medical culture in Wolverhampton was different without published evidence of practice does not mean innovation did not take place. New methods of treatment were introduced in other workhouses, for instance, the medical officer in Leicester workhouse treated leg ulceration by skin grafting in the early 1870s, only a few years after the method was published in *The Lancet*.[210]

Workhouse patients were provided with a range of sick diets, tailored to specific conditions and the severity of the illness, as was the case in voluntary hospitals. With medical extras, additional nutrition, usually in the form of meat or fish, could be provided to suit individual patients. Alcohol was regarded as one of the most potent forms of drug therapy in the nineteenth century. Despite becoming less popular toward the century's end, few leading practitioners of the day advocated dispensing with it completely, since they believed it to be effective even if they were in dispute over its mode of action. It was used therapeutically in workhouse infirmaries, the extent of its prescription depending on the medical officer's stance within the alcohol debate. Whether it was the guardians or the medical officers who paid for drugs and whatever the degree of influence of the local temperance movement, these factors had only a limited effect. Historians' allegation that the main reason for the prescription of alcohol was evasion by the medical officer of the cost of drug therapy does not appear justified. Rather, the evidence in this chapter suggests it was the strongly held belief in its power to effect a cure that determined how much it was used. There is some evidence from Wolverhampton that guardians also believed in the therapeutic benefits of alcohol, although they continually strove to restrict consumption. In this respect, they were no different than managers at voluntary hospitals, where restrictions on the medical use of alcohol were put in place. However, they do not appear to have had much success in Wolverhampton and Birmingham in curtailing its use. The evidence from these workhouses suggests that medical officers continued to prescribe food, alcohol, drugs, and other treatments despite pressure for restriction by guardians or outside agencies. The task of ensuring that patients were given the medication that was prescribed was the responsibility of the nursing staff and we look at how well they carried out their duties in the final chapter.

Chapter Six

Poor Law Nursing

The dominance of the Nightingale reforms in the history of nursing has overshadowed improvements within poor law nursing. Indeed, studies of nursing within poor law institutions have been sparse, possibly because of the uncertainty surrounding the nature of those carrying out nursing duties.[1] Accounts included in general studies of nursing history have concentrated on the improvement in conditions of service and the increasing involvement of poor law nurses with acutely ill patients. Christopher Maggs describes nurse recruitment in the late nineteenth century in one voluntary hospital and three poor law infirmaries and notes that the most significant quantitative change over the period was the rapid expansion in the number of nurses in the poor law sector.[2] In a general text on the history of nursing, the poor law sector receives minimal attention, even in the section on midwifery, although the majority of births in institutions took place in the workhouse.[3] For instance, 1 percent of the 1.3 percent of births in institutions in 1890 is estimated to have taken place in workhouses.[4] Rosemary White has provided the one dedicated account of poor law nurses, in which she points out that, despite the lack of interest by historians and the nursing profession, they nursed 75 percent of all hospital patients.[5] Moreover, the nature of the nursing tasks they performed and their interaction with the patients they cared for has been relatively neglected. White has been praised for doing much to rehabilitate the image of the poor law nursing service by showing that its members often achieved relatively high standards of nursing care.[6] Their status was on par with those trained in voluntary hospitals as a substantial number of poor law probationers have been shown to find employment in the voluntary hospital sector.[7] Although Brian Abel-Smith and Anne Digby contend that nursing staff disliked the tedium of caring for the chronic sick, Rosemary White maintains that poor law nurses developed expertise in the nursing care of those with chronic illnesses and incurable diseases and played a major part in retaining the caring role within nursing.[8]

The historiography of the nursing profession prior to 1980 has been written for the most part as a conventional, congratulatory discourse and only since the late 1980s has it developed into a more critical and reflective area of scholarship. The most recent accounts place the history of nursing within a wider historical context and focus on the reality of practicing as a nurse in the nineteenth century and the nature of the women who chose to be nurses.[9] Little research has been carried out on the period before the nineteenth century or in its early decades. One of the early initiatives to offer training to nurses was by the Institution of Nursing Sisters, set up by the Quaker philanthropist, Elizabeth Fry, in 1842. The institute's nurses gained experience by means of short attachments in London voluntary hospitals. Thereafter, the majority went into private practice. Fourteen years later, the Anglican Sisters of St. John's House spearheaded reform of hospital nursing in England. They devised a system of training and took over the nursing at King's College Hospital, London.[10] On Nightingale's return from Crimea in 1856, a national appeal raised sufficient funds to establish a training institution for nurses. Four years later, the first probationers from the school arrived at St. Thomas' Hospital, London. Although the Nightingale School achieved little in its first ten years, the surrounding publicity encouraged other hospitals to copy the system. Additionally, the school attracted motivated recruits, who carried the banner elsewhere.[11] Throughout the second half of the nineteenth century, nursing developed as a profession and nursing registration was eventually achieved in 1919.

This chapter will compare nursing practice at the workhouses in Wolverhampton and Birmingham between 1834 and 1914 and analyze whether the levels of nurse staffing were sufficient to meet the needs of the increasing numbers of patients. In the process, it will address the following questions. To what extent were pauper nurses utilized and paid nurses employed, especially in the early decades of the New Poor Law? Was the turnover of nursing staff as high in these two workhouses as has been suggested by other studies and, if so, what were the reasons for their resignations or dismissals? How did the introduction of training influence the standard of nursing care, and what effect did the erection of an infirmary as a separate institution from the workhouse have on the training of probationer nurses? To what extent were men involved in nursing in the workhouse infirmaries and how were they affected by the nursing reforms? Was the reputation of nurses for maltreating their patients justified and to what extent did they exhibit a caring attitude toward their patients? In other words, was Anne Crowther justified in remarking that "the records of almost any union will produce a dreary tale of nursing inefficiency, neglect and cruelty"?[12] In the process of answering such questions, the chapter will also attempt to draw out the experience of being a poor law nurse in the Victorian period.

Poor Law Nursing Reform

During the nineteenth century, nursing practice underwent major reform. At the time the New Poor Law was enacted in 1834, the majority of nursing care in workhouses and their infirmaries was carried out by inmates, who were predominantly older women. They were rewarded for their work with extra rations, which often included beer and gin, gaining them the reputation of working frequently in a state of intoxication. Pauper nurses were prone to be unreliable, incompetent, at times cruel, and liable to steal food and medication meant for patients. It was acceptable in the nineteenth century to imbibe alcohol while at work. Nurses in voluntary hospitals were also supplied with alcohol, often as part of their remuneration, and drunkenness among these nurses was also not uncommon.[13] It was unusual for nonpauper personnel to be paid to carry out nursing duties in workhouses prior to the New Poor Law and for several decades afterwards. The Fourteenth Annual Report of the Poor Law Commissioners in 1847 listed the nurse as one of the officers of workhouses, giving guardians the right to appoint remunerated nurses. Eighteen years later, the Poor Law Board issued a circular to metropolitan guardians advising the employment of paid nurses to promote better nursing in workhouses and stressing that they be adequately remunerated.[14] In the same year, *The Lancet* set up an investigation into the state of workhouse infirmaries and subsequently campaigned for the employment of paid nurses to ensure "a thorough and genuine performance of [nursing] duties."[15] In 1892, Dr. Downes, medical inspector for the Local Government Board, issued a letter stating that paupers were not suitable for employment on nursing duties and suggested a paid nurse-to-patient ratio between 1:15 and 1:10, but the board only advised guardians that they should feel satisfied that the number of nursing staff was adequate for the care of those inmates who were sick. Three years later, the board issued a circular letter stressing that a nurse was required to have experience in the treatment of the sick, was to be competent, and requesting guardians to discontinue the use of inmates as assistant nurses "as far as possible."[16] Finally, in 1897, the board issued an order banning inmates from carrying out nursing duties, but continued to sanction their employment as attendants, working under the supervision of a paid nurse, who required only practical experience in nursing, and with the approval of the medical officer. After the New Poor Law, guardians were slow to appoint paid nurses, so that by 1849 there were only 171 employed in England and Wales.[17] As a result of the 1866 circular, there was a considerable expansion in their numbers in metropolitan workhouses, from 111 in that year to 748 in 1883–84, while in the country as a whole, the 884 paid nurses employed in 1870 represented a large increase in their number five years previously.[18] By 1896, their number had risen to 3,715 nationwide, with around 40 percent in London. The national ratio was 15.6 patients per nurse, being lower (11.6) in London and higher (18.5) in the provinces. Birmingham's ratio of 12.6 was nearer to that of a metropolitan rather than a provincial workhouse.[19] However, in the 1890s, inmates were still being employed as paid attendants to supplement the nonpauper nursing staff. Patient-to-nurse ratios were higher in poor law infirmaries than in voluntary hospitals; for instance, in 1909, the number of beds per nurse in infirmaries ranged between 7.2 and 22.2, while in voluntary hospitals it was between 2.1 and 4.7, depending on how much surgery was carried out in an institution.[20]

The next development to influence the standard of nursing care in workhouse infirmaries was the introduction of trained nurses. Five years after the Nightingale School of Nursing opened at St. Thomas' Hospital, London, in 1860, twelve nurses from the school were sent to Brownlow Hill infirmary in Liverpool on a trial basis. The scheme was regarded as successful in improving the nursing standards and trained nurses were gradually introduced throughout the country. However, the introduction of training was slower and more difficult in workhouses than voluntary hospitals because of the Local Government Board's stance that all staff must be accountable to the guardians.[21] One result was a severe shortage of trained nurses to satisfy the requirements of the infirmaries. To ease the problem of nurse recruitment, the Association for Promoting Trained Nursing in Workhouse Infirmaries and Sick Asylums (also known as the Workhouse Training Association) was set up in 1879 and began financing nurses' training, following which it placed them in workhouses.[22] The Departmental Committee on Nursing the Sick Poor in 1902 also addressed the shortfall of trained nurses and recommended that individual poor law training schools should be coordinated into a national scheme, with major and minor schools providing a three-year or one-year course respectively. The shortened length of training in the minor schools would provide more nurses more quickly with sufficient skills to be competent. One reason for the scarcity was that infirmaries could not attract nurses trained in voluntary hospitals as infirmary nurses were less well paid, worked longer hours, and had poorer working conditions than hospital nurses, plus their patients were of a lower social class. All this left poor law nurses with a lower status within the nursing profession.

Nursing Recruitment and Duties

To understand the level of care a nurse would be able to perform, it is necessary to be acquainted with her previous occupational and social background. Hospital nurses in the early part of the nineteenth century were drawn mainly from domestic servants (see table 6.1), although nursing formed the lowest rung on the domestic service ladder. In voluntary hospitals, sisters, who supervised the nurses, often came from a higher social class, while the matron, topping the nursing hierarchy, originated from an even higher social standing, although she was usually employed as a housekeeper rather than a nurse.[23] Paid nurses in workhouses were equivalent to sisters in that they supervised the pauper nurses, but they did not share a common class background. Table 6.1 demonstrates the domestic service backgrounds of applicants for the post of nurse in the female infirmary wards in Birmingham in 1852, with those already employed as nurses the next most common after domestic service. Surprisingly, one of the two candidates recommended to the board of guardians by the Visiting and General Purposes Committee was Sarah Davis, who had no obvious previous occupation, but they were impressed by her testimonial from a minister of religion. The other was Elizabeth Manton, who was already employed at the workhouse as night nurse and had a testimonial from Mr. Humphrey, the workhouse medical officer. When she had been relieved from her post of nurse at the workhouse at the time the guardians reduced the nursing complement, she obtained employment as nurse at the Queen's Hospital in Birmingham, but had subsequently applied successfully for the post of night nurse at the infirmary. She was upgraded to infirmary nurse and Sarah Davis was given her previous post as night nurse, although the latter resigned for unknown reasons seven months later.[24] The majority of the candidates were middle-aged, widowed, or separated from their husbands, similar to the eleven applicants a decade previously, where only one was a spinster.[25] Surprisingly, when twenty-seven-year-old Ellen Spencer was appointed as night nurse in Birmingham in 1877, she was described as a "trained nurse," since training was still in its infancy at that time. Nurses appointed at the General Hospital in Birmingham at this time came from similar backgrounds, but this changed in the second half of the nineteenth century, with younger and more unmarried women being appointed, as occurred in other voluntary hospitals.[26] By early the next century, eleven of the applicants for posts as charge nurses at Wolverhampton workhouse were working as nurses and the other five were not in employment.[27] This recruitment pattern relates to female nurses as nursing was a female-dominated occupation and men were rarely employed in voluntary hospitals.[28]

Table 6.1. Applicants for the post of nurse in the female infirmary wards at Birmingham workhouse, 1852

Name	Age	Place of abode	Comments
Ann Jones	35	At Mrs. Parsons, Cottage Yard, Hospital Street	Domestic servant; married, but not living with husband, one little girl in service; 1 testimonial
Elizabeth Manton	41	At present night nurse in infirmary at new workhouse	Widow, no dependent children; 2 testimonials, one from Mr. Humphrey
Mary Minshull	45	Night nurse at the General Hospital, which she leaves tomorrow	Widow, no children; 4 testimonials, from Dr. Wright and others
Elizabeth Withers	57	32 Tark Street	Deserted by husband; 2 children with her, under 12 years of age; no testimonials
Margaret Morris	47	22 Latimer Street West	Widow, no family; has been private nurse for years, formerly nurse at Infant Poor Asylum and at Queen's Hospital; testimonial private
May Larkin	52	At Mr. Roberts, Kent Street	Widow; 2 daughters, both married; has been cook and housekeeper in various private families; 4 testimonials, from Lady Sligo and others
Sarah Frances Davis	27	2 House, 24 Court High Street, Bordesley	Married; husband in the 40th Regiment Foot, now in service in Australia; no family 3 testimonials, including one from the minister of Zion Chapel, Newhall Street

Note: All addresses were in Birmingham.

Source: BCL, VGPC, GP/B/2/8/1/1, December 17, 1852.

The occupational background of men before they took up nursing was different from women, although John Warder, who was appointed assistant keeper in the insane wards in Birmingham workhouse in 1846, had been a gentleman's servant. Edward Harwood, aged fifty-one years, who was employed as male nurse the same year, had previously worked as a farmer before posts as porter and nurse in other workhouses.[29] One of the other two keepers had worked as a butcher and the other as a gunsmith.[30] Thomas Gale, appointed as attendant in the epileptic ward in 1851, had been a corporal in the 54th Regiment of Infantry.[31] The social origins of male keepers were likely to be a reflection of the local employment situation, as was the case for their equivalent in lunatic asylums.[32] Between 1881 and 1914, the most common previous occupations of the all-female probationers appointed at Portsmouth and Leeds workhouse infirmaries, other than nursing, were in domestic and personal services.[33] At times, employees performing nonnursing duties in Birmingham workhouse were selected as nurses. For instance, Fanny Giles, who was appointed as nurse of the women's infirmary ward in 1844, had been employed as cook for at least three years beforehand.[34] Domestic tasks formed a major part of a nurse's duties, which Brian Abel-Smith has described as a "specialised form of charring."[35] However, Anne Borsay contests this description on the grounds that nonchild nursing was being recognized as an activity in its own right by the beginning of the nineteenth century.[36] Nevertheless, responsibility for the good order of the wards and the cleaning not only of the wards, but also of all the rooms and passages of Westminster Hospital, London, was included in the nursing regulations in 1835. Carol Helmstadter and Judith Godden have described hospital nurses in the early nineteenth century as "essentially cleaning women."[37] Nurses gave minimal personal attention, although they assisted those patients who were required to be in bed by day and those who were unable to wash themselves. In addition, they carried out such treatments as bleeding with leeches, blistering using poultices, which they would prepare themselves, and administering emetics and enemas, all of which required supervision and care of patients for a period following treatment.[38] The Poor Law Commissioners issued a General Consolidated Order in 1847, defining the duties of the nurse as attending upon those in the sick wards, administering all medicines and medical applications as directed by the medical officer, and ensuring that a light was kept on at night in the wards. The only qualification required was the ability to read the directions for giving the medicines.[39]

As was the case with nursing in voluntary hospitals, a workhouse nurse's working life was arduous, with long hours and a requirement to be available both day and night. Living conditions were extremely harsh and many nurses ate and slept in the wards with the patients. Protests, albeit infrequent, against the poor quality of living, accommodation, and food occurred in both voluntary hospitals and workhouse infirmaries.[40] Evidence for the exact tasks that nurses undertook is sparse. In the early nineteenth century, Birmingham guardians' main requirement was that they kept the wards in "that state of cleanliness which is essential to the welfare of the sick."[41] In Wolverhampton in 1890, nursing duties still included housekeeping tasks, such as keeping the porter's book in his absence and assisting the matron "in the stores." They were also responsible for personally supervising the bathing of all female children prior to examination by the medical officer.[42] Bathing patients was the activity that took up most of the nurses' time in Birmingham workhouse in

Table 6.2. Weekly average hours worked by sisters and nurses in 1911

Infirmary/hospital	Sisters	Nurses
Birmingham infirmary	61½	64¼
Marylebone infirmary	61¾	73¼
Manchester infirmary	64¾	69¾
Liverpool infirmary	71¾	74½
General Hospital, Birmingham	56¼	72½
Queen's Hospital, Birmingham	61½	61¼

Source: BCL, Infirmary Management Committee, GP/B/2/4/4/6, February 27, 1911.

1907.[43] One of their main tasks in the General Hospital in Birmingham was cleaning the wards, although they also assisted those patients who needed personal care. By 1878, they were allowed to take patients' temperatures, but it was not until the early twentieth century that they had the responsibility for measuring patients' pulse and respiratory rates.[44]

No information is available on the hours of work in Birmingham or Wolverhampton workhouses in the nineteenth century, but in the latter, nurses were granted leave on one Sunday per month in 1870.[45] Early in the twentieth century, nurses were on duty from 7:00 a.m. until 8:00 p.m. daily except Sunday, when they had leave for half a day once a month. However, they were only on "active duty" for two-thirds of this time and for the remainder, they needed only to be on call on the premises. As a result, their time on active work did not exceed eight hours daily.[46] In the early 1910s, Birmingham guardians admitted that the nurses' hours were long, but compared favorably with other infirmaries and the local voluntary hospitals (table 6.2). Sisters worked from 8:00 a.m. until 1:00 p.m., 1:30 p.m. until 4:15 p.m., and 7:15 p.m. until 9:15 p.m., and had a whole day of leave each month. Nurses worked from 7:00 a.m. until 8:30 a.m., 9:15 a.m. until 1:30 p.m., and 4:15 p.m. until 9:00 p.m.[47] However, by the following year, sisters' hours had been reduced from sixty-one and a half to fifty-four and a half per month.[48]

Nursing Turnover in Wolverhampton, 1839–90

The high turnover of paid nurses in workhouses, while generally accepted as being the norm, has not received detailed attention in the literature to date and there are no accounts of nurse employment over a continuous time period. In her study of Leicester workhouse, Angela Negrine cites only one example of a brief length of tenure, when five nurses appointed in 1886 all resigned at the same time the following year.[49] The nurse appointed by the Reading Union workhouse in 1870 resigned within days and her replacement was asked to leave within six months because of inefficiency, including giving patients the wrong medication.[50] Furthermore, few accounts of poor law nursing include the early decades of the New Poor Law or attempt to analyze why turnover was so high. It may have been the result of the long hours of work, the heavy workload, or the fact that the nurses often ate and slept in the wards with their patients. An additional factor may have been the loss of women to marriage, a feature of women's employment at the time, although the extent of this factor is debatable.

The main problem for Wolverhampton guardians was not recruitment but the retention of the paid nurses they had appointed. Nursing staff turnover was high in the fifty years after the first nurse was appointed in 1839, with the guardians needing to employ eighteen female nurses (table 6.3). Excluding Nurse Elizabeth Careless, who remained in post for twenty-six years, the average length of stay was less than two years. The nineteen male nurses and superintendents of the male insane patients employed over that time had similar lengths of stay of one year and six months and one year and eleven months respectively, but ten of the nurses were in post for less than a year. The exceptions were the seven superintendents for the female insane who served three years on average (table 6.4). This contrasts with the tenure of the medical officers, which ranged between seven and twenty-two years after tendering had been abolished in 1841. However, continuity of nursing staff was better than it appears from these figures, as many of the nurses appointed were chosen from the superintendents of the insane and their assistants.

Two months after the union workhouse opened in 1839, the guardians advertised for a nurse for the sick, the only requirement being "persons willing to undertake the situation." Sarah Keeling was subsequently appointed as "Head Nurse" at the workhouse at a salary of twelve pounds per annum.[51] Within a month they were again advertising for a nurse and appointed Elizabeth Davies on a trial basis for one month, on an annual salary of fifteen pounds, prior to a permanent arrangement if found suitable, suggesting that Sarah Keeling had not been so. However, by November that year, Davies had been replaced by thirty-five-year-old Maria Carphew.[52] Over the next two years, she was reprimanded over her conduct, on the first occasion for failing to bathe a child, as instructed by the medical officer, and on the second for being described by him as "disorderly and riotous in the lying-in ward."[53] With only one paid nurse in the workhouse, pauper nurses were

Table 6.3. Nurses appointed to the infirmary wards in Wolverhampton workhouse, 1839–90

Female wards			Male wards		
Name	Date of appointment	Length of service	Name	Date of appointment	Length of service
Sarah Keeling	December 1839	6 months	Mrs. Poole	May 1856	4 years, 2 months
Elizabeth Davies	February 1840	8 months	Edward Shubotham	July 1860	4 years, 9 months
Maria Carphew	November 1840	4 years, 6 months	Thomas Alldridge	April 1865	1 year, 4 months
Jane Frost	May 1845	2 years	William Barley	August 1866	5 months
Elizabeth Careless	August 1847	4 years	John Jennings	February 1867	11 months
Mary Ann Sharratt	July 1851	8 months	William Ward	January 1868	8 months
Sarah Cox	March 1852	1 year	William Stokes	September 1868	1 month
Mary Leeson	March 1853	1 year, 6 months	Francis Evenson	October 1868	4 months
Martha Gettings	September 1854	7 months	William Ward	February 1869	8 months
Catherine Cox	April 1855	1 year, 6 months	Edwin Ladbrook	October 1870	9 months
Sarah Mercer	September 1856	ca. 3 years, 9 months	William Humphreys	September 1871	4 months
Sophia Siddons	mid-1860	ca. 2 years	Edwin Ladbrook	February 1872	3 years, 3 months
Mrs. Shelley	August 1862	3 years, 7 months	Joseph Downward	July 1875	3 months
Elizabeth Careless	March 1866	7 years, 3 months	Joseph Smith	October 1875	4 years, 5 months
Ellen Ward	June 1873	1 year, 2 months	Robert Clinton	April 1880	7 months
Mary Wedgebarrow	August 1874	11 months	Llewellin Harris	December 1880	1 year
Mary Daly	July 1875	5 years, 2 months	Charles Cattrell	December 1881	2 years, 3 months
Elizabeth Clarke	September 1880	1 year, 9 months	George Thomas	March 1884	5 years, 5 months
Martha Trow	July 1882	1 year, 9 months	Samuel Austin	August 1889	Not known
Clara Lyne	March 1884	1 year, 3 months			
Sarah Stringer	May 1885	11 years, 10 months			

Source: WALS, WBG, PU/WOL/A/2–22, 1839–90.

Table 6.4. Appointments as superintendents of the insane in Wolverhampton workhouse, 1861–90

Male insane			Female insane		
Name	Date of appointment	Length of service	Name	Date of appointment	Length of service
William Parker	January 1861	1 year, 4 months	Mary Parker	January 1861	1 year, 4 months
Mr. Lack	mid-1862	ca. 4 years, 6 months	Mrs. Lack	mid-1862	ca. 4 years, 6 months
Henry Pretty	February 1867	1 year, 3 months	Margaret Yeomans	February 1867	6 years
Mr. J. Wright	May 1868	1 year, 2 months	Sarah Lowe	February 1873	1 year, 4 months
James Akrigg	July 1870	8 months	Mrs. Hollowell	May 1874	7 months
Gerard Carroll	March 1871	1 month	Maria Cartwright	December 1874	10 months
Joseph Kenney	April 1871	9 months	Mary Ann Stanley	November 1875	4 years, 4 months
Joseph Downward	February 1872	3 years, 6 months	Sarah Owen	April 1880	12 years, 9 months
Daniel Johnson	August 1875	4 years, 8 months			
Richard Owen	April 1880	14 years, 4 months			

Source: WALS, WBG, PU/WOL/A/11–18, 1860–81.

responsible for delivering babies in the ward. When Sarah Porter's illegitimate baby died shortly after such a delivery, the subsequent coroner's verdict was that the lying-in ward was "perversely misconducted." The pauper nurses in question were deemed no longer fit to carry out such duties, as they had not informed the medical officer in the Porter case. Despite the master and matron expressing their disquiet at pauper nurses acting as midwives, the guardians took no action.[54] Two years later, the master again reported Nurse Carphew for behaving with "gross indecency" in the lying-in ward, and she must have been dismissed or resigned as the records show four applicants for her post.[55] Reasons for nurses leaving or resigning their posts were not recorded for the majority of nurses. However, Edward Shubotham, who resigned in 1865, was on a list of nurses at Birmingham workhouse one year later.[56] A married man in his mid-thirties, he had been appointed in May 1860 when the workhouse medical officer requested the appointment of a male nurse. He considered that a man would have better control of the male patients, as well as being "better for the sake of morality." The guardians questioned whether he would be as sympathetic as a female nurse, to which the medical officer responded that he had "never observed sympathy between nurses and patients in public institutions."[57] As a result, men were employed as nurses in the male ward for the next thirty years (table 6.3).

Two nurses were dismissed for being unable to carry out their duties efficiently. Jane Frost, who had previously been a "housekeeper for invalids" and a children's nurse, was the first in 1847, after two years of service. At this time, there were fifty-seven patients in the infirmary, infectious disease, and lying-in wards, all of which would have been under her care.[58] She wrote to the guardians requesting they reconsider their decision, but they upheld it on the grounds that she was "far advanced in years" when she was appointed (although only sixty-three years old at the time) and considered that her inability to supervise pauper nurses "amounted to insubordination."[59] The guardians decided that her successor "should be able to write" and appointed Elizabeth Careless, who was in her early fifties.[60] The Poor Law Board did not sanction the appointment of Catherine Thompson as night nurse in Birmingham workhouse in 1852 because she would not be able to read the directions of the medical officer although the guardians considered her competent to fulfil the office of nurse.[61] Wolverhampton guardians dismissed Sophia Siddons in 1860 after a complaint by the medical officer of her inefficiency, "harshness," and neglect of her duties. She was given an ultimatum of resigning within the week or being dismissed and chose the former.[62] The following year, she was appointed nurse at Dudley workhouse and remained there until her death in 1876.[63] Although she was not dismissed for her inefficiency, Mrs. Martha Gettings tendered her resignation in 1855, within seven months of appointment, following investigation into a complaint by Benjamin Lane, an inmate, regarding his medical treatment. The nurse admitted she had failed to carry out the doctor's order to apply a poultice to Lane's chest and admitted she had "a bad memory," which resulted in her frequently forgetting directions. At that time, she had had the assistance of six wardsmen and seven wardswomen, who were provided with a better diet than the other inmates.[64] Surprisingly, Mrs. Gettings was among the nine applicants when the post became vacant again in the following year, but was not appointed.[65] Another common reason for dismissal was taking leave without consent and failing to return to the workhouse, as happened with four male nurses during 1868 and early 1869. William Barley, appointed in 1866, was unfortunate to be given one month's notice after only six months in post because he was unable to work due to a chronic leg ulcer.[66] The only instance of nurses returning from leave "drunk" occurred in 1881 when male nurse, Llewellin Harris, and the assistant superintendent of the male insane, Henry Jenkins, arrived back intoxicated on consecutive Saturday and Sunday evenings. Harris was dismissed, but Jenkins was only required to resign.[67]

Another who was coerced into resigning was Joseph Darnward when it was discovered, in October 1875, that he had married Maria Cartwright, the assistant superintendent of the female insane without permission of the guardians; Cartwright resigned a few weeks later. He had been appointed keeper of the male insane inmates three years before and subsequently as male nurse only a few months before his resignation.[68] Marriage was also the reason for the resignation of two officers in March 1880, when Daniel Johnson, superintendent of the male insane, married Jane Moore, assistant superintendent of the female insane. The Johnsons were reemployed as a married couple in charge of temporary workhouse accommodation. Joseph Smith, the male nurse of over four years' standing, and Mary Stanley, the recently appointed superintendent of the female insane, also resigned on exactly the same date, though the reasons were not recorded in the minutes. Mrs. Stanley, a widow in her early forties, was reemployed six months later as the assistant in the female insane wards.[69] Men, as well as women, were required to resign on getting married, as nurses were required to live in the workhouse and had very little leave. The only opportunity for a married couple was joint employment, for instance, William and Mary Parker, husband and wife in their early forties, appointed in January 1861 as superintendents of the male and female insane respectively. They resigned sixteen months later to become master and matron of another workhouse.[70] Their successors as superintendents of lunatics, Mr. and Mrs. Lack, resigned when he was appointed "Collector of Local Rates" for Wednesfield Heath.[71] Thirteen years later, another married couple, Richard and Sarah Owen, were chosen as superintendents of the insane. When Mrs. Owen died in 1893 in her mid-fifties, her husband continued in his post.[72] In 1873, Mrs. Elizabeth Careless retired in her eightieth year as nurse in the female infirmary, suffering from "partial paralysis." She had been an officer in the workhouse since 1847 and had also worked briefly on the fever ward (during the smallpox epidemic in 1849) and as matron's assistant. The guardians approved a superannuation allowance for her of twenty pounds per annum.[73]

Catherine Cox, appointed nurse in the female infirmary in 1855, resigned after eighteen months in post when her request for an increase in her annual salary of fifteen pounds was refused.[74] The female nurse's salary was increased to twenty pounds seven years later and Thomas Alldridge, the male nurse, had his annual salary increased in 1865 to thirty pounds after dispensing had been added to his other duties.[75] In light of the difficulties in retaining nursing staff at that time, one of the guardians, Mr. Sidney, intended to propose

Table 6.5. Salary schedule for officers in Wolverhampton workhouse, 1876

Officer	Present annual salary	Minimum salary	Maximum salary
Male nurse	£30	£30	£35
Female nurse	£25	£20	£25
Superintendent of male insane	£30	£30	£35
Superintendent of female insane	£30	£25	£30
Assistant superintendent of female insane	£26	£20	£25

Source: WALS, WBG, PU/WOL/A/16, February 11, 1876.

a motion to replace pauper nurses with paid employees. Regrettably, he died before he could bring the motion before the board.[76] Two years later, the workhouse medical officer suggested that all the nurses should be paid, but the master judged the nursing situation satisfactory "considering the class of nurses employed." The guardians took no action, as appointing extra nurses would involve providing extra accommodation for them.[77] Around this time, recruitment of nursing staff began to be problematic. When Edwin Ladbrook, who had commenced work in October 1870, resigned nine months later, the guardians had no response to their initial advertisement for his replacement, but were able to appoint William Humphreys two months later.[78] When he contracted smallpox the following year, the master was unable to find a temporary replacement, but he recovered and resumed his duties after a few weeks.[79] Four years later, the guardians adopted a new schedule of officers' salaries, after obtaining information from forty-seven other unions. This involved increasing the starting salaries by an increment of one pound every second year to a fixed maximum, obviating the necessity for officers to apply at intervals for an increase (table 6.5).[80] The maximum salaries differed little from those they were paying at the time and were in line with wages in other poor law institutions and in the General Hospital, Birmingham.[81] Although the guardians paid the superintendents of the insane the same wages as the nurses, they disagreed with the Local Government Board that they were on "the same footing" as the nurses, as they did not consider that they performed nursing duties.[82] In the early 1880s, there were twenty-seven applications for the post of male nurse and thirteen for that of assistant superintendent of the male insane, demonstrating that recruitment was no longer a difficulty and it would remain as such throughout that decade.[83]

From the time the workhouse opened, the nursing staff consisted of only 1 nurse until 1856, when a second was appointed. Two superintendents of the insane were added to the nursing complement eleven years later and 2 assistant superintendents five years after that. By comparison, inmates had increased from just over 300 to almost 1,000 and patients from 55 in 1842 to 423 in 1888.[84] In 1874, one of the guardians considered it a disgrace that there was only 1 female paid nurse, Mrs. Mary Wedgebarrow, as she had over 100 sick inmates under her care.[85] The 2 nurses employed to care for patients with physical illnesses saw their patients increase from 87 each in 1866 to 157 each 22 years later.[86] There is no evidence from Wolverhampton that the increasing number of sick inmates influenced length of service, as there was a tendency for nurses to stay in post longer after 1880. Nor were the salaries a deterrent, as they were comparable to most other medium-sized and large workhouses in the third quarter of the century.[87] Of those who resigned, only a few took up nursing posts elsewhere and a substantial proportion may have left out of a dislike for the type of work they were required to carry out.[88] The impact of loss due to marriage would have been lessened to a degree in Wolverhampton by the guardians' preference for appointing older widows, and male nurses left employment after a short period as frequently as their female counterparts. A major factor causing the high turnover was the exhausting nature and the demanding pace of the work, which applied also to nursing in voluntary hospitals. For instance, the average length of stay of 7 nurses at St. Thomas' Hospital in 1847–48 was eight weeks.[89]

Paying Nurses and Paupers in the First Birmingham Workhouse

Although the New Poor Law facilitated the employment of paid nurses, many boards of guardians were slow to implement the new arrangements while some large workhouses included remunerated nurses among their servants under the Old Poor Law arrangements. In 1818, Birmingham guardians gave the surgeons they employed instructions to appoint "one chief nurse" to each ward in the Town Infirmary and resolved that the nurses were to be "entirely under the direction of the Surgeons." Furthermore, each nurse would be allowed as many assistants as was necessary from among the female paupers in order to keep the wards clean. Five years later, they increased the nurses' salaries to two shillings and six pence and the assistants to one shilling per week when they discovered the "pernicious custom" of the nurses receiving gratuities from patients due to the inadequacy of the salaries.[90] The nurses' annual pay at that time of six pounds, ten shillings was better than that of four pounds, thirteen shillings paid to the nurses at the General Hospital in Birmingham.[91] The nursing arrangements continued unchanged after 1834, but in 1842, they advertised for "several females as nurses in the Town Infirmary," with the requirements that the women were "of good character, of assiduity and determination, and possessed of kind feelings towards sick patients." The House Committee interviewed eleven applicants, some of whom were already employed, while others were pauper nurses. For instance, Elizabeth Higgs, a pauper nurse, who was forty-one years of age and had a boy in the guardians' facility for pauper children, was continued as nurse in the lying-in ward at an annual salary of ten pounds. Ann Rose, a spinster aged forty-six years, remained as nurse of the old and infirm women's wards on eight pounds per annum. Six other appointments, all widows, were made to the infirmary wards, women's fever, venereal and insane wards, and the bedridden ward. The annual salaries ranged from eight pounds to thirteen pounds and the nurses were allowed a ration of tea, sugar, and butter.[92]

The matron was instructed to appoint fit, able-bodied women as assistants, but the house surgeon considered only Elizabeth Harrington, a widow "with no encumbrances," competent to perform the duties required. In addition, he pointed to the need for night nurses, as many of the more disabled patients required as much attention at night as by day. Mary Mills, aged twenty-two years, who was retained as nurse in the women's fever ward, was later considered to be too young after accusations of her misbehavior with William Purnell, the male nurse on the fever wards. As a pauper, she could not be dismissed, but was transferred to duties elsewhere in the workhouse. Purnell was retained, although, one month later, he was dismissed for further misconduct.[93] Table 6.6 shows those acting in nursing roles in August 1842 and nearly all the nonpauper nurses were employed on the female side, while some of the male wards, for instance, venereal, did not have any pauper assistance. It is also interesting to note that Elizabeth Higgs's payment had been reduced by half. Three years later, the guardians appointed midwives for the districts and one, Mrs. Edge, was also required to attend midwifery cases in the workhouse on the payment of four shillings per case.[94] Elizabeth Vincent, a widow aged thirty-seven and nurse in the women's infirmary ward in August 1842, resigned in July the following year, was reappointed to the same post in the following April, but resigned a month later to become matron of the Lying-in Hospital at Islington in London.[95] The clinical activity, for which the 7 paid nurses and 14 paupers acting in a caring role were responsible, involved 264 admissions to the Town Infirmary in the relevant quarter of 1842, with 158 inpatients on average.[96]

In July of the same year, the Poor Law Commissioners advised the guardians that paying gratuities to inmates for employment appeared to be an illegal charge on the poor rates and recommended the practice cease

Table 6.6. Paid and pauper nurses in Birmingham workhouse, 1842

	Name	Position	Salary
Officers:	Ann Howlett	Nurse in men's infirmary	£10 per annum
	Elizabeth Vincent	Nurse in women's infirmary	£10 per annum
	Mary Ann Raven	Nurse in women's bedridden ward	£8 per annum
	Elizabeth Line	Nurse in women's venereal ward	£8 per annum
	Ann Titley	Nurse in women's insane ward	£10 per annum
	Ann Rose	Nurse in aged and infirm women's ward	£8 per annum
	Thomas Lamb	Assistant keeper in men's insane ward	£8 per annum
Paupers:	Joseph Gregory	Attendant in men's venereal ward	1s per week
	Joseph Galey	Night attendant in men's sick ward	1s.9d per week
	George Baker	Attendant in men's fever ward	1s.6d per week
	Isabella Taylor	Nurse in women's fever ward	£1.10s per quarter
	Elizabeth Higgs	Nurse in lying-in ward	£1.5s per quarter
	William Ware	Keeper in men's insane ward	4s.6d per week
	Catharine Tipton	Nurse in children's ward	1s per week
	Mary Johnson	Nurse in women's insane ward	£1.7s.6d per quarter
	Elizabeth Atherley	Nurse in women's dayroom	1s per week
	Maria Horton	Nurse in old and infirm men and boys' rooms	£1.5s per quarter
	William Percival	Wardsman to able-bodied men	1s per week
	Joshua Haywood	Wardsman to partially disabled men	1s per week
	Mary Knight	Nurse in children's ward	1s per week
	Stephen Bridge	Leech bleeder	1s per week
	John Dawson	Leech bleeder	1s per week
	M. A. Harriman	Assistant to Nurse Rose	5s per quarter
	Isabella Taylor, jun.	Assistant to Nurse Johnson	5s per quarter

Source: BCL, House Committee, GP/B/2/3/1/1, August 9, 1842; BPP, 1843 [491], 139–40.

forthwith. The guardians reviewed a list of 15 "servants employed" in nursing duties, which included those classed as both paupers and nonpaupers (table 6.6). They had been receiving salaries ranging from eight pounds to twenty pounds yearly. The guardians resolved that inmates who were employed in tasks in the workhouse should receive extra rations of meat at dinner and a daily beer allowance, presumably instead of monetary remuneration.[97] However, four years later, the allowances for pauper assistant nurses were reduced to the ordinary diet of the workhouse, plus one pint of tea with bread and butter twice daily.[98] This decision may have been the consequence of new and replacement appointments increasing the nursing establishment to 19, of which only 7 had remained in post from 1842.

They included a few who had been pauper nurses in that year, but as they were continuing to receive an annual salary, they would now be designated as officers. At this time, the daily number of inmates varied between 470 and 500, with around one-third needing medical attention.[99] Taking into consideration only those nurses directly involved with sick inmates and lunatics reveals that there was 1 nurse for every 11 patients. This was similar to the situation at the General Hospital in 1851, with 220 beds and 17 nurses, giving a ratio of 1 nurse to 13 beds.[100] Despite the greater number of nurses to care for patients in Birmingham workhouse, staff turnover appears almost as high as in Wolverhampton, although fewer were dismissed for misconduct. The misbehavior of the 2 nurses in the fever wards in 1842 has already been mentioned and, two years later, Mary Williams and William Fitzer, both nurses in the fever wards, were dismissed because of "gross misconduct."[101] Of the other dismissals, George Bates had used violent language when intoxicated; the nurse in the women's sick ward was declared inefficient by the medical officer; Charlotte Greasley had acted "most improperly" to her patients on the female venereal ward; and 2 nurses were dismissed in 1849 without reasons being recorded. Ann Rose, the nurse in the old women's ward, was reprimanded for selling the tea, sugar, and butter provided for the inmates, but resigned of her own accord.[102] However, these incidences involved a very small proportion of the total nursing staff over sixteen years. With further resignations and the release of 3 nurses, the nursing complement was reduced to 7 nurses, including 1 night nurse, plus 1 "Insane Keeper" in early 1851. Only 4 nurses in employment two years before had been retained, indicating a high turnover of staff in a short period of time.[103]

Maintaining Nursing Care in the Second Birmingham Workhouse

The smaller number of nurses was unlikely to be able to cope with the increasing incidence of sickness among paupers in the expanded new Birmingham workhouse. Three months after it opened in 1852, the 8 paid nurses who were providing care were increased by 3 when the children were transferred to the workhouse from the Asylum for the Infant Poor.[104] When Charlotte Davis, nurse in the women's sick ward resigned four years later, Fanny Giles, a nurse on the equivalent male ward, was put in charge of both, a move that was challenged by the central authority. However, the guardians defended the action by claiming she could manage both wards efficiently

Table 6.7. Paid nurses in selected English workhouses, 1856

Union/parish	Capacity: Number of inmates	Nursing staff	Salary range
Birmingham	1,663	12 nurses 1 attendant on epileptic ward	£6–£26
Bethnall Green	1,016	2 nurses	£15–£20
City of London	1,010	1 superintendent nurse 2 nurses	£20–£31
Clifton	1,180	4 lunatic keepers	£13–£23
Greenwich	1,044	18 paid nurses	Not recorded
Lambeth	1,100	1 nurse	£50
Leicester	1,000	2 nurses 2 attendants on insane	£15–£20
Liverpool	2,345	4 nurses 1 superintendent of lunatics	£12.10s–£20
Manchester	2,000	12 nurses	£2.12s–£22
Marylebone Street	2,000	1 head nurse 1 midwife 11 nurses	£6–£50
Nottingham	1,150	3 nurses	£20–£31.4s
Portsea Island	1,150	1 matron of hospitals 1 nurse 2 keepers of lunatics	£5.4s–£40

Source: BCL, Returns relating to the number of officers and servants, GP/B/16/2/1, October 15, 1856.

and the Poor Law Board sanctioned it for a period of six months, following which it expected a report on her performance.[105] Perhaps it was this issue that prompted the guardians to request the clerk to ascertain staffing levels and salaries from other workhouses built to accommodate 1,000 inmates or more (table 6.7). As Birmingham came out well, no changes were made.[106] Ten years later, pauper help was still being used, with 45 assisting in the infirmary wards by day and 15 at night, so relieving the paid nurses of household tasks, such as cleaning the wards (table 6.8).[107]

A further comparison of nursing standards is possible from the surveys conducted by Edward Smith, medical officer to the Poor Law Board, of forty metropolitan and forty-eight provincial workhouses in 1866–67.[108] He commented that the appointment of paid nurses had been generally accepted as appropriate, as only four workhouses in the capital were without them. Furthermore, workhouse medical officers found pauper nurses "old, ill-trained and unreliable," necessitating salaried nurses. The provinces fared less well, as eleven workhouses had no paid nurses, but these were

Table 6.8. Day nurses, attendants, pauper nurses, and patients in Birmingham infirmary on March 21, 1866

Name of wards	Nurses and attendants	Pauper assistants		Number of patients
		Day	Night	
Male epileptic	Thomas Bevan	3	2	57
Female epileptic No. 1	Ann Giles	2	1	39
Female epileptic No. 2	Bridget Driscoll	2	1	24
Male infirmary	Fanny Giles	3	2	51
Female infirmary	Catherine Latouche	4	1	63
Smallpox and fever	Jane South	5	1	21
Female venereal	Amelia Orgill	2	–	28
Women and children's infirmary	Mary Barber	4	1	49
Lying-in ward	Ann Latouche	3	–	24
Female bedridden	Jane Smith	3	1	64
Male bedridden	Edward Shubotham	8	–	77
Male bad leg and venereal	Edward Shubotham	4	–	43
Male convalescent	Edward Shubotham	1	–	15
Boys' sickroom	None	1	–	16
Total	11	45	10	571

Source: BCL, VGPC, GP/B/2/8/1/5, March 23, 1866.

usually the smaller institutions, with less than 100 beds. The ratio of the number of inmates on the medical officers' books to that of paid nurses at the time of the visit varied greatly, from 15 patients to 1 nurse in one workhouse to as high as 255 in London and between 4 and 132 in the rest of the country. Paradoxically, the workhouses where few nurses were employed produced the highest ratios in London, but the lowest in the provinces, as this occurred in the smallest workhouses, usually with fewer than 150 inmates.[109] The ratios available for the workhouses in table 6.7 are: Birmingham, 26 (22 nurses for 582 patients); City of London, 17; Greenwich, 98; Lambeth, 166; Leicester, 14; Liverpool, 38; Manchester, 59; Marylebone Street, 22; Nottingham, about 75; and Portsea Island, 49.[110] Birmingham came out best in terms of paid nurse staffing of the provincial workhouses with more than 500 inmates and only three London workhouses were better staffed. The contrast with Wolverhampton is stark, with 4 paid nurses, 238 patients, and a ratio of 1 nurse to 60 patients, with only eight provincial workhouses having a higher rate. Smith found it impossible to believe that the number of paid nurses was sufficient, with 2 nurses for around 160 cases of "ordinary sick" and 2 attendants for nearly 70 lunatics.[111]

Table 6.9. Increases in annual salaries for nurses in Birmingham workhouse, 1875

Nurse's department	Annual salary	
	Before increase	After increase
Female bedridden	£20	£25
Male infirmary	£18	£20
Female infirmary	£18	£20
Fever ward	£21	£24
Lying-in ward	£22	£25
Female epileptics	£18	£20
Venereal ward	£15	£20
Old women's ward	£18	£20
Nights	£15	£22

Source: BCL, House Sub Committee, GP/B/2/3/3/4, February 23, 1875.

Despite Birmingham's level of nurse staffing being among the best in the country, the guardians became concerned in 1874 over the large number of nurses' resignations. They consulted one nurse, Martha Gilbert, and the master and decided there was no one particular reason, but it was possible that the salaries they were offering were lower than in other poor law institutions. Furthermore, there was by this time more alternative nursing work as the town had around seven voluntary hospitals. They requested information from six large workhouses and subsequently increased salaries by between two pounds and seven pounds, with the largest increase for those on night duty (table 6.9).[112] These salaries were in line with those at the General Hospital in the 1870s, where a head nurse received between twenty pounds and twenty-five pounds and an undernurse between thirteen pounds and eighteen pounds.[113] However, some nurses remained loyal to the workhouse for many years. When Jane Smith, nurse in the female bedridden ward, was forced to resign because of long-standing ill health and "advancing age" (although only in her mid-fifties), she was granted "an annual emolument" of forty pounds in light of her twenty-five years' service.[114] In late 1877, a subcommittee was set up to consider the medical and nursing arrangements in the workhouse. On the medical officer's advice, the subcommittee recommended appointing additional nurses for the female venereal ward, female bedridden ward, male infirmary, and the male and female epileptic wards. Members of the inquiry agreed to recommend appointing a superintendent of the nursing staff, who would be "well qualified by training and education" and who would supervise the "whole of the Nursing of the Sick," despite the senior medical officer's view that a professional nurse was not necessary. Kate

Nicholson, who was in her mid-twenties and younger than most of her nursing staff, was appointed to the post in the following year.[115]

However, turnover of staff remained high, with twenty-one nurses and attendants leaving over a fifteen-month period out of a nursing establishment of twenty-eight. Two were dismissed for misconduct and two men because they were married, the guardians preferring single men. As a result, Edward Marshall was replaced by thirty-one-year-old Samuel Bradburn, who had worked as a nurse at Manchester and Sheffield unions after a period as a rubber worker.[116] Edward Riley, nurse in the male surgical and venereal wards, resigned in December 1881 because the work was "too much" for him.[117] Thirty years before, William Key, attendant on the male epileptic ward, resigned in similar circumstances as he found the "confinement prejudicial to his health," and joined the Birmingham police force.[118] The most common reasons for female nurses resigning in 1880–81 were to get married and to join or accompany their husbands (table 6.10).[119] Thus, marriage was an important factor in the loss of nurses in Birmingham at that time, at variance with Sue Hawkins's claim that it was not a significant drain on nursing departments based on finding less than 3 percent annually resigning for this reason at St. George's Hospital, London.[120] Despite the medical officer's and Nicholson's request for more nursing staff, the guardians agreed only to a temporary increase, as the number of sick inmates had "considerably decreased."[121] However, the following year, Nicholson managed to get the newly constituted "Infirmary Sub Committee" to agree to five additional nurses for the male and female surgical wards, the male venereal ward, and for night duty on the male and female epileptic wards. The committee also agreed to provide uniforms for nursing staff, as a means of controlling the spread of infection during the current smallpox epidemic, although it is not clear if this was a temporary measure. However, when probationers were appointed for the first time a year later, uniforms consisting of print dresses, aprons, collars, and caps were provided, but were supplied only after probationers had completed their trial period of four weeks. Assistant nurses and charge nurses were also provided with uniforms that would distinguish their grade from each other and from the probationers.[122] In 1899, Wolverhampton guardians were spending around eighty pounds annually on uniforms.[123] The appointment of probationers in Birmingham increased the nursing staff to thirty-seven, although the number of patients had remained static.[124] Although pauper nurses were still employed at night, their main duties were keeping the fires burning, giving ordinary drinks to patients, and being present on the wards while the night nurses undertook rounds. Consequently, skilled temporary nursing staff were required at times

Table 6.10. List of nurses and attendants leaving office in Birmingham workhouse, July 1880–October 1881

Name	Designation	Reason for resignation
E. G. Gibbons	Nurse	Dismissed for misconduct
Julia Phillips	Nurse on lock ward	To join husband
Sarah Madden	Temporary nurse	Incompetent
George Bebbington	Attendant aged men's ward	Services dispensed with as they
Edward Marshall	Male nurse	were married and single men were preferred
E. Spencer	Nurse	To get married
M. Burley	Night nurse	To join husband
Florence Petty	Nurse	To join husband
M. Rich	Nurse	To get married
M. Launsbury	Nurse	To get married
E. Edward	Night nurse	Misconduct
M. A. Hudson	Nurse	To get married
M. Hadew	Nurse	Given notice
George White	Attendant, aged men's ward	Given notice
E. White	Nurse	Resigned with husband
E. Astley	Nurse	Resigned with husband, (tramp master)
S. Bradburn	Male nurse	Obtained more lucrative situation
Fanny Tulkington	Nurse	LGB refused to ratify appointment
Caroline Wiggett	Nurse	Resigned with husband (watchman, opening own business)

Note: Three other nurses resigned, but no reason was given.

Source: BCL, VGPC, GP/B/2/8/1/8, October 28, 1881.

of increased demand; for instance, two nurses were employed in the female infirmary in 1883 at the visiting physician's request to provide adequate nursing care to a large number of "extremely dangerous cases of pneumonia" who needed "unremitting attention."[125] At the end of 1885, the guardians took the unusual step of appointing Lydia Rogers as "Head Night Nurse." She was a twenty-eight-year-old unmarried nurse working in St. Bartholomew's Hospital in London before her appointment in Birmingham.[126]

Between January 26 and March 11, 1889, thirty-three nurses were transferred to the new infirmary, as the relevant patients were gradually moved.[127] However, not all patients were transferred and those with venereal disease and in the bedridden wards remained in the workhouse. Similarly, chronic and venereal patients were not transferred from the body of Blackburn workhouse to the new hospital wards in 1888. John Pickstone claims that the exclusion of patients requiring careful and intensive nursing from the "hospital section" of the workhouse was common.[128] When a nurse in the workhouse died two years later, the master, supported by the matron and medical officer, claimed three other nurses were incompetent and "not fit to trust old people with." They requested that trained nurses be appointed in their place, to which the guardians agreed, but decided to advertise for "attendants trained in nursing, ages not to exceed thirty-five years."[129] Within two months, the master complained that none of the newly appointed "attendants" would remain long in post unless they were placed on the same footing as the nurses in the infirmary, with their better diet and other privileges. The guardians approved this request and also reverted to the designation of nurses.[130] In the early twentieth century, the post of assistant matron at the workhouse was advertised as requiring a qualified nurse and attracted forty-five applications. Emma King, the assistant matron at West Ham workhouse, was appointed with an annual salary of fifty pounds, increasing over five years to sixty pounds.[131] She died two years later of typhoid fever despite being admitted to the infectious disease hospital and was succeeded by Maud Plant.[132] However, the appointment of a trained nurse as assistant matron did not mean that nursing in all the workhouse wards was of a high standard. Mr. E. B. Wethered, a Local Government Board inspector, was critical of the fact that only one nurse was employed on each of two of the female bedridden wards, with thirty-four patients in each ward who were "actually bedridden." He considered there should be seven nurses on each ward to prevent the pauper assistants from having to perform nursing duties.[133]

The chronic nature of the majority of the patients in the workhouse may have contributed to the paucity of nurses and the difficulty with their retention. Several historians have commented on the less interesting nature of patients with chronic disability and the restricted variety of illnesses that their nurses experienced.[134] Concurrent with the development of scientific medicine, there arose the view that the "chronic sick" did not need skilled nursing.[135] However, Anne Gibson, matron of Birmingham Infirmary, in her evidence to the Departmental Committee inquiring into the Nursing of the Sick Poor in Workhouses, stated that the "nursing of the chronic and aged sick" was most important, "one of the highest and best proofs of a good nurse that she is able to deal with that type of care."[136] Unfortunately, she had authority only over nursing in the infirmary and not in the workhouse itself.

Introducing Nurse Training into Workhouses

The earliest attempt to provide formal training to pauper nurses was made by the Epidemiological Society in the mid-1850s, with the award of certificates for satisfactory completion (see appendix E). It foundered because of the inmates' inability to benefit from training and the opposition of Florence Nightingale. The trial scheme of introducing trained nurses into Liverpool Union's infirmary, Brownlow Hill, was led by Agnes Jones, Florence Nightingale's "best pupil."[137] They were employed to work on the male wards only and were funded for three years by a local merchant and leading nursing reformer, William Rathbone. He had been dissatisfied with the standard of nursing he had encountered on his visits to workhouses and approached Nightingale for assistance. One year after their introduction, the workhouse master reported a marked improvement in the standard of nursing and rehabilitation of the patients, and a better demeanor among the male patients. The visiting physician preferred the new system as it convinced him of the nurses' ability to implement medical orders, as well as promote good morale on the wards.[138] Although the scheme foundered after Jones's death from typhus in 1868, similar training initiatives were subsequently set up at Highgate by St. Pancras Union and at St. Marylebone Union in London with funding from the Nightingale Fund.[139]

However, trained nurses could not be employed without the supervision of an officer who had undergone training. Such appointments were facilitated by a Local Government Board order of 1897, which required the appointment of a superintendent nurse, who had undergone three years' training in any workhouse where 3 or more nurses were employed, and that matrons in the separate infirmaries be trained nurses and have overall control of the nursing staff. Five years after the appointment of a superintendent of nurses at Birmingham workhouse in 1878, 3 probationer nurses were appointed at an initial annual salary of ten pounds, increasing over three years to eighteen pounds, plus the provision of a uniform. The superintendent, Kate Nicholson, suggested that those who passed the medical officer's examination, which consisted of a written paper and viva voce, should be rewarded by being appointed to the first substantive nursing post to become available. More probationers were taken on over the next four years and in November 1887 their number was increased to 20 in light of the anticipated opening of the new infirmary and the total abolition of pauper nursing.[140] The guardians sought the central authority's permission to engage up to 20 staff nurses (annual salary of twenty to twenty-five pounds), 10 assistant nurses (twenty pounds), and 50 probationers (ten to eighteen pounds) in the new infirmary with a total bed complement of 1,665.[141]

They appointed as matron to the new infirmary Miss Annie Gibson, who held the appointment of superintendent at Brownlow Hill Infirmary in Liverpool and was, therefore, one of Agnes Jones's successors. She was paid £130 per annum and given the remit to "take control of the sick in the wards" under the supervision of medical staff and to maintain good order among the nurses and inmates.[142] According to Rosemary White, Gibson became a powerful figure, with well-considered ideas, and one of the most influential members of the poor law medical service.[143] She instigated a scheme for training paying probationers within the infirmary and the fee per trainee of twenty-eight pounds per annum generated £900 in revenue for the guardians in 1893, with up to 25 pupils at a time undergoing training.[144] As a result, assistant nurses were no longer employed, with charge nurses increased by 2 to 22.[145] Gibson may have obtained the idea for the scheme from that of the Nightingale School in London in the late 1860s as she had trained at St. Thomas' Hospital, where women from the higher social classes could pay for training. It was these "lady-pupils" who later were at the forefront of reform.[146] By 1896, Birmingham infirmary was training 32 paying probationers. In a return of nursing staff in workhouses in England and Wales in 1896, Birmingham was the only one that declared additional fee-paying nurses and it is likely the scheme was unique within the poor law nursing service, although a similar scheme had been in operation at the General Hospital for at least two decades. Of the 73 paid nurses, 35 had received training prior to their appointment, in contrast to Wolverhampton workhouse, where none of the 3 nurses, caring for 165 sick and bedridden inmates, had received prior training and where 43 inmates assisted in the personal care of patients.[147] The nurse-to-patient ratio in Birmingham infirmary was 1:13, compared with 1:55 in Wolverhampton workhouse (table 6.11). In Birmingham, it was almost as good as at Withington Infirmary in Manchester (1:10), where the nursing was described in a report in the *British Medical Journal* as of the same standard as in general hospitals, but it was poor by comparison with the General Hospital, Birmingham (1.4 in 1898).[148] However, a few years later, the training scheme was discontinued, but Birmingham infirmary continued to take pupils from the Workhouse Nursing Association, receiving a solitary fee of twenty pounds for each trainee.[149] The General Hospital had also discontinued its intake of paying probationers two years previously.[150] In 1902, Birmingham was training 88 probationers, with 27 in their first year, 32 in their second, and 29 in their third and final year.[151] After the Central Midwives Board was established

Table 6.11. Number of patients and paid nurses in selected urban workhouses in England and provincial England, 1896

Union or parish	Number of sick inmates	Number of paid nurses	Number of patients per nurse
St. Pancras	1,686	98	17
Holborn	917	69	13
Birmingham	917	73	13
Liverpool	1,202	100	12
West Derby	1,237	110	11
Manchester	981	95	10
All England	56,628	3,625	16
Provincial England	39,083	2,111	19

Source: HCPP, 1896 (371), *The number of sick* persons occupying the wards for the sick, 2–4, 6–7, 28–29, 32–33.

that year, lectures by a medical authority were introduced to allow nurses to qualify for its diploma and training was extended to four years to allow for the additional number of deliveries required by the board to be carried out.[152]

Nurse training could not commence in Wolverhampton workhouse before a superintendent nurse had been appointed and the guardians did not decide to do so until 1893, when they advertised for a "thoroughly competent" woman as "Head Nurse" to be responsible for nursing throughout the workhouse and to "re-model" the nursing arrangements. From 14 applicants, they selected Miss Anna Menon, remunerating her annually with thirty-five pounds.[153] At the time of her application, she was a staff nurse at Walsall Cottage Hospital, but had received her training at Whitechapel Infirmary, London.[154] When the Local Government Board approved the appointment of probationer nurses early the following year, it added the rider that the nurse staffing should be reevaluated to ensure it was "put upon an efficient footing." From the 105 applications, the board interviewed 10 candidates and appointed 4 probationers to serve two-year appointments at a salary of ten pounds annually. An additional 2 were appointed five months later, but only because of pressure exerted on the guardians by the central authority to improve staffing levels.[155] The board voted against Miss Menon being allowed to be present during the interviews, a factor that may have played a part in the large number of probationers leaving before completing their training. However, this was not peculiar to Wolverhampton; for instance, 30 percent of probationers left before completing their training in Kensington poor law infirmary between 1890 and 1915.[156] The difficulty the guardians experienced in making appointments was that there were no criteria of suitability to assist them. The Departmental Committee into the Nursing of the Sick Poor in Workhouses in 1902 faced a similar problem and could only recommend that potential probationers should be of a minimum age of twenty-one years, of good character and health, and have intelligence.[157] From the initial appointment of probationers to the opening of the new workhouse ten years later, 12 resigned, although reasons were only given on two occasions. Nurse O'Reilly was accused of "neglect of duty," while Gertrude Hill suffered an accident during a gale.[158] In addition, 2 probationers were deemed not fit to carry out their duties because of their state of health and 1 was assessed as unsuitable for nurse training by the medical officer. Early the next century, the surgeon in Birmingham workhouse reported that Dora Copeland had a cardiac murmur and "must give up nursing."[159]

The training complement of probationers in Wolverhampton workhouse had been increased to 12 by 1896 and the length of training increased to three years. Two years later, 3 additional probationers were accepted from the Trained Nurses Institution, each with a payment of ten pounds.[160] In the same year, the superintendent nurse resigned and her appointed successor did likewise before taking up her appointment. They were replaced by Miss Maud Carter, in her late twenties, at an annual salary of forty pounds. There was also difficulty in appointing trained nurses at this time, with no applications for the post of charge nurse, so one of the probationers was upgraded.[161] This was not unique to Wolverhampton, as about a quarter of poor law medical institutions reported difficulty in recruitment around this time.[162] At the end of the century, the nurses not in training had been increased to 10 for day duty and 5 for night duty to care for 226 physically ill patients (nurse-to-patient ratio of 1:15, one of the lowest in Staffordshire).[163]

For adequate staffing at the infirmary of the new workhouse (opened in 1903), it was agreed that 6 charge nurses and 18 probationers would be required, an increase of 3 and 4 respectively.[164] Within four years, an additional 2 charge nurses and 9 probationers were needed.[165] In 1904, the Local Government Board approved Wolverhampton infirmary as a training school for nurses and, six years later, the Central Midwives Board recognized it as suitable for training in midwifery, allowing it to be included in the trainees' program.[166] Because of the guardians' concern that 2 probationers had resigned within three months due to physical incapacity to perform their duties, they required that all applicants pass a medical examination before appointment, carried out by the medical officer.[167] Another issue hindering training was the conscientiousness of the trainees. In 1903, the superintendent nurse, Miss Carter, complained of "carelessness and neglect" by several probationers, who were exhorted by the guardians to make more effort in the best interest of the patients. Two years later, the situation was reversed and after a two-hour meeting with the guardians, Miss Carter, and probationers, she agreed to carry out her duties to the satisfaction of the guardians and the benefit of the nursing staff.[168] The second complaint against probationers for not taking an interest in lectures or studying as they ought was made by the resident medical officer. Once again, a meeting with the interested parties resolved the situation.[169] One probationer in particular, Annie Coyle, had neglected her studies, in addition to returning to duty late, making tea when on duty, and leaving the ward unattended. She had previously been shown leniency, but was now dismissed.[170] Dismissals of probationers had been rare since transfer to the new workhouse, with only 1 other nurse so disciplined. The next year, Miss Carter resigned and was succeeded by Miss Annie Tyers, who had been night superintendent.[171] Certificates of completion of training included an assessment of probationers' proficiency; for example, in 1908 nurses Wain and Prescott were both rated as good for surgical nursing, medical nursing, and obstetrical nursing. Prescott was given good for conduct, but Wain was rated very good.[172]

The Conduct of Nurses and Patients

Was the reputation of workhouse nurses for inefficiency, negligence, and being frequently under the influence of alcohol while on duty justified? There were a few instances of nurses returning to the workhouse from leave in a drunken state, as in the 1850s in Birmingham, and this usually led to their resignation. The workhouse medical officer complained on a number of occasions of nurses not carrying out his orders or exhibiting rudeness. Prior to the transfer to the new workhouse, the only report of drunkenness was that of George Bates, the nurse of the men's fever ward in 1843, but his dismissal may have resulted more from his use of "violent language to the master."[173] Subsequently, only one nurse was dismissed after returning "drunk from leave" in 1882. Surprisingly, four months after Nurse Jane Thompson's dismissal, Nurse Cherton was merely reprimanded for the same offense.[174] The only other incident involving alcohol consumption was Nurse Rogers's contention that the superintendent nurse, Kate Nicholson, was "tight" on the night that Nurse Harrison died in 1885. The guardians found the accusation was "without foundation," and Nurse Rogers resigned.[175] The only incident in Wolverhampton workhouse in the nineteenth century of a nurse being reprimanded because of "a state of intoxication" was in 1873 and involved the male nurse, Edwin Ladbrook, on his return to the workhouse one evening.[176] The only dismissals took place in the early decades of the twentieth century. Richard Newell, the attendant in the male mental wards, also returned from leave intoxicated at 11:00 a.m. and was still in the same state at 7:30 p.m.[177] Wheeley, the attendant on the male skin ward, did not pay his usual visit to the wards at 11:00 p.m. because of the "influence of drink."[178] It is impossible to know if alcohol was a factor in the many resignations by nurses, but the findings in Birmingham and Wolverhampton would support Anne Borsay and Billie Hunter's assertion that tales of drunken and disorderly nurses are exaggerated.[179]

However, nurses were also dismissed for taking unapproved leave and returning late from leave without the consumption of alcohol being involved. After being in office only three weeks, male nurse William Stokes stayed away from Wolverhampton workhouse for two days in September 1868 and offered his resignation when asked for an explanation. His replacement, Francis Eveson, repeated the offense by taking one day's leave within three months and he also resigned.[180] Thomas Lamb, underkeeper of the men's insane ward, and Ann Sholton, nurse of the lying-in ward, in the infirmary in Birmingham were more fortunate. Although they stayed out of the workhouse overnight in January 1844, they were merely reprimanded after expressing their contrition.[181] Leaving work without permission and patients unattended was one of the most severe problems in voluntary hospitals, but Helmstadter and Godden consider that such behavior was characteristic of the early nineteenth-century workforce in general.[182]

Nursing staff were also charged with the more serious offense of assaulting patients. In 1854, Mrs. Sarah Pugh, attendant in the female epileptic wards in Birmingham workhouse, resigned after she had severely beaten Caroline Morris in a dispute about the amount of money Morris had given to her for safekeeping.[183] Ten years later, Thomas Armitage, superintendent over the aged men, pushed Edward Heap over and dislocated his hip.[184] There were no further reports of assault in Birmingham after the separate infirmary opened the following year. In Wolverhampton workhouse in 1843, an inmate, Hannah Deakin, complained that Nurse Careless had beaten one of her children. When evidence of violence was found to be visible on the child, the nurse was reprimanded and removed from the nursery.[185] However, John Moore, a pauper attendant in the insane wards, who assaulted Thomas McDonald, was taken before the magistrates, suggesting that male inmates were treated more severely than officers and female inmates in incidences of assault.[186] Miss Steward, one of the assistants on the female insane ward, was reported in 1899 by the superintendent to have treated a patient roughly. The wardswoman, Elizabeth Thomas, said she had seen Steward strike a patient several times and place a pillow on her face. Steward denied this, but admitted she had had difficulty pacifying the patient. No action was taken, as Thomas's account could not be corroborated.[187] Patients' behavior could put staff members at risk of injury. For instance, in Wolverhampton workhouse in 1907, there was an unprovoked assault by a patient on three nurses, two of whom sustained serious injuries. The patient was charged with unlawful wounding and intent to do grievous bodily harm. Nurses Blackmore and Walker were allowed an additional two weeks' leave after they had made a satisfactory recovery.[188] The few reported incidents of nurses' maltreatment of sick inmates suggest that general callousness toward patients was not prevalent in the workhouses of Wolverhampton and Birmingham.

The Reality of Poor Law Nursing

The deeply entrenched historiographical view of poor law nursing prior to the development of Nightingale nurses is that of the workhouse reformers of the 1860s of idle, drunk, incapable, indifferent, inhumane, and untrained pauper nurses.[189] This depiction has been enhanced by Kim Price's claim that the standards of care practiced by poor law nurses was below the expected level for the time.[190] Poor law historian Steven King has questioned this viewpoint in relation to nursing under the Old Poor Law, suggesting that professional networks developed long before the later nineteenth century. He points out that workhouse nursing was not provided only by other pauper inmates.[191] The analysis in this chapter provides a perspective that contradicts much of the traditional narrative of early New Poor Law workhouse nursing. The connotation of "untrained" to workhouse nurses is often used to imply that standards of care practiced by nurses in voluntary hospitals were higher, although training was not available for them either. However, the material presented here demonstrates that working conditions, hours of duty, salaries, and staffing levels in the workhouses were similar to those of the local voluntary hospitals, especially in Birmingham, where nurses moved between the two types of institutions. Helmstadter and Godden have shown that the behavior of nurses in voluntary hospitals was at times as undisciplined as workhouse nurses have been portrayed in poor law literature.[192] However, in the evidence presented here, only a small proportion of nurses needed to be reprimanded or dismissed for misdemeanors. Although staffing levels were low in some workhouses, for instance, Wolverhampton,

Birmingham infirmary's ratio of nurses to patients was as good as the leading local voluntary hospital during most of the study period. Thus, workhouse nursing was not invariably of poorer quality than that in voluntary hospitals. What has become clear from the situation in Birmingham is that there was often little distinction between paid and pauper nurses other than a salary differential, and pauper nurses could move into the higher paid bracket, particularly after guardians were prevented from paying them in cash. Some of the nurses appointed in 1849 had children resident in Birmingham's poor law institution for children and paid toward their keep from their wages. It is likely that they themselves would have been inmates if not employed as nurses. King found that a large proportion of women who were not paupers when they took on a nursing role subsequently became so.[193] The situation in Birmingham workhouse up to the mid-nineteenth century supports King's view that the relationship between pauper status and nursing is complex.

According to Christopher Maggs, there was a qualitative change in attitude to those caring for the sick from 1881.[194] It was accompanied by nurses' demand for greater professional recognition, resulting in greater status for nursing as a suitable occupation for single, middle-class women. However, it had become closely associated with the qualities of caring that were considered to be the hallmark of femininity.[195] Nursing reform had not accommodated male participation in general nursing and male nurses were deemed suitable only for mental health nursing.[196] For instance, no training school in London in the late nineteenth century would accept men.[197] Probationers appointed in Birmingham and Wolverhampton were exclusively female, and from that time men were retained only on the male lunatic wards. Historically, male nurses have been relatively neglected by researchers as a source of study, possibly because they have been regarded as a "social anomaly."[198] In the workhouses of Birmingham and Wolverhampton, they had a prominent place in the nursing complement and participated in general nursing prior to the introduction of training. Thereafter, their numbers dwindled, so that there was only one male nurse among a nursing staff of thirty-three in Birmingham workhouse in 1883.[199] Consequently, their contribution to general nursing prior to the reforms has not been given due recognition.

It is generally accepted that nurse turnover was high in the nineteenth century in both workhouse and voluntary hospitals and this is borne out in both Wolverhampton and Birmingham, although more so in the former. However, no one specific reason could be identified for the frequent resignations, but the heavy workload and harsh conditions may have led to many nurses resigning without wishing to disclose their reasons. With a greater number of nurses employed in the infirmary, Birmingham workhouse records did not detail routine replacement of nurses, but the larger complement would have had less impact on continuity of care when compared with Wolverhampton. The introduction of nurse training in workhouses did not resolve the problem of high turnover, as many left before completing their training. Guardians accepted probationers readily after pauper nursing was prohibited, for they were less costly than trained nurses. Initially, they may have been regarded as a form of cheap labor as formal theoretical learning was not introduced until early in the twentieth century. As Sue Hawkins has emphasized, nurse training in the nineteenth century had as much to do with building character and instilling discipline as with acquiring nursing skills.[200] However, Birmingham workhouse did subject its early probationers to an examination in 1883.

There is no doubt that nurse training improved the standard of nursing in the late nineteenth and early twentieth century. One direct result of appointing a trained matron in Birmingham infirmary in 1889 was the introduction of an innovative scheme whereby probationers paid for their training (along the lines of that in the Nightingale School) and so were supernumerary to salaried staff. It is more difficult to judge if training influenced the caring nature of nurses and improved the overall quality of care provided under the New Poor Law. We will now turn to the issue of general standards of care in the concluding chapter.

Chapter Seven

"Every Care and Kindness"

The Standard of Workhouse Medicine

The traditional narrative of poor law medical care emphasized a sharp divide between the old and new poor laws that has allowed historians to make broad-brush comparisons of the quality of care before and after 1834. Those who regard care as better under the Old Poor Law focus mainly on outdoor medical relief, whereas those who favor New Poor Law medicine concentrate on workhouse care. However, a new appreciation of workhouse medicine has emerged that stresses the continuity from the old to the new forming a continuous line of development throughout the nineteenth century.[1] Utilizing letters written by paupers requesting relief, Steven King has demonstrated that medical welfare was a significant call on poor law resources. While the workhouse was a relatively small element, it was the single most important form of institutional provision for the sick poor. By the end of the Old Poor Law, there had grown a substantial patchwork of support for sick paupers and this core function of the old continued to grow under the new.[2] Assessing quality of the care from a single parameter is problematic as care is multifactorial, involving adequate staffing levels of suitably trained personnel, the provision of adequate facilities, nourishment and treatments, and safety from harm. Thus, it is from these perspectives that the standard of care in Birmingham and Wolverhampton workhouses will be examined.

The preceding chapters clearly demonstrate that both workhouse infirmaries played an important part in the provision of medical care for paupers after the New Poor Law. This included those with short-term acute illnesses and those who had sustained accidents, the type of patients that historians have suggested were not to be found in workhouses. In Birmingham this also took place before 1834 and changed little afterwards as the parish continued as before under its local act. In Birmingham and Wolverhampton, almost one-third of patients had acute medical and surgical conditions in 1869, a greater proportion than in inner London workhouses.[3] Another group of patients who needed admitting urgently were those with disturbed behavior due to mental illness. Both Wolverhampton and Birmingham arranged transfer to asylums for the majority of these patients as best they could against a background of the lack of availability of local institutions and a lack of available beds within them. There is no evidence that financial considerations were implicated in preventing asylum admission. When restraint was in use in the early years, guardians imposed conditions on its use and restrictions on the availability of restraint equipment. Regulations were also introduced to control the use of the padded cell. When epileptic fits came under better control with drug therapy later in the century, more progressive policies were introduced and Birmingham was in the forefront of setting up an epileptic colony to provide specialist care. Inmates with venereal disease fared less well, often having the least satisfactory living conditions. Although notorious for misbehaving, only a minority did so, but clearly they were not afraid to challenge authority. Toward the end of the century, Birmingham referred many to the Lock Hospital for the newly introduced treatment with salvarsan.

A significant element of acute care was provided for patients with infectious and epidemic diseases, as these patients were usually "unwanted" by nonpoor law medical institutions. Indeed, for patients in Birmingham and Wolverhampton suffering from a wide range of communicable diseases, there was little alternative but admission to workhouse infirmaries and this did not change after isolation hospital development occurred. Even after the Public Health Act (1875) allowed compulsory isolation of infectious patients, the need for isolating sufferers was met by workhouse facilities and it was one area where the principle of less eligibility did not apply.[4] When epidemics struck, it was boards of guardians who had to respond by erecting temporary facilities. Isolation was seen as one of the "major weapons" in containing the spread of infection within a community and, in this regard, guardians were providing a beneficial service to the locality that went beyond the requirements of the poor law system. On some occasions, guardians and the local sanitary authorities cooperated in providing isolation premises. Birmingham was an outstanding example of this cooperation, which resulted in the joint management of facilities for infectious disease. Thus, poor law medical facilities were an essential component of the management and treatment of communicable diseases in the nineteenth and early twentieth centuries. With regard to tuberculosis, guardians did more than merely provide accommodation for isolation, but under the guidance of the medical officers, attempted to adopt methods of medical management similar to those used in use in sanatoriums.

Whether Birmingham and Wolverhampton guardians limited the treatments that inmates could receive and overruled medical officers' prescriptions and advice was raised in chapter 4. The incontrovertible answer is that they did not. Despite the constraints imposed upon them, medical officers kept control of pharmaceutical treatments and medical extras, even when guardians were paying the drugs bill. The change in Wolverhampton in the 1870s, when the medical officer no longer had to meet the cost of drugs out of his salary, appeared to have no effect on prescribing, confounding the general assumption that medical extras were ordered in preference to drugs to protect the medical officers' salaries. At times, workhouse medical officers introduced new treatments, both medical and surgical, and used anesthetic agents for operations on inmates soon after they became generally available, with the guardians paying an additional doctor for administering them. Patients appeared satisfied if they received from the medical officer the type of treatment they expected and within a reasonable time.

Some of the medical officers employed in both towns strove to provide as high a standard of medical care as was possible and at times succeeded despite their heavy workload. On the other hand, others were content to carry out their duties in a manner that satisfied the guardians and were content to accept increases in salary as patient numbers increased, rather than request additional professional assistance. Birmingham's example indicates that sufficient medical staffing was provided in the early period after the New Poor Law as a legacy of the previous system, and later when the infirmary was aligned with voluntary hospitals, but it was barely sufficient in the interim period. The workhouse infirmary attracted medical officers of high quality at times throughout the century and visiting physicians and a surgeon of high standing within the profession. At least one of the physicians tailored his treatment of sick inmates to match that offered to patients in the voluntary hospital. In Wolverhampton, the single, part-time medical officer could hardly be expected to provide more than basic attention because of the excessive workload, but at times care provided was exemplary.

Conflict between guardians and medical officers may have had a bearing on standards of care. As John Stewart and Steven King point out, a "war of attrition" between guardians and medical officers would hardly be conducive to effective patient care.[5] In addition, Price considers the frequency of occurrence of charges of negligence to be some measure of the quality of medical practice.[6] However, many of the charges of negligence were not brought about by the practice of poor standards of patient treatment, although that is not to say that poor medical practice did not occur. Doctors were charged more often because of failure to complete the voluminous amount of paperwork required by the guardians. By preferring to give priority to their patients, many benefited from the administrations of their medical attendants, the extent depending on how conscientious and caring an individual doctor was rather than his relationship with the guardians. Thus, the standards of the medical officers were one of the indicators of the quality of care in workhouse infirmaries.

Just as important was nursing care, although nurses in the first half of the nineteenth century were required to carry out mainly household tasks rather than give personal attention to patients. Wolverhampton workhouse was typical of many in relying heavily on pauper nursing throughout the nineteenth century. Although Birmingham employed a greater proportion of remunerated nurses, the differentiation between them and pauper nurses was indistinct in the years shortly after 1834, as inmates were often taken on as paid nurses. The high turnover of nursing staff was not the result of any one factor, but the heavy workload and harsh conditions may have led to many nurses resigning without wishing to disclose their reasons. Once training was introduced and it became more formalized toward the end of the century, standards of nursing care improved in terms of attitude to patient management, rather than the acquisition of specific nursing skills. One disadvantage of the nursing reforms was to drive men away from general nursing in workhouses and diminish their role within the developing nursing profession. General nursing standards were less than acceptable in workhouses such as Wolverhampton, which relied on pauper assistance to supplement a few paid nurses. In contrast, standards in Birmingham workhouse appeared to be similar to those in the voluntary hospitals, and nursing staff moved between the two types of institutions.

Price maintains that the crusade in the early 1870s against outdoor relief extended the less-eligibility principal to medical care in the workhouse and put pressure on guardians to cut costs. The result was lower care standards, brought about in part by the reduction in medical staffing.[7] However, the crusade had no detrimental effect on the number of medical officers in either Wolverhampton or Birmingham; indeed, they were increased in the mid-1870s in the latter's workhouse. Another influence of the crusade on workhouses was the influx of the most vulnerable groups among paupers, namely those with mental and physical chronic illnesses.[8] However, there was no sudden and sustained increase in the total number of inmates or in older or disabled inmates in either Wolverhampton or Birmingham over the period of the campaign, despite Birmingham guardians being aggressive crusaders. By the early 1890s, poor law infirmaries were providing sufficiently high standards of care to attract nonpauper patients. In this regard, Wolverhampton workhouse lagged behind the general picture, as standards did not improve substantially, including the appointment of a resident medical officer, until the move to the new workhouse in the first decade of the twentieth century. This delay is surprising, as the guardians had accepted the responsibility of providing for sick paupers as early as the mid-1840s.

One of the important medical roles of the workhouse was the care and treatment of paupers suffering from chronic illnesses and disabilities, as they had access to few other avenues of institutional care. They were rarely identified as a distinct group of inmates, and Wolverhampton workhouse was typical in this respect. The opportunity to discern their nature and care needs arose in Birmingham due to its designation of some wards as "the bedridden wards." The majority were in the older age group, resulting in the workhouse gaining the reputation as the institution of the aged by the late nineteenth century. The inclusion of disabled paupers among those in the care of the workhouse medical officer in the mid-nineteenth century was a reflection of disability becoming medicalized. However, later in the century, those requiring less in the way of direct medical care, for example, those needing few or no drug prescriptions, were seen as requiring less medical care and thus acquired a lower status in medical eyes. As a result, the quality of care received by inmates with chronic medical conditions declined, coinciding with acute medical treatment becoming more predominant within the institution. This situation did not alter until medical interest in the care of older people took place in the 1930s, arising directly from workhouse medical care and leading to the birth of the medical specialty of geriatric medicine and to improved standards of care and treatment for frail older patients.[9]

The traditional narrative of poor law medical care is one of progressive improvement toward the establishment of the National Health Service, no doubt because the majority of the hospital beds taken over in 1948 were in former poor law institutions. This study advances a new perspective of workhouse medicine by demonstrating the complex nature of institutional medical care for the destitute. It has shown the variability of medical care both within the same workhouse over time and between two institutions in adjacent towns. It can be argued that medical and nurse staffing in Birmingham workhouse was of a good standard immediately after the New Poor Law, deteriorated for certain periods thereafter, but improved toward the end of the nineteenth century to lessen the difference between it and the local voluntary hospitals. Furthermore, the two workhouse infirmaries emerge as the providers of an important element of medical care for the poor in their own right in the nineteenth and early twentieth centuries and not merely stepping-stones to later developments. The pattern of admissions and discharges in Birmingham and Wolverhampton suggest a significant number of those receiving indoor medical relief were able to return to their communities in an improved condition, if not cured. Furthermore, despite the stigma of being paupers and subjection to authoritarian discipline, sick inmates experienced conditions that were better than those portrayed by the pessimistic interpretations of the older historiography of the New Poor Law. The Local Government inspector, Murray Browne, was impressed by the standard of care in Birmingham infirmary in 1893 after conducting a formal inquiry into the treatment of patients. Addressing the guardians, he said that the infirmary had come out of the investigation reflecting the greatest credit on it and its management. "He could not see how rich people in sickness could be any better off or so well provided for and he knew perfectly well he could not die in a better place or have better nursing in sickness."[10]

However, we have little understanding of the effect of medical care on the lives of sick inmates, as their voices have largely remained unheard except when complaints are made. So we shall end, as we began, with some of their expressions of appreciation for the care they received that have come to light during this investigation. In 1884, Birmingham guardians received a letter of thanks from the vice-consul of Sweden and Norway on behalf of one of his countrymen, F. Broderson, for the "extreme kindness" with which he had been treated while a patient in the epileptic ward, especially by the lady superintendent. While visiting Broderson, he had been surprised when he saw what could be done for the patients. He was "extremely thankful" for the treatment of his countryman, "who might have perished in the streets if it had not been for the workhouse."[11] Early in the twentieth century, Henry Yarwood also expressed his gratitude to the staff in Birmingham infirmary, where he had spent sixteen weeks in ward 3B in 1902 receiving treatment for Bright's disease, in what would have been an acute episode of a long-term renal disease. He had received "every care and kindness from doctor and nurses" and would "never forget the doctor who pulled me through my long and dangerous illness." He had recovered sufficiently to return to playing his "organette" and "out of sheer gratitude," offered to do so without charge in the wards on Christmas Day.[12]

In 1895, the chairman of Wolverhampton guardians read a letter at a meeting of the board from a resident at Blakenhall, who "wished to tender his sincere thanks for their kindness in supporting him and his family during the five years he had been unable to work." Presumably he had received intermittent outdoor relief over that time. He "had kept at work as long as he was able." He "had been an inmate in the infirmary for some weeks and came into workhouse infirmary as he thought to die." He had been discharged "completely cured after a few weeks and been able to resume work to support his family."[13]

Appendix A

Prevalence of Selected Infectious Diseases in Birmingham Workhouse on the Last Day of the First Week of Each Quarter for the Years 1877–80 and 1894–1911

Quarter and year	Whooping cough	Measles	Diphtheria	Typhoid	Itch
Lady Day 1878	16	3		1	
Midsummer 1878	33			2	
Michaelmas 1878	29				
Christmas 1878	17			2	26
Lady Day 1879	10			2	23
Midsummer 1879	8	40			18
Michaelmas 1879	13				27
Christmas 1879	4	3			
Lady Day 1880	5			1	56
Midsummer 1880		18			28
Michaelmas 1880	35	2			37
Christmas 1880	35			3	24
Midsummer 1894		9		1	4
Christmas 1894	1				4
Lady Day 1895					4
Midsummer 1895	2			3	1
Michaelmas 1895	16			2	3
Christmas 1895	7			5	
Lady Day 1896	3	6		6	1
Midsummer 1896	1			2	4
Michaelmas 1896	9			3	
Christmas 1896	4			1	1
Lady Day 1897	1	3		4	
Midsummer 1897	2		3	3	
Michaelmas 1897		4			1
Christmas 1897	2	1		2	1

Quarter and year	Whooping cough	Measles	Diphtheria	Typhoid	Itch
Lady Day 1898	2			4	
Midsummer 1898	2	2		3	
Michaelmas 1898	3			2	
Christmas 1898	3				1
Lady Day 1899		20		4	1
Midsummer 1899	1	1			4
Michaelmas 1899	2				2
Christmas 1899	1	1			4
Lady Day 1900	3	3			6
Midsummer 1900	24				
Michaelmas 1900	17	2			6
Christmas 1900		1			1
Lady Day 1901					1
Midsummer 1901	1	11	1		2
Michaelmas 1901	5		2		3
Christmas 1901	4		3		4
Lady Day 1902	6	15	3		10
Midsummer 1902	10	5	2		6
Michaelmas 1902	10	2	1		13
Christmas 1902	9	2			14
Lady Day 1903		1	2		5
Midsummer 1903	7				6
Michaelmas 1903	1	9			7
Christmas 1903	1				6
Lady Day 1904			1		6
Midsummer 1904	5	20	2		9
Michaelmas 1904	16	1			3
Christmas 1904	8		7	1	6
Lady Day 1905	10	1	1		6
Midsummer 1905	4	3			10
Michaelmas 1905		5	1		7
Christmas 1905	5	8			9
Lady Day 1906	7				10
Midsummer 1906	3				12
Michaelmas 1906	1	1	2		5
Christmas 1906					14
Lady Day 1907	1	9			18
Midsummer 1907	1	1	1		14
Michaelmas 1907	5				8
Christmas 1907					8
Lady Day 1908	12		2		20
Midsummer 1908	17	2	1		13
Michaelmas 1908	7				8
Christmas 1908					13
Lady Day 1909	7	5	3		15

Quarter and year	Whooping cough	Measles	Diphtheria	Typhoid	Itch
Midsummer 1909	5	18			10
Michaelmas 1909		1	2		9
Christmas 1909	2		2		12
Lady Day 1910	2				12
Midsummer 1910	35		1		12
Michaelmas 1910	25				27
Christmas 1910	19				15
Lady Day 1911	13	14			19

Source: Birmingham Central Library, Local Government Board Returns, GP/B/5/1/1–8, 1877–1911.

Appendix B

Medical Relief in Birmingham Workhouse for Selected Weeks, 1851–56

Week Ending	No. on Medical Relief	All Infectious diseases	Cutaneous Diseases	Fever (mild)	Fever (typhus)	Diarrhea	Consumption
October 25, 1851	246	25	0	7	2	8	2
December 6, 1851	124	16	1	4	2	4	3
January 3, 1852	134	9	4	5	0	2	1
April 3, 1852	139	16	1	2	3	3	6
July 3, 1852	176	33	13	5	1	5	8
October 2, 1852	172	33	12	5	11	5	0
December 25, 1852	154	26	12	8	1	5	9
April 2, 1853	202	42	14	4	0	7	13
July 9, 1853	191	34	15	5	0	4	8
October 1, 1853	166	32	7	3	1	6	5
January 7, 1854	246	35	10	2	0	10	7
April 1, 1854	249	44	20	4	1	0	9
July 1, 1854	246	53	18	6	1	7	16
October 7, 1854	226	42	12	2	1	10	11
December 16, 1854	280	44	20	3	1	4	12
March 15, 1856	385	65	28	7	0	0	9

Note: Diarrhea is included in the total number of infectious diseases as it appeared this way in the records; fever labeled as typhus would have included the infection later separately identified as typhoid.

Source: TNA, MH12/13297–99, 13300.

Appendix C

List of Drugs Kept in the Wards of Birmingham Infirmary in 1896

Drug	Comment
Carbolic (1 in 20)	Lotion
Boracis	Astringent, used for diarrhea
Plumbi	Astringent, used for constipation and in neurological conditions
Belladonna	For pain relief, as muscle relaxant, to reduce bronchial secretions
Saponis	Soap, for dyspepsia and purging
Terebenth Acetum	Turpentine, as diuretic and cathartic internally; in plasters externally
Lime Water	Tonic, astringent; used for bladder stones
Olive Oil	Laxative, expectorant
Castor Oil	Laxative
Brandy or Whisky	Stimulants
Mist Terrae Co	Mixture
Mist Stimulant	Mixture of iron, strychnine, phosphoric acid
Mist Ammon et Senegae	Mixture, used for coughing and to promote sweating
Pil Cal cum Col	Pill, containing colocynth and calomel; purgative
Pulv Calomelanos	Powder, of mercurous chloride; purgative
Ung Zinci	Ointment for eyes and ulcers
Ung Boracis	Ointment containing borax
Silv Amyli et Zinci Oxide	Contains zinc; tonic, antispasmodic
Pig Iodi	Possibly ointment; contains iodine; used for ringworm
Mist Alba	Mixture, possibly containing soap, ammonia, turpentine, or magnesium; cathartic

Sources: BCL, WIMC, GP/B/2/4/4/2, May 15, 1896; comments collated from Buchan, *Domestic Medicine*; Graham, *Modern Domestic Medicine*; *The British Pharmacopoeia 1932*; Bentley, *A Text-book of Pharmaceutics*, London, 1933; Risse, *Hospital Life in Enlightenment Scotland*.

Appendix D

Pauperism Rates and Institutionalization Rates for Birmingham Parish, Wolver-hampton Union, and England and Wales, 1840–1911

	Birmingham				Wolverhampton				England and Wales	
Year	Total paupers	Pauperism rate	Indoor paupers	Institutionalization rate	Total paupers	Pauperism rate	Indoor paupers	Institutionalization rate	Pauperism rate	Institutionalization rate
1840	7,476	6.7%	716	10%	1,102	2.3%	409	37%	7.7%	16%
1861	8,889	4.2%	1,404	16%	3,563	3.2%	663	19%	4.3%	14%
1871	9,768	4.2%	1,701	17%	5,332	4.5%	696	13%	4.3%	15%
1881	7,586	3.1%	2,320	31%	7,815	6.1%	912	12%	3.0%	22%
1891	4,495	1.8%	2,672	59%	5,312	3.9%	915	17%	2.5%	24%
1901	3,599	1.5%	2,290	64%	4,581	3.0%	1,142	25%	2.4%	21%
1911	5,319	2.4%	3,091	58%	3,962	2.4%	1,203	30%	2.1%	35%

Note: Data for 1840 for Birmingham is based on the average weekly number of paupers for the year ending Lady Day; and for Wolverhampton the number for the quarter ending Lady Day. Pauper numbers for all other years are one-day counts on July 1.

Source: Williams, *From Pauperism to Poverty*, 158; House of Commons Parliamentary Papers, 1840 (629), 6, 1840 (543), 2, 1861 (324B), 3, 42–43, 1871 (140 B.I.), 5, 6, 32–33, 1881 (60 B.I.), iii, 30–31, 1890–91 (130 B.I.), ii, iii, 34–35, 1901 (73–I), ii, iii, 30–31, 1911 (263–I), ii–iv, 14.

Notes

Introduction

1. Wolverhampton Archives and Local Studies (hereafter WALS), Wolverhampton Board of Guardians (hereafter WBG), PU/WOL/A/3, July 23, Aug. 6, 1841.
2. Price, "A Regional, Quantitative and Qualitative Study," 266, 339, 345; Marland, *Medicine and Society*, 93; Digby, *Making a Medical Living*, 244.
3. Driver, *Power and Pauperism*, 18–19.
4. Bynum, *Science and the Practice of Medicine*, 25.
5. Pickstone, *Medicine and Industrial Society*, 223.
6. King, "Regional Patterns," 63; italics in original.
7. Digby, *Pauper Palaces*, 166.
8. Gestrich, Hurren, and King, "Narratives of Poverty and Sickness," 24; Tomkins, "Labouring on a Bed of Sickness," 52.
9. Fissell, *Patients, Power and the Poor*, 99–100.
10. Gestrich, Hurren, and King, "Narratives of Poverty and Sickness," 21.
11. Tomkins, "Labouring on a Bed of Sickness," 52.
12. King, "Poverty, Medicine and the Workhouse," 229, 245; Gestrich, Hurren, and King, "Narratives of Poverty," 21; Negrine, "Practitioners and Paupers," 193.
13. Siena, "Contagion, Exclusion," 19.
14. Boulton and Schwarz, "The Medicalisation of a Parish Workhouse," 122, 130.
15. Butler, "Disease, Medicine and the Urban Poor," 270–72.
16. King, "Poverty, Medicine and the Workhouse," 230–35, 241.
17. King, "Thinking and Rethinking the New Poor Law," 10.
18. Stewart and King, "Death in Llantrisant," 69; King, "Poverty, Medicine and the Workhouse," 228.
19. King, "Thinking and Rethinking the New Poor Law," 5–6.
20. King and Tomkins, "Introduction," 1.
21. Pinker, *English Hospital Statistics*, 57; Woodward, *To Do the Sick No Harm*, 36.
22. Reinarz, "Investigating the 'Deserving' Poor," 111–33.
23. Riley, *Sick, Not Dead*, 30–34, 132.
24. Hennock, *The Origins of the Welfare State*, 143, 177–78.
25. Hamlin, *Public Health and Social Justice*, 2–3, 28–29.
26. Driver, *Power and Pauperism*, 25–26.

27. House of Commons Parliamentary Papers (hereafter HCPP), 1834 XXVII [C. 44], *Report from His Majesty's Commissioners for Inquiring into the Administration and Practical Operation of the Poor Laws* (hereafter *Administration and Practical Operation of the Poor Laws*), 25, 146, 170, 176.
28. Driver, *Power and Pauperism*, 20–21.
29. Hamlin, *Public Health*, 29.
30. Digby, *The Poor Law*, 9.
31. Driver, *Power and Pauperism*, 147; Morrison, *The Workhouse*, 43, 54.
32. Kidd, *State, Society, and the Poor*, 34–35.
33. Driver, *Power and Pauperism*, 64; Hamlin, *Public Health*, 20.
34. Crowther, *The Workhouse System*, 3.
35. Crowther, *The Workhouse System*, 3, 6.
36. Morrison, *The Workhouse*, 1999, 43.
37. Crowther, *The Workhouse System*, 193–221; Higgs, *Life*, 18–21.
38. The aim of moral regulation was to improve the self-discipline of individuals. Driver, *Power and Pauperism*, 11.
39. Driver, *Power and Pauperism*, 10, 71; Lees, *The Solidarities of Strangers*, 147.
40. Crowther, *The Workhouse System*, 211–12; Driver, *Power and Pauperism*, 64.
41. Green, "Pauper Protests," 1371–59.
42. King, "Thinking and Rethinking the New Poor Law," 5–9.
43. Driver, *Power and Pauperism*, 28, 34.
44. Driver, *Power and Pauperism*, 29.
45. Hennock, *The Origins of the Welfare State*, 27.
46. Tolley, "The Birmingham, Aston and Kings Norton Boards of Guardians," 190; Rothery, "'Who Do They Think They Are?,'" 30.
47. Rothery, "'Who Do They Think They Are?'" 30; King, "Thinking and Rethinking the New Poor Law," 11, 15.
48. Pickstone, *Medicine and Industrial Society*, 35.
49. Flinn, "Medical Services," 49.
50. Morrison, *The Workhouse*, 171.
51. Fraser, *The Evolution*, 100; Hodgkinson, *The Origins of the National Health Service*, 451; Ashforth, "The Urban Poor Law," 148.
52. Hodgkinson, "Poor Law Medical Officers," 300.
53. Crowther, "Paupers or Patients?," 33–34, 40, 53; Brand, *Doctors and the State*, 85.
54. Price, *Medical Negligence*, 99.
55. Brand, *Doctors and the State*, 88.
56. Crowther, *The Workhouse System*, 167.
57. Lawrence, *Medicine in the Making of Modern Britain*, 42–43.
58. Loudon, *Medical Care and the General Practitioner*, 228.
59. Sands Cox also founded Queen's College, which developed into the medical school and ultimately the University of Birmingham.
60. Barling, *The History of the Birmingham Medical School*, 74–89.
61. Negrine, "Practitioners and Paupers," 196–97, 200–201.
62. Railton and Barr, *Battle Workhouse*, 90.

63. Sheen, *The Workhouse and Its Medical Officer*.
64. Barling, *The History of Birmingham Medical School*, 2.
65. Finer, *The Life and Times*, 157–59.
66. Price, *Medical Negligence*, 72.
67. Price, *Medical Negligence*, 103–13; Hurren, "Poor Law versus Public Health," 401–2.
68. Price, *Medical Negligence*, 14.
69. Flinn, "Medical Services," 61.
70. Crowther, "Paupers or Patients?," 37; Brand, *Doctors and the State*, 234; Hodgkinson, *The Origins of the National Health Service*, 680–82.
71. Hodgkinson, *The Origins of the National Health Service*, xv–xvi; Brand, *Doctors and the State*, 234.
72. Crowther, "Paupers or Patients?," 53.
73. Flinn, "Medical Services," 61.
74. Price, "A Regional, Quantitative and Qualitative Study," 2, 336.
75. Lees, *Solidarities of Strangers*, 279.
76. Hodgkinson, "Poor Law Medical Officers," 338.
77. Shave, *Pauper Policies*, 26, 214.
78. Ayers, *England's First State Hospitals*, 28.
79. Hodgkinson, *The Origins of the National Health Service*, 521.
80. Hodgkinson, *The Origins of the National Health Service*, 545.
81. Fowler, *Workhouse*, 150.
82. Levene, "Between Less Eligibility and the NHS," 323.
83. Finer, *The Life and Times*, 340–46; Pelling, *Cholera, Fever*, 64.
84. Pelling, *Cholera, Fever*, 83–84, 111, 301.
85. Hamlin, *Public Health*, 74–76, 132–37, 142, 215–17, 288.
86. Hardy, *Health and Medicine*, 30.
87. Fraser, *The Evolution*, 48.
88. Brand, *Doctors and the State*, 203–4.
89. Brand, *Doctors and the State*, 230, Price, *Medical Negligence*, 151.
90. Tolley, "The Birmingham, Aston and Kings Norton Boards of Guardians," 396.
91. Booth, *The Aged Poor*, 96.
92. Hopkins, *Birmingham*, 94; Woods, "Mortality and Sanitary Conditions," 177.
93. Mayne, *The Imagined Slum*, 60.
94. Ward, "Birmingham: A Political Profile," 169.
95. Gehrke, "A Radical Endeavor," 24–25.
96. Dick, "The City of a Thousand Trades," 127.
97. Briggs, *History of Birmingham*, 1.
98. Hennock, *Fit and Proper Persons*, 61–62.
99. Hennock, *Fit and Proper Persons*, 119–20.
100. Woods, "Mortality and Sanitary Conditions," 177.
101. Gehrke, "A Radical Endeavor," 23.
102. Bunce, "The Social and Economical Aspects of Birmingham," 688.

103. Timmins, "The Industrial History of Birmingham," 216.
104. Peyton, "Manufacture of Iron and Brass Bedsteads," 624.
105. Aitken, "Brass and Brass Manufactures," 363.
106. Hopkins, *Birmingham*, 10, 17, 144; Woods, "Mortality and Sanitary Conditions," 178; Briggs, *History of Birmingham*, 1, 5–6.
107. Wright, "The Jewellery and Gilt Toy Trades," 454.
108. Timmins, "The Industrial History of Birmingham," 211; Aitken, "Brass and Brass Manufactures," 255.
109. Barnsby, *Social Conditions in the Black Country*, 3–4; Cockin, *The Staffordshire Encyclopaedia*, 567.
110. Barnsby, *Social Conditions in the Black Country*, 3–4.
111. Dick, "The City of a Thousand Trades," 127.
112. Smith, "The Governance of Wolverhampton," 22–325.
113. Smith, "The Governance of Wolverhampton," 3, 74, 127, 134.
114. Smith, "The Governance of Wolverhampton," 101; Barnsby, *Social Conditions in the Black Country*, 61–62.
115. Anonymous, "The Lancet Sanitary Commission," 555.
116. Smith, "The Governance of Wolverhampton," 101–20; Barnsby, *Social Conditions in the Black Country*, 67–69, 79–80.
117. Smith, "The Governance of Wolverhampton," 223–25.
118. Barnsby, *Social Conditions in the Black Country*, 55–56, 59, 808–1.
119. Barnsby, *Social Conditions in the Black Country*, 55–56.
120. HCPP, 1842 (006), *Report to Her Majesty's Principal Secretary of State for the Home Department, from the Poor Law Commissioners, on an Inquiry into the Sanitary Condition of the Labouring Population of Great Britain*, 15.
121. Tildesley, *A History of Willenhall*, 83, 92.
122. Barnsby, *Social Conditions in the Black Country*, 247.
123. Loveridge, "Wolverhampton Trades," 117; Tildesley, "Wolverhampton Trades. Addenda," 122.
124. Upton, *A History of Wolverhampton*, 87–88; Cockin, *The Staffordshire Encyclopaedia*, 597–98.
125. Driver, *Power and Pauperism*, 42–48.
126. Tolley, "The Birmingham, Aston and Kings Norton Boards of Guardians," 323–38.
127. Hutton, *An History of Birmingham*, 375; Upton, *The Birmingham Parish Workhouse*, 23–26.
128. Birmingham Central Library (hereafter BCL), Birmingham Board of Guardians' Minute Book (hereafter BBG), GP/B/2/1/1, May 30, 1785; GP/B/2/1/2, Mar. 2, 1813.
129. BCL, BBG, GP/B/2/1/1, Mar. 30, 1796.
130. Reinarz and Ritch, "Exploring Medical Care," 143.
131. Langford, *Modern Birmingham*, 381–82.
132. Hodgkinson, *The Origins of the National Health Service*, 530–31.
133. HCPP, 1867–68 (4), *Provincial Workhouses. Report of Dr Edward Smith, Medical Officer to the Poor Law Board, on the Sufficiency of the Existing*

Arrangements for the Care and Treatment of the Sick Poor in Forty-Eight Provincial Workhouses in England and Wales (hereafter *Provincial Workhouses*), 261-57.

134. HCPP, 1870 (468-I), *Poor Relief. Returns "Showing the Numbers and Ages of the Paupers on the District and Workhouse Medical Officers' Relief Books in the Several Unions and Parishes in England and Wales, on the Last Day of the Twelfth Week of the Half Year Ended at Lady-Day 1870"* (hereafter *Poor Relief*), 4-25.

135. Ritch, "English Poor Law Institutional Care," 76-78.

136. Wolverhampton City Council, "The Workhouse," The History of Wolverhampton: The City and Its People, 2005, www.wolverhampton-history.org.uk/work/the_workhouse; The National Archives (hereafter TNA), MH12/11674, Apr. 2, 1836; Aug. 27, 1838.

137. WALS, *Wolverhampton Chronicle* (hereafter *WC*), Mar. 14, 1838; WBG, PU/WOL/A/2, Sept. 27, 1839.

138. TNA, MH12/11674, Nov. 30, 1837.

139. WALS, WBG, PU/WOL/A/3, July 22, 1842; TNA, MH12/11675, Nov. 9, 1842.

140. WALS, *Wolverhampton Journal* (hereafter *WJ*), LS/L07/79, liv.

141. Tolley, "The Birmingham, Aston and Kings Norton Boards of Guardians," 117-19, 133-34.

142. Tolley, "The Birmingham, Aston and Kings Norton Boards of Guardians," 45.

143. Barnsby, *Social Conditions in the Black Country*, 105.

144. Rothery, "'Who Do They Think They Are?,'" 20-23.

145. Eden, *The State of the Poor*, 655, 739; Lane, *A Social History of Medicine*, 69.

146. Humphreys, "The Poor Law and Charity," 31, 151, 248, 411.

147. Pinches, "Charities in Warwickshire," 257-59, 264-65.

148. Gorsky, Mohan, and Willis, "A 'Splendid Spirit of Co-operation,'" 170, 176-77.

149. Tomkins, "'Labouring on a Bed of Sickness,'" 99.

150. Sheard, "Reluctant Providers?," 117.

151. Price, "A Regional, Quantitative and Qualitative Study," 2, 326.

152. Crowther, *The Workhouse System*, 169; Hodgkinson, "Poor Law Medical Officers," 325.

153. Brand, "The Parish Doctor," 97-122, 106; Hodgkinson, "Poor Law Medical Officers," 308.

154. Flinn, "Medical Services," 55; Price, *Medical Negligence*, 115.

155. Flinn, "Medical Services," 56; Digby, *Pauper Palaces*, 171.

156. Price, "A Regional, Quantitative and Qualitative Study," 237.

Chapter One

1. Shave, *Pauper Policies*, 6.
2. Hodgkinson, *The Origins of the National Health Service*, 147, 465–67; Crowther, *The Workhouse System*, 89.
3. Jackson, "The Medway Union Workhouse," 19.
4. Ashforth, "The Urban Poor Law," 148; Hodgkinson, *The Origins of the National Health Service*, 451.
5. Abel-Smith, *The Hospitals*, 200.
6. King, *Poverty and Welfare*, 29; Hodgkinson, *The Origins of the National Health Service*, 60.
7. Higgs, *Life*, 72.
8. Williams, *From Pauperism to Poverty*, 97.
9. Hodgkinson, *The Origins of the National Health Service*, 542; Brand, "The Parish Doctor," 110.
10. Brand, "The Parish Doctor," 98; Reinarz and Schwarz, *Medicine and the Workhouse*, 4.
11. Quoted in Woodward, *To Do the Sick No Harm*, 47.
12. WALS, House Committee (hereafter HC), PU/WOL/E/1, May 7, 1903.
13. BCL, Infirmary Sub Committee (hereafter ISC), GP/B/2/4/1/2, May 16, 1884.
14. Reinarz, *The Birth of a Provincial Hospital*, 24.
15. Edwards, "Age-Based Rationing in Nineteenth-Century England," 227–65, 240–41.
16. Pinker, *English Hospital Statistics*, 61–62.
17. Williams, *From Pauperism to Poverty*, 203.
18. Turner, "Introduction," 6; Hughes, "Disability and the Body," 58–76.
19. Hughes, "The Constitution of Impairment," 155–72.
20. Hughes, "Disability and the Body," 60–62.
21. Borsay, "History, Power and Identity," 104–6; Hughes, "The Constitution of Impairment," 157.
22. Edwards, "Age-Based Rationing," 263; Bergen, "The Blind, the Deaf and the Halt," 371.
23. Weisz, *Chronic Disease*, 2–7.
24. Timmerman, "Chronic Illness," 394; Weisz, *Chronic Disease*, 176.
25. Burch and Sutherland, "Who's Not Yet Here?," 128; Anderson and Carden-Coyne, "Enabling the Past," 447.
26. For example, Borsay, *Disability and Social Policy*.
27. Bergen, "The Blind, the Deaf and the Halt," 22, 115.
28. Boulton, Davenport, and Schwarz, "'These ANTE-CHAMBERS OF THE GRAVE?,'" 58–60.
29. Upton, *The Birmingham Parish Workhouse*, 134–35.
30. BCL, BBG, GP/B/2/1/1, June 6, 1785, Mar. 23, 1789; June 3, 1793.
31. BCL, BBG, GP/B/2/1/2, Aug. 11, 1818; GP/B/2/1/5, Oct. 12, 1847.

32. BCL, BBG, GP/B/2/1/3, Apr. 7, 1835; Nov. 15, 1837; GP/B/2/1/5, Apr. 20, 1847.
33. Pickstone, *Medicine and Industrial Society*, 86–87.
34. Griffith, *History of the Free-Schools*, 165, 233.
35. Hodgkinson, *The Origins of the National Health Service*, 539.
36. Langford, *Modern Birmingham*, 383.
37. Pickstone, *Medicine and Industrial Society*, 123.
38. BCL, Visiting and General Purposes Committee (hereafter VGPC), GP/B/2/8/1/4, Jan. 1, Dec. 16, 1864; GP/B/2/8/1/5, Nov. 10, 1865.
39. BCL, VGPC, GP/B/2/8/1/5, July 27, Aug. 10, 1866.
40. Anonymous, "Dr. Edward Smith's Reports," 166.
41. Richardson, *English Hospitals*, 72.
42. BCL, BBG, GP/B/2/1/59, May 7, 1890.
43. Hearn, *Dudley Road Hospital*.
44. Barnsby, *Social Conditions in the Black Country*, 115.
45. WALS, Master's Journal (hereafter MJ), PU/WOL/U/2, Apr. 16, 1842.
46. TNA, MH12/11682, Oct. 27, 1855.
47. Anonymous, "The Lancet Sanitary Commission," 555–56.
48. WALS, WBG, PU/WOL/A/22, Jan. 13, 1888; PU/WOL/A/23, Nov. 7, 1888; Nov. 4, 1890.
49. HCPP, 1890–91 (365), *Workhouses, &c. Return Showing, in Respect of Each Workhouse, Workhouse Infirmary, and Sick Asylum in England and Wales, the Number of the Beds in the Wards for the Sick; the Average Number of Sick Persons Occupying Those Wards during the Months of September, October, and November in the Present Year; the Number of Paid Officers Acting as Nurses; and the Number of Such Officers Who, Prior to Their Appointment by the Guardians or Managers, Had Received Any Training in Nursing* (hereafter *The Number of the Beds in the Wards for the Sick*), 11.
50. HCPP, 1909 [Cd. 4835], *Royal Commission on the Poor Laws and Relief of Distress. Appendix volume IV. Minutes of Evidence* (hereafter *Royal Commission on the Poor Laws*), 339.
51. Booth, *The Aged Poor*, 88, 92.
52. HCPP, 1834, XXVII [C.44], *Administration and Practical Operation of the Poor Laws*, 172.
53. Digby, *Pauper Palaces*, 144.
54. MacKinnon, "The Use and Misuse," 6.
55. MacKinnon, "The Use and Misuse," 6.
56. HCPP, 1866 (372), *Metropolitan Workhouse Infirmaries, &c. Copy of the Report of Dr. Edward Smith LL.B., F.R.S., Poor Law Inspector and Medical Officer to the Poor Law Board, on the Metropolitan Workhouse Infirmaries and Sick Wards* (hereafter *Metropolitan Workhouse Infirmaries*), 1; 1867–68 (4), 21.
57. MacKinnon, "The Use and Misuse," 7.
58. BCL, BBG, GP/B/2/1/5, Aug. 14, 1845; GP/B/2/1/6, Apr. 24, 1849.
59. BCL, House Committee (hereafter HC), GP/B/2/3/1/1, Aug. 9, 1842.
60. HCPP, 1867–68 (4), *Provincial Workhouses*, 45–46.

61. WALS, MJ, WOL/PU/U/2, Apr. 16, 1842.
62. HCPP, 1867–68 (4), *Provincial Workhouses*, 153.
63. BCL, Workhouse Management Committee (hereafter WMC), GP/B/2/3/2/2, Feb. 28, 1896.
64. Anonymous, "The Lancet Sanitary Commission," 555; WALS, *WJ*, LS/ LO7/79, lvi.
65. King, "Poverty, Medicine and the Workhouse," 232.
66. BCL, BBG, GP/B/2/1/2, June 2, 1818; TNA, MH12/13287, Dec. 28, 1842.
67. HCPP, 1841 [327], *Seventh Annual Report of the Poor Law Commissioners*, 135–36.
68. BCL, BBG, GP/B/2/1/3–5; Hodgkinson, *The Origins of the National Health Service*, 147.
69. Griffith, *History of the Free-Schools*, 165, 233, 293.
70. BCL, BBG, GP/B/2/1/5, Mar. 8, 1847; "loathsome" disease or disorder was a term often applied to leg ulceration: Loudon, "Leg Ulcers," 264.
71. BCL, BBG, GP/B/2/1/6, Jan. 2, Apr. 9, 1849.
72. BCL, BBG, GP/B/2/1/15, Feb. 28, 1855; Griffith, *History of the Free-Schools*, 173, 233–34.
73. WALS, WBG, PU/WOL/A/3, Mar. 24, Apr. 1, 1842; PU/WOL/A/4, Oct. 28, 1842; Jan. 6, 1843.
74. WALS, WBG, PU/WOL/A/4, Jan. 27, Feb. 17, May 5, June 16, July 14, Sept. 29, 1843; Mar. 29, 1844.
75. WALS, *WC*, Dec. 2, 1846.
76. WALS, *WC*, Aug. 14, 1867; BCL, BBG, GP/B/2/1/30, Nov. 11, 1863.
77. WALS, *WC*, Nov. 20, 1872.
78. TNA, MH12/11675, June 2, 1841; HCPP, 1843 (144), *Poor Law Amendment Act. Poor relief. Returns of sums expended in every union in England and Wales, in each of the years ended Lady-Day 1841 and 1842*, 9.
79. BCL, BBG, GP/B/2/1/12, Mar. 23, 1853.
80. TNA, MH12/11711, Medical Officer of Health's annual report for 1891.
81. HCPP, 1870 (468–I), *Poor Relief*.
82. The others were Liverpool, Manchester, Chorlton, Portsea Island, Bristol, Preston, West Derby.
83. HCPP, 1870 (468–I), *Poor Relief*, 2–24.
84. HCPP, 1867–68 (4), *Provincial Workhouses*, 56–157.
85. HCPP, 1882 (100B.1), *Poor Rates and Pauperism. Return (B.). Paupers Relieved on 1st July 1882*, 30; HCPP, 1883 (68B), *Poor Rates and Pauperism. Return (B). Paupers Relieved on 1st July 1883*, 30; BCL, VGPC, GP/B/2/8/1/9, Aug. 14, 1885.
86. BCL, Workhouse Infirmary Admission and Discharge Book, HC/ DR/2/1/1, Dec. 16, 1899, to June 9, 1900.
87. BCL, Local Government Board (hereafter LGB) Returns, GP/B/5/1/2, June 6, 1896.
88. HCPP, 1870 (468–I), *Poor Relief*.

89. HCPP, 1870 (468–I), *Poor Relief,* 2–3, 18–21, 54–63, 83, 87, 112–13, 116–17, 146–47, 172–73, 176–77, 202–3, 206–7, 232–33, 236–37.
90. Reinarz, *Health Care in Birmingham,* 18; Loudon, "Leg Ulcers," in which he discusses the possibility of a connection with vitamin C deficiency, 263–73.
91. HCPP, 1861 (490), *Paupers in Workhouses. Returns from Each Workhouse in England and Wales, of the Name of Every Adult Pauper Who Has Been an Inmate of the Workhouse during a Continuous Period of Five Years* (hereafter *Paupers in Workhouses*), ii, 168–69, 194–95.
92. BCL, VGPC, GP/B/2/8/1/3, Jan. 11, 1861.
93. WALS, WBG, PU/WOL/A/28, Feb. 2, Mar. 16, 1900.
94. WALS, *WJ,* LS/LO7/79, lvi.
95. WALS, *WJ,* 80; WALS, WBG, PU/WOL/A/32, Feb. 9, 1906.
96. Pickstone, *Medicine,* 214–15.
97. HCPP, 1867–68 (4), *Provincial Workhouses,* 5.
98. HCPP, 1870 (468–I), *Poor Relief,* 2–3, 63.
99. HCPP, 1870 (468–I), *Poor Relief,* 2–3, 17, 21, 23; 1867–68 (4), 35.
100. HCPP, 1870 (468–I), *Poor Relief,* 2–3, 21, 23; Wolverhampton workhouse contained only one surgical patient diagnosed with an acute condition.
101. HCPP, 1870 (468–I), *Poor Relief,* 2–3, 63.
102. HCPP, 1895 [C.7684], *Royal Commission on the Aged Poor. Report of the Royal Commission on the Aged Poor Appointed to Consider Whether Any Alterations in the System of Poor Law Relief Are Desirable, in the Case of Persons Whose Destitution Is Occasioned by Incapacity for Work Resulting from Old Age, or Whether Assistance Could Otherwise Be Afforded in Those Cases* (hereafter *Royal Commission on the Aged Poor*), xxxvi.
103. Ritch, "English Poor Law," 76–78.
104. Borsay, *Disability,* 8.
105. HCPP, 1904 (113), *Boards of Guardians (Persons in Receipt of Relief). Boards of Guardians (Persons in Receipt of Relief). Return "Showing, in Respect of Each Union and Parish under a Separate Board of Guardians in England and Wales the Number of Persons of Each Sex in Receipt from Boards of Guardians (a) of Indoor Relief or (b) of Outdoor Relief, on the 1st Day of September 1903, Who Were over 60 Years of Age, Distinguishing Those Who Were over 60 and under 65, 65 and under 70, 70 and under 75, 75 and under 80, and 80 Years of Age and Upwards; Lunatics in Asylums, Licensed Houses and Registered Hospitals; Vagrants and Persons Who were Only in Receipt of Relief Constructively by Reason of Relief Being Given to Wives or Children, Not Being Included (in Continuation of Parliamentary Paper, no. 36, of Session 1891); and Showing in Regard to (a) the Number of Those Who in the Opinion of the Medical Officer of the Workhouse Could Not Satisfactorily Take Care of Themselves Owing to Mental or Physical Infirmity,"* iii, iv, 127, 132.
106. HCPP, 1866 (372), *Metropolitan Workhouse Infirmaries,* 37, 73, 106, 153.
107. HCPP, 1867–68 (4), *Provincial Workhouses,* 7.
108. Bosworth, "Public Healthcare in Nottingham," 215–16.

109. Railton and Barr, *Battle Workhouse*, 49.
110. BCL, HC, GP/B/2/3/1/1, Apr. 5, June 7, 1842.
111. BCL, BBG, GP/B/2/1/7, Apr. 2, 1850.
112. BCL, BBG, GP/B/2/1/6, Apr. 9, 1849.
113. BCL, VGPC, GP/B/2/8/1/3, Jan. 27, Nov. 2, 1860; June 14, 1861.
114. BCL, VGPC, GP/B/2/8/1/4, May 22, 1865.
115. BCL, VGPC, GP/B/2/8/1/5, Mar. 23, 1866; HCPP, 1867–68 (4), 45–46, 48.
116. BCL, House Sub-committee (hereafter HSC), GP/B/2/3/3/3, June 3, 1873.
117. BCL, HSC, GP/B/2/3/3/2, Oct. 25, 1870; LGB Letters, GP/B/1/2/1/1, Feb. 18, 1871.
118. BCL, VGPC, GP/B/2/8/1/9, Aug. 14, 1885.
119. BCL, BBG, GP/B/2/1/57, June 19, 1888.
120. BCL, VGPC, GP/B/2/8/1/9, Aug. 14, 1885; HSC, GP/B/2/3/3/13, Dec. 8, 1891.
121. BCL, Birmingham Union Board Minutes (hereafter BUB), GP/B/2/1/83, Sept. 23, 1914.
122. Negrine, "Medicine and Poverty," 134.
123. HCPP, 1867–68 (4), *Provincial Workhouses*, 45.
124. BCL, HSC, GP/B/2/3/3/13, Dec. 8, 1891.
125. Census Enumerator's Books (hereafter CEB), 1891.
126. Jones, "Disability in Herefordshire," 34, 39.
127. BCL, HSC, GP/B/2/3/3/4, Nov. 25, 1873.
128. BCL, WMC, GP/B/2/3/2/6, June 16, 1911.
129. BCL, WMC, GP/B/2/3/2/3, Dec. 7, 1900.
130. BCL, BUB, GP/B/2/1/83, Sept. 23, 1914.
131. HCPP, 1867–68 (4), *Provincial Workhouses*, 5; 1870 (468–I), 53–54, 57.
132. BCL, BBG, GP/B/2/1/57, June 19, 1888.
133. BCL, HSC, GP/B/2/3/3/15, Mar. 21, 1893.
134. BCL, GP/B/addnl.ACC.2009/109 Box 49, Visiting Surgeon's Report, Nov. 26, 1900.
135. BCL, WMC GP/B/2/3/2/6, Apr. 28, 1911.
136. BCL, WMC, GP/B/2/3/2/1, Apr. 11, 1890.
137. BCL, HSC, GP/B/2/3/3/22, Feb. 27, 1906.
138. BCL, WMC, GP/B/2/3/2/6, Apr. 28, 1911.
139. HCPP, 1896 (371), *Workhouses, &c. Return Showing, in Respect of Each Workhouse and Separate Workhouse Infirmary in England and Wales, the Number of Sick Persons Occupying the Wards for the Sick on 1st June 1896. (Distinguishing the Sick and Bedridden from Those Who Are Aged and Infirm Only)* (hereafter *The Number of Sick Persons Occupying the Wards for the Sick*), 28; BCL, LGB Returns, GP/B/5/1/2, May 30, 1896.
140. Railton and Barr, *Battle Workhouse*, 132–33.
141. BCL, WMC, GP/B/2/3/2/1, July 10, 1891; HSC, GP/B/2/3/3/13, Sept. 8, 1891.

142. BCL, Workhouse Infirmary Management Committee (hereafter WIMC), GP/B/2/4/4/3, Mar. 18, 1898.
143. BCL, HC, GP/B/2/3/14/1, Sept. 16, 1914.
144. Weisz, *Chronic Disease*, 7.
145. Negrine, "Medicine and Poverty," 217–20.
146. Denham, "The History of Geriatric Medicine," 60–61.
147. Ritch, "English Poor Law," 84.
148. Denham, "The Surveys of the Birmingham Chronic Sick Hospitals," 282.
149. Weisz, *Chronic Disease*, 181.
150. Gorsky, "Creating the Poor Law Legacy," 442. Similarly, voluntary and municipal hospitals in the United States sought to eliminate patients with chronic disease, Weisz, *Chronic Disease*, 58–59.
151. WALS, MJ, PU/WOL/U/2, Apr. 16, 1842.
152. WALS, WBG, PU/WOL/A/3, Mar. 24, 1842; PU/WOL/A/8, Oct. 29, 1852.
153. WALS, WBG, PU/WOL/A/6, Aug. 14, 1846.
154. WALS, *WC*, Nov. 18, 1843.
155. WALS, *WC*, Nov. 28, 1866.
156. Anonymous, "The Lancet Sanitary Commission," 555.
157. WALS, *WC*, July 14, 1886.
158. HCPP, 1867–68 (4), *Provincial Workhouses*, 153.
159. WALS, *WC*, May 3, 1882.
160. WALS, WBG, PU/WOL/A/25, Jan. 25, 1895; *WC*, Apr. 1, 1896.
161. TNA, MH12/11715, July 8, 1898; the most likely diagnosis in this case was tuberculosis.
162. WALS, *WJ*, LS/L07/79, liv.
163. WALS, Special Committees (hereafter SC), PU/WOL/P/1, Apr. 2, 1906.
164. WALS, HC, PU/WOL/E/4, Apr. 25, 1912.
165. Abel-Smith, *The Hospitals*, 209.
166. HCPP, 1909 [Cd. 4835], *Royal Commission on the Poor Laws*, 773.
167. Hearn, *Dudley Road Hospital*, 35.
168. BCL, Infirmary Management Committee (hereafter IMC), GP/B/2/4/4/5, Apr. 8, 1907; Hearn, *Dudley Road Hospital*, 24.
169. BCL, IMC, GP/B/2/4/4/6, Jan. 9, 1911.
170. HCPP, 1909 [Cd. 4835], *Royal Commission on the Poor Laws*, 342.
171. Negrine, "Practitioners and Paupers," 202–3.
172. WALS, MJ, PU/WOL/U/2, Aug. 16, 1845.
173. WALS, WBG, PU/WOL/A/4, Oct. 14, 1842.
174. TNA, MH12/11682, Feb. 2, 1855.
175. WALS, WBG, PU/WOL/A/25, Mar. 13, 1896; HC, PU/WOL/E/1, Dec. 13, 1902.
176. BCL, WMC, GP/B/2/3/2/1, June 15, 1884; GP/B/2/3/2/5, Sept. 17, 1908.
177. BCL, Incident Book, GP/B (ACC2009/109), Box 15, Feb. 4, 1886.
178. Youngson, *The Scientific Revolution*, 212.

179. Tröhler, "Surgery (Modern)," 980.
180. Stanley, *For Fear of Pain*, 318.
181. Price, "A Regional, Quantitative and Qualitative Study," 233; Brand, "The Parish Doctor," 120.
182. Davies, "Birmingham Workhouse Infirmary," 284.
183. TNA, MH12/11682, Feb. 2, 1855.
184. WALS, WBG, PU/WOL/A/11, May 3, 1861; HC, PU/WOL/E/1, Oct. 30, 1900.
185. HCPP, 1870 (468–I), *Poor Relief*, 3, 19, 21.
186. HCPP, 1870 (468–I), *Poor Relief*, 4; Railton and Barr, *Battle Workhouse*, 44.
187. BCL, VGPC, GP/B/2/8/1/2, Jan. 8, 1858; BBG, GP/B/2/1/22, Feb. 9, 1859.
188. BCL, BBG, GP/B/2/1/9, July 23, 1851; GP/B/2/1/14, Feb. 24, 1854.
189. BCL, BBG, GP/B/2/1/23, June 22, 1859.
190. HCPP, 1867–68 (4), *Provincial Workhouses*, 45.
191. BCL, ISC, GP/B/2/4/1/4, Nov. 25, 1887.
192. BCL, Infirmaries Committee (Hospitals) (hereafter IC(H)), GP/B/2/4/8/1, July 9, 1913.
193. BCL, IMC, GP/B/2/4/4/6, Oct. 23, 1911.
194. Riley, "Operation for Strangulated Femoral Hernia," 110.
195. TNA, MH12/13357, May 20, 1888.
196. BCL, IMC, GP/B/2/4/4/5, July 11, 1910.
197. WALS, WBG, PU/WOL/A/29, Nov. 22, 1901; Jan. 3, June 6, Nov. 14, Dec. 5, 1902; July 17, 1903.
198. Price, *Medical Negligence*, 124.
199. Marland, *Medicine and Society*, 91.
200. HCPP, 1870 (468–I), *Poor Relief*, 24–25.
201. Webb and Webb, *The State and the Doctor*, 99.
202. As portrayed by Borsay, *Disability*.
203. HCPP, 1861 (490), *Paupers in Workhouses*, 194–95.
204. Edwards, "Age-Based Rationing," 230, 238; Levene, "Between Less Eligibility," 322–45.
205. Stone, *The Disabled State*, 29–30, 51.
206. Sneyder and Mitchell, "Afterword—Regulated Bodies," 182; Turner, "Introduction," 8; Stone, *The Disabled State*, 28.
207. Siena, *Venereal Disease*, 136; Thomas, "The Old Poor Law and Medicine," 1.
208. Crowther, "Health Care and Poor Relief," 209.
209. Siena, *Venereal Disease*, 136, 178.
210. Siena, "Contagion, Exclusion," 20.
211. Green, "Icons of the New System," 265–68.
212. BCL, BBG, GP/B/2/1/2, 27 Oct. 1818; January 19, 1819; no information is available for Wolverhampton workhouse under the Old Poor Law.
213. Ritch, "New Poor Law Medical Care," 48–50.

Chapter Two

1. Logan, "Mortality in England and Wales," 138–40.
2. Mooney, "Infectious Diseases and Epidemiologic Transition," 600.
3. Wohl, *Endangered Lives*, 3–4; Woods and Woodward, "Mortality, Poverty," 20.
4. Hardy, *The Epidemic Streets*, 1.
5. Anonymous, "Reports of the Old Cholera Haunts," 656.
6. Logan, "Mortality in England and Wales," 138–41.
7. Omran, "The Epidemiological Transition," 509–38.
8. Omran, "The Epidemiological Transition," 534.
9. McKeown and Record, "Reasons for the Decline of Mortality," 94–122.
10. Szreter, "The Importance of Social Intervention," 2.
11. Hardy, *The Epidemic Streets*, 290–92.
12. Mercer, *Infections, Chronic Disease*, ix, 11, 33, 220.
13. Wohl, *Endangered Lives*, 138; Pickstone, *Medicine and Industrial Society*, 156, 158; Currie, *Fever Hospital*, 13, 125–26.
14. Mooney, *Intrusive Interventions*, 12.
15. Mooney, *Intrusive Interventions*, 71, 73.
16. Smith, *The People's Health*, 241.
17. BCL, BBG, GP/B/2/1/33, May 23, 1866.
18. Mooney, Luckin, and Tanner, "Patient Pathways," 244.
19. Siena, "Contagion, Exclusion," 28; Hodgkinson, *The Origins of the National Health Service*, 161.
20. Bynum, "Cullen and the Study of Fevers," 138.
21. Keele, "Clinical Medicine in the 1860s," 7.
22. By contrast, only 2 percent of patients in Birmingham had fever and all were grouped under the generic term; there were no fever patients in Wolverhampton workhouse. HCPP, 1870 (468-I), *Poor Relief*, 3, 52–53, 57, 82, 86, 232, 236.
23. Morrison, *The Workhouse*, 156, 169.
24. Railton and Barr, *Battle Workhouse*, 57–59.
25. Wildman, "'He's Only a Pauper Whom Nobody Owns,'" 30–31.
26. WALS, MJ, PU/WOL/U2, Mar. 20, 1842.
27. WALS, WBG, PU/WOL/A/6, Jan. 29, 1847; *WC*, Sept. 20, 1847.
28. WALS, WBG, PU/WOL/A/12, Sept. 1, 1864; DX/673/66, "Wolverhampton Union Workhouse."
29. BCL, BBG, GP/B/2/1/5, Mar. 8, Oct. 12, Oct. 28, 1847; *Aris's Birmingham Gazette*, Aug. 14, 1848.
30. Langford, *Modern Birmingham*, 381–82.
31. BCL, VGPC, GP/B/2/8/1/4, June 17, 1864; GP/B/2/8/1/5, May 22, 1865; HCPP, 1867–68 (4), *Provincial Workhouses*, facing 46.
32. WALS, *WJ*, vol. 2, LS/LO7/79, liv; DX/120/10/4; DX/120/10/8; DX/120/10/9, "New Wolverhampton Workhouse."

33. BCL, B. Col. 41.11, Miscellaneous Documents, vol. 4, "Report in Reference to the New Workhouse Infirmary," 18.
34. Mercer, *Infections*, 101.
35. The infecting organism is a paramyxovirus, causing respiratory infection, with fever and a rash; secondary bacterial complications affected the lungs and ears.
36. Hardy, *The Epidemic Streets*, 9, 29, 43.
37. BCL, BBG, GP/B/2/1/19, Dec. 17, 1856.
38. BCL, VGPC, GP/B/2/8/1/6, Oct. 6, 1876; TNA, MH12/13326, "Medical Officer of Health's Report for 1876."
39. BCL, LGB Returns, GP/B/8/5/1/1, Mar. 29, 1879.
40. BCL, Incident Book, GP/B/(Acc 2009/109), Box 15, May 12, 1886; LGB Returns, GP/B/5/1/7, Jan. 5 to Mar. 30, 1907.
41. BCL, IMC, GP/B/2/4/4/5, July 11, 1910.
42. WALS, *WC*, Feb. 10, 1864; Mar. 18, 1891.
43. TNA, MH12/11721, "Annual Report of Health of Wolverhampton for 1898, 1899–1900"; Smith, *The People's Health*, 143.
44. Crompton, *Workhouse Children*, 90.
45. Smith, *The People's Health*, 146; Hardy, *The Epidemic Streets*, 28.
46. Hardy, *The Epidemic Streets*, 9.
47. The causative organism is a small rod-shaped bacterium, *Bordetella pertussis*. The paroxysmal coughing is mediated via the production of toxin and can result in apneic attacks in infants.
48. WALS, MJ, PU/WOL/U2, Nov. 18, 1843.
49. TNA, MH12/11721, "Annual Report"; Hardy, *The Epidemic Streets*, 10.
50. WALS, *WC*, Oct. 17, 1893.
51. Crompton, *Workhouse Children*, 90–91.
52. It is caused by a hemolytic streptococcal bacterium, *Streptococcus pyogenes*, which can also produce tonsillitis and erysipelas. Scarlet fever is the response to the toxin produced by the organism and results in widespread erythema of the skin.
53. Worboys, *Spreading Germs*, 262.
54. Hardy, *The Epidemic Streets*, 59.
55. Smith, *The People's Health*, 137.
56. Smith, *The People's Health*, 65.
57. Creighton, *A History of Epidemics*, 727–28.
58. Smith, *The People's Health*, 137.
59. Hardy, *The Epidemic Streets*, 56.
60. Pickstone, *Medicine and Industrial Society*, 158–59; Gray, *The Edinburgh City Hospital*, 148–49.
61. Woodward, "Medicine and the City," 68.
62. WALS, WBG, PU/WOL/A/17, Oct. 19, 1877; PU/WOL/A/20, Mar. 26, 1886.
63. WALS, *WC*, Nov. 28, Dec. 5, 1877.
64. WALS, WBG, PU /WOL/A/25, Dec. 13, 1895.

65. HCPP, 1895 (28), *Sanitary Districts (Accommodation for Infectious Diseases)*. *Return to an Order of the Honourable the House of Commons, Dated 27 February 1893; for, Return "Showing the Area and Population According to the Last Census of Every Urban and Rural Sanitary District in England and Wales, and Also Showing, as Regards Every Such District and Every Port Sanitary District in England and Wales, Whether the Sanitary Authority Had, on or before the 31st Day of December 1892, Made Special Provision for Any Accommodation of the Nature of an Isolation Hospital (Other than in Connection with Workhouses) for Cases of Infectious Disease Arising in Their District, and, if So, Giving Further Particulars Relating to the Provision of Isolation Hospitals* (hereafter *Sanitary Districts [Accommodation for Infectious Diseases]*), 354.

66. WALS, *WC*, Nov. 27, 1895.

67. BCL, WMC, GP/B/2/3/2/1, May 28, 1889.

68. HCPP, 1895 (28), *Sanitary Districts (Accommodation for Infectious Diseases)*, 402; TNA, MH/13365, "Health of the City," 49−51.

69. BCL, Incident Book, GP/B (ACC2009/109), Box 15; IMC, GP/B/2/4/4/5, July 11, 1910.

70. BCL, ISC, GP/B/2/3/2/3, Jan. 24, 1902.

71. Creighton, *A History of Epidemics*, 736; Hardy, *The Epidemic Streets*, 80. The causative organism is *Corynebacterium diphtheriae*, which affects the pharynx and larynx, with resultant membrane formation, and produces a toxin, causing cardiac damage and neurological lesions. There were three strains of the bacterium, namely *gravis*, *intermedia*, and *mitis*, with case fatality being highest in the first and lowest in the last.

72. Pickstone, *Medicine and Industrial Society*, 159.

73. Smith, *The People's Health*, 151; Hill, "Reports of Medical Officers of Health," 178.

74. Pickstone, *Medicine and Industrial Society*, 159.

75. Hill, "Remarks on the Incidence of Diphtheria in Birmingham," 342.

76. BCL, BBG, GP/B/2/1/81, Nov. 20, 1912.

77. Smith, *The People's Health*, 151.

78. TNA, MH12/11721, "Annual Report."

79. WALS, *WC*, Nov. 27, 1895.

80. WALS, WBG, PU/WOL/A/26, Jan. 29, Feb. 5, 19, 26, 1897; TNA, MH12/11715, Jan. 6, Feb. 10, Mar. 1, 1897.

81. Hardy, *The Epidemic Streets*, 84.

82. Hill, "Remarks on the Incidence of Diphtheria," 342−43; Kenwood, "Notes on the Origin of Diphtheria," 344.

83. WALS, Workhouse Visiting Committee (hereafter WVC), PU/WOL/H/2, Jan. 1, 1897.

84. WALS, WVC, Nov. 25, 1898.

85. Worboys, *Spreading Germs*, 262.

86. TNA, MH12/11711, "Medical Officer of Health's Report for 1891."

87. Loudon, *The Tragedy*, 6; Dobson, *Disease*, 72.

88. Bynum, *Science and the Practice*, 205; Loudon, *The Tragedy*, 5.
89. Loudon, *The Tragedy*, 13, 32.
90. Loudon, *The Tragedy*, 92–93, 106.
91. WALS, WBG, PU/WOL/A/3, Feb. 18, 1842.
92. BCL, VGPC, GP/B/2/8/1/1, Apr. 7, 1854.
93. BCL, VGPC, GP/B/2/8/1/3, Feb. 25, 1859.
94. BCL, BBG, GP/B/2/1/42, Jan. 21, 1874.
95. BCL, ISC, GP/B/2/4/1/1, May 4, 1883.
96. BCL, ISC, GP/B/2/4/1/2, Oct. 16, 1885; HCPP, 1886 (19–Sess. 2), 3–11.
97. BCL, Incident Book, GP/B/(ACC2009/109), Box 15, L.
98. BCL, VGPC, BP/B/2/8/1/9, Aug. 13, 1886; ISC, GP/B/2/4/1/4, Nov. 4, 1887.
99. BCL, LGB Returns, GP/B/5/1/4–5, 1899–1912.
100. Luckin, "Evaluating the Sanitary Revolution," 118.
101. The causative organism, *Rickettsia prowazekii*, is excreted in the feces of the body louse and can survive there for many months.
102. Hardy, *The Epidemic Streets*, 192, 210.
103. Hardy, *The Epidemic Streets*, 194.
104. Creighton, *A History of Epidemics*, 195.
105. Hardy, *The Epidemic Streets*, 204; Luckin, "Evaluating the Sanitary Revolution," 111.
106. Dobson, *Disease*, 36; Siena, "Contagion, Exclusion," 27.
107. Bradley, Jones, and Somerwell, "Who Cared?," 94–96.
108. WALS, WBG, PU/WOL/1/15, Mar. 24, 1842; MJ, Mar. 26, 1842; Oct. 26, 1844.
109. HCPP, 1870 (468–I), *Poor Relief*, 52, 63, 82, 86, 233, 286.
110. Anonymous, "Reports of the Old Cholera Haunts," 656.
111. Creighton, *A History of Epidemics*, 213; Worboys, *Spreading Germs*, 132.
112. The rash is typically rose-colored and spotted and appears later in the course of the disease. It is associated with diarrhea and may be followed by intestinal ulceration.
113. Wohl, *Endangered Lives*, 278; Pelling, *Cholera, Fever*, 197, 283; Woods, "Mortality and Sanitary Conditions," 197–98.
114. Known as *Salmonella typhi*, it is excreted in human feces.
115. Worboys, *Spreading Germs*, 268–69.
116. Smith, *The People's Health*, 245; Luckin, "Evaluating the Sanitary Revolution," 107.
117. Woods, "Mortality and Sanitary Conditions," 181; Hardy, *The Epidemic Streets*, 152.
118. Hardy, *The Epidemic Streets*, 152–53, 159, 165; Wohl, *Endangered Lives*, 128.
119. Anonymous, "Reports of Medical Officers of Health," 178.
120. WALS, *WC*, Nov. 24, 1869.

121. WALS, WBG, PU/WOL/A/20, Aug. 21 and 28, 1885; WALS, L614, "Report on the Health of the Borough of Wolverhampton, for the Year 1887," 12.
122. WALS, WBG, PU/WOL/A/24, Aug. 12, 1892.
123. WALS, *WC*, Mar. 20, 1895; Nov. 27, 1895.
124. BCL, VGPC, GP/B/2/8/1/8, Apr. 28, May 12, 1882.
125. BCL, VGPC, GP/B/2/8/1/9, Aug. 14, 1885.
126. BCL, VGPC, GP/B/2/8/1/9, Dec. 17, 1886.
127. BCL, IMC, GP/B/2/4/4/5, Jan. 13, 1908.
128. BCL, WMC, GP/B/2/3/2/5, Jan. 10, Feb. 5, 1908.
129. Shave, "'Immediate Death or a Life of Torture,'" 170.
130. Boulton, Davenport, and Schwarz, "'These ANTE-CHAMBERS OF THE GRAVE?,'" 77.
131. Morris, *Cholera 1832*, 17.
132. Wohl, *Endangered Lives*, 118.
133. Smith, *The People's Health*; Pelling, *Cholera, Fever*, 2; HCPP, *Metropolitan Sanitary Commission. Second Report*, 1847–48 [921], 1.
134. WALS, *WC*, Oct. 3, 1848.
135. The infecting organism is the bacillus *Vibrio cholerae*, which causes sudden severe watery diarrhea, associated with abdominal pain and vomiting.
136. Worboys, *Endangered Lives*, 248, 252; Pelling, *Cholera, Fever*, 305.
137. Smith, *The People's Health*, 232–33.
138. WALS, WBG, PU/WOL/A/2, Aug. 13, 18, 21, 28, 1849.
139. BCL, BBG, GP/B/2/1/6, Sept. 11, 1849.
140. WALS, WBG, PU/WOL/A/8, Sept. 21, 1853.
141. Bynum, *Science and Practice*, 74. No specific organism has been identified with this disease.
142. Wohl, *Endangered Lives*, 23.
143. WALS, WBG, PU/WOL/A/13, Aug. 14, 1866.
144. TNA, MH12/13297–99, 13300.
145. WALS, WBG, PU/WOL/A/29, Nov. 22, 1901. Dysentery is caused by bacilli of the *Shigella* family and results in fever and bloody diarrhea.
146. BCL, BBG, GP/B/2/1/32, July 19, 1865.
147. Wohl, *Endangered Lives*, 132; Hardy, *The Epidemic Streets*, 149.
148. It is caused by a diminutive, brick-shaped virus, *Variola major*. The rash begins with flat, reddish spots, first on the face, then spreads throughout the body. It becomes raised with blisters, which dry to form crusts or scabs, accompanied with general swelling of the body.
149. Hopkins, *Princes and Peasants*, 4.
150. Known as *Variola minor*.
151. Hopkins, *Princes and Peasants*, 7, 47; Razell, *The Conquest of Smallpox*, 20–21. However, it was less than 1 percent using the Suttonian method of superficial inoculation, Razell, *The Conquest of Smallpox*, 22–23.
152. Worboys, *Endangered Lives*, 117–18.
153. Hardy, *The Epidemic Streets*, 10.

154. Creighton, *A History of Epidemics*, 604, 606, 614.
155. WALS, MJ, PU/WOL/U/2, June 7, 1845.
156. WALS, *WC*, Sept. 30, 1863, to Sept. 13, 1865; Nov. 18, 1863.
157. WALS, *WC*, Feb. 24, 1864.
158. BCL, BBG, GP/B/2/1/31, May 25, 1864.
159. BCL, VGPC, GP/B/2/8/1/4, Dec. 2, 1864.
160. Creighton, *A History of Epidemics*, 614.
161. Hardy, *The Epidemic Streets*, 126.
162. BCL, BBG, GP/B/2/1/40, Dec. 27, 1871; Jan. 10, 1872.
163. BCL, VGPC, GP/B/2/8/1/6, May 10, 1872.
164. BCL, BBG, GP/B/2/1/41, Mar. 19, 1873.
165. The number of admissions in December is different in the written account in the minutes and the table copied into them.
166. BCL, HSC, GP/B/2/3/3/3, Jan. 28, 1873.
167. Pickstone, *Medicine and Industrial Society*, 165.
168. BCL, HSC, GP/B/2/3/3, June 3, 1873; GP/B/2/3/4, Nov. 25, 1873.
169. WALS, WBG, PU/WOL/1/14, Mar. 10, Apr. 14, 1871.
170. WALS, *WC*, July 5, 1871; Nov. 3, 1871.
171. WALS, WBG, PU/WOL/1/15, Dec. 29, 1871; Jan. 5, 1872.
172. Creighton, *A History of Epidemics*, 614.
173. WALS, WBG, PU/WOL/A/19, Sept. 15, Nov. 3 and 17, 1882.
174. WALS, WBG, PU/WOL/A/19, Apr. 27, May 4, July 27, 1883; *WC*, Apr. 25 to June 20 1883.
175. BCL, BBG, GP/B/2/1/47, Apr. 7, 1880.
176. BCL, WIMC, GP/B/2/4/4/2, Apr. 28, 1893; Visiting Surgeon's Report to Infirmary Management Committee, GP/B/addnl.ACC.2009/109, Box 49, Apr. 28, June 3 and 6, 1893; June 12, 1894; Feb. 15, 1895.
177. Worboys, *Endangered Lives*, 118; Mooney, "'A Tissue of the Most Flagrant Anomalies,'" 261–90.
178. Hopkins, *Princes and Peasants*, 92; Hardy, *The Epidemic Streets*, 113; Pickstone, *Medicine and Industrial Society*, 158.
179. Hopkins, *Princes and Peasants*, 95.
180. Hill, "The Epidemic of Small-Pox," 6.
181. Hardy, *The Epidemic Streets*, 137; Hopkins, *Princes and Peasants*, 96.
182. WALS, WBG, PU/WOL/A/24, Feb. 3, 1893; *WC*, Feb. 8 and 15, 1893.
183. WALS, WBG, PU/WOL/A/24, Sept. 23, 1892; *WC*, June 28, 1892; Mar. 8, 1893.
184. WALS, WBG, PU/WOL/A/25, Feb. 7, 1896; WVC, PU/WOL/H/2, Mar. 17, 1896.
185. WALS, HC, PU/WOL/E/1, Dec. 31, 1902; Jan. 15, 1903.
186. BCL, WMC, GP/B/2/3/2/1, Jan. 13, 1893; WIMC, GP/B/2/4/4/2, Apr. 28, 1893; WMC, GP/B/2/3/3/2, Oct. 27, 1873.
187. BCL, WIMC, GP/B/2/4/4/4, Feb. 17, 1902; WMC, GP/B/2/3/2/3, July 10, 1903.
188. Hardy, *The Epidemic Streets*, 123.

189. WALS, WBG, PU/WOL/A/15, Jan. 8, Apr. 5, 1872.
190. WALS, WBG, PU/WOL/A/19, Aug. 3, Sept. 7, 1883.
191. WALS, WBG, PU/WOL/A/24, Feb. 10, 1893.
192. BCL, BBG, GP/B/2/1/33, May 23, 1866.
193. BCL, HSC, GP/B/2/3/3/3, Jan. 28, 1873.
194. BCL, VGPC, GP/B/2/8/1/6, Jan. 31, Feb. 14, 1873.
195. BCL, BBG, GP/B/2/1/43, Aug. 9, Dec. 9, 1874.
196. BCL, VGPC, GP/B/2/8/1/9, Nov. 9, 1883.
197. BCL, VGPG, GP/B/2/8/1/7, July 25, 1878; GP/B/2/8/1/9, Dec. 7, 1884; BBG, GP/B/2/11/52, Mar. 19, 1884.
198. BCL, WMC, GPB/2/3/2/1, Mar. 17, 1888.
199. Hill, "The Epidemic of Small-Pox," 5.
200. BCL, BBG, GP/B/2/1/62, Nov. 15, 1893; Apr. 4, 1894.
201. Kerr, "Sites of Complaint," 205–6.
202. Kerr, "Sites of Complaint," 208; Worboys, Endangered Lives, 240.
203. BCL, BBG, GP/B/2/1/64, July 1, 1896.
204. Woods, "Mortality and Sanitary Conditions," 181.
205. Hopkins, Princes and Peasants, 303, 317.
206. Pickstone, Medicine and Industrial Society, 160, 165–68.
207. Smith, The People's Health, 389.
208. Railton and Barr, Battle Workhouse, 57–59.
209. WALS, HC, WOL/PU/E/4, Jan. 18, 1912.
210. HCPP, 1895 (28), Sanitary Districts (Accommodation for Infectious Diseases), 352–55, 400–403.

Chapter Three

1. Clark, "The Rejection of Psychological Approaches," 354.
2. Scull, "The Social History of Psychiatry," 5; Walton, "The Treatment of Pauper Lunatics," 166.
3. Scull, "The Social History of Psychiatry," 6.
4. Scull, The Most Solitary of Afflictions, 18–19, 24.
5. Walton, "The Treatment of Pauper Lunatics," 167.
6. Smith, "Cure, Comfort and Safe Custody," 6, 24.
7. Hodgkinson, "Provision for Pauper Lunatics," 142.
8. Scull, The Most Solitary of Afflictions, 267.
9. Scull, The Most Solitary of Afflictions, 362.
10. Smith, "'A Sad Spectacle of Hopeless Mental Degradation,'" 103.
11. Morrison, The Workhouse, 162.
12. Scull, The Most Solitary of Afflictions, 46.
13. WALS, MJ, PU/WOL/U/2, Oct. 8, 1842.
14. TNA, MH12/11676, Aug. 12, 1844; WALS, MJ, PU/WOL/U/2, Aug. 17, 1844.

15. WALS, WBG, PU/WOL/A/6, Feb. 13, 1846.
16. WALS, WBG, PU/WOL/A/8, Jan. 2, 1852.
17. HCPP, 1859, Session 1 (228), *Lunacy. Return to an Address of the Honourable the House of Commons, Dated 11 April 1859;—for, "Copy of the Supplement to the Twelfth Report of the Commissioners in Lunacy to the Lord Chancellor,"* 61, 69, 8–10.
18. WALS, *WC,* May 25, 1859.
19. WALS, *WC,* Dec. 11 and 25, 1867; HCPP, 1867–68 (4), *Provincial Workhouses,* 153; BCL, VGPC, GP/B/2/8/1/4, May 22, 1865; HCPP, 1870 (468–I), *Poor Relief,* 24–25, 54.
20. WALS, *WC,* Mar. 28, 1860; Dec. 11, 1861.
21. For example, Hodgkinson, "Provision for Pauper Lunatics," 149–50.
22. WALS, *WC,* July 11, 1860; Apr. 25, 1877.
23. WALS, WBG, PU/WOL/A/15, Apr. 12, 1872.
24. WALS, *WC,* Nov. 20, 1872.
25. WALS, *WC,* June 21, 1876.
26. WALS, *WC,* Dec. 1, 1875; June 28, 1882.
27. Smith, "The Pauper Lunatic Problem," 106.
28. Smith, "'A Sad Spectacle,'" 107.
29. BCL, BBG, GP/B/2/1/3, Apr. 7, 1834; Nov. 15, 1837.
30. BCL, HC, GP/B/2/3/1/1, Aug. 13, 1844.
31. Smith, "The Pauper Lunatic Problem," 114; Smith, "'A Sad Spectacle,'" 111–12; BBG, GP/B/2/3/1/1, HC, Oct. 30, 1843; Apr. 23, 1844.
32. BCL, BBG, GP/B/2/1/4, Jan. 27 and July 27, 1845.
33. BCL, BBG, GP/B/2/1/5, Dec. 23, 1845.
34. BCL, BBG, GP/B/2/1/5, June 15, 1846; July 6 and Oct. 13, 1846.
35. TNA, MH12/13297, Oct. 7, 1851.
36. BCL, LGB Letters, GP/B/1/2/1/4, Feb. 13, 1888; HCPP, 1888 (74 B.I.), *Pauperism (England and Wales). Return (B.I.),* 30.
37. BCL, HSC, GP/B/2/3/3/2, Oct. 25, 1870; LGB Letters, GP/B/1/2/1/6, Feb. 7, 1899.
38. WALS, WBG, PU/WOL/A/28, Feb. 2 and June 8, 1900.
39. Smith, "*Cure, Comfort,*" 113.
40. Hodgkinson, "Provision for Pauper Lunatics," 139, 149.
41. WALS, MJ, PU/WOL/U/2, Apr. 8, Aug. 13, 1842, and Dec. 31, 1842.
42. WALS, WBG, PU/WOL/A/11–12, June 17, 1862; Nov. 10, 1865.
43. TNA, MH12/11690, Oct. 18, 1873.
44. WALS, WBG, PU/WOL/A/18 and 22, Dec. 31, 1880; Dec. 23, 1887.
45. WALS, WBG, PU/WOL/A/22, May 24, 1889.
46. BCL, HC, GP/B/2/3/1/1, Aug. 13 and Sept. 3, 1844.
47. BCL, Register of Insane (hereafter RI), MS/344/12/1, 1845–50.
48. BCL, BBG, GP/B/2/1/5, June 15, 1846.
49. BCL, LGB Letters, GP/B/1/2/1/1, Feb. 18, 1871; HSC, GP/B/2/3/3/2, May 16, 1871.
50. Smith, "*Care, Comfort,*" 248–55.

51. Scull, *The Most Solitary of Afflictions*, 38.
52. Hodgkinson, "Provision for Pauper Lunatics," 147.
53. BCL, BBG, GP/B/2/1/4, Jan. 2 and 15, 1844.
54. BCL, RI, MS/344/12/1, 1845–50.
55. BCL, RI, MS/344/12/1, 1845–50.
56. WALS, WBG, PU/WOL/A/8, Jan. 2 and May 7, 1852; *WC*, May 12, 1852.
57. BCL, VGPC, GP/B/2/8/1/2, Apr. 3, 1857.
58. BCL, VGPC, GP/B/2/8/1/3, Dec. 6, 1861.
59. BCL, VGPC, GP/B/2/8/1/7–8, Mar. 19, 1880; July 7, 1882.
60. WALS, *WC*, June 22, 1881.
61. WALS, WVC, PU/WOL/H/2, Feb. 16, 1900; HC, PU/WOL/E/1, May 9, 1901.
62. Smith, *"Care, Comfort,"* 149, 273–75.
63. BCL, HSC, GP/B/2/3/3/6, Nov. 13, 1877; Apr. 30, 1878.
64. WALS, WBG, PU/WOL/A/16, June 9, 1876; July 9–30, 1875.
65. WALS, WBG, PU/WOL/A/17, Dec. 27, 1878; Jan. 3, 1879.
66. BCL, VGPC, GP/B/2/8/1/4, Aug. 1, 1862.
67. BCL, HC, GP/B/2/3/1/1, July 4, 1844.
68. BCL, HC, GP/B/2/3/1/1, Aug. 13, 1844.
69. WALS, WBG, PU/WOL/A/17, Jan. 12, 1877; PU/WOL/A/19, Mar. 30, 1883; *WC*, June 28, 1881.
70. BCL, BBG, GP/B/2/1/6, Apr. 24, 1849; BCL, VGPC, GP/B/2/8/1/6, Aug. 1, 1873; GP/B/2/8/1/9, July 4, 1883; LGB Letters, GP/B/1/2/1/9, Apr. 12, 1906.
71. Friedlander, *The History of Modern Epilepsy*, 2.
72. Eadie and Bladin, *A Disease Once Sacred*, 4, 147.
73. Clouston, *Unsoundness of Mind*, 237–39.
74. Scott, *The History of Epileptic Therapy*, 37–38.
75. Scott, *Epileptic Therapy*, 49–50; Friedlander, *Modern Epilepsy*, 277.
76. WALS, *WC*, Dec. 25, 1867; July 11, 1866; June 22, 1881.
77. TNA, MH12/11690, Oct. 8, 1873; WALS, *WC*, Jan. 3, 1877.
78. TNA, MH12/13365, Feb. 26, 1892.
79. BCL, VGPC, GP/B/2/8/1/6, Aug. 1, 1873.
80. BCL, RI, MS/344/12/1, 1845–50.
81. WALS, *WC*, Dec. 25, 1867.
82. BCL, HSC, GP/B/2/3/3/2, May 16, 1871.
83. BCL, IMC, GP/B/2/4/4/1, Feb. 11, 1889.
84. WALS, HC, PU/WOL/E/1, Mar. 12, 1901.
85. BCL, WIMC, GP/B/2/4/43, July 10, 1896.
86. BCL, LGB Letters, GP/B/1/2/1/6, Feb. 7, 1899; WIMC, 2/4/4/3, Feb. 4, 1901.
87. BCL, LGB Letters, GP/B/1/2/1/7-8, Apr. 12, 1904; June 16, 1905.
88. BCL, IHSC, GP/B/2/4/5/1, July 24, 1899; LGB Letters, GP/B/1/2/1/9, Apr. 12, 1906.
89. WALS, WBG, PU/WOL/A/18, Oct. 1, 1880; *WC*, Oct. 6, 1880.

90. WALS, WVC, PU/WOL/H/1, Apr. 20, 1894.
91. HCPP, 1900 (362), *Lunatics and Epileptics in Workhouses. Return of the Number of (a) Lunatics, and (b) Epileptics, Not Classed as Insane, Who Were Inmates of Workhouses in England and Wales on the 1st Day of January 1900, Showing the Numbers Admitted from Each Administrative County and County Borough* (hereafter *Lunatics and Epileptics in Workhouses*), 2–3; WALS, WBG, PU/WOL/A/28, Feb. 2 and June 8, 1900.
92. HCPP, 1908 [Cd. 4202], *Royal Commission on the Care and Control of the Feeble-Minded*, 8:302–6.
93. WALS, WBG, PU/WOL/A/26, May 14 and 21, 1897; PU/WOL/A/35, Mar. 15, 1912.
94. Hutchings, *Monyhull*, 11–12.
95. The Royal Commission on the Care and Control of the Feeble-Minded defined *feeble-minded* as people who may be capable of earning a living under favorable circumstances, but who are incapable from mental defect existing from birth or from an early age (a) of competing on equal terms with their normal fellows or (b) of managing themselves and their affairs with ordinary prudence. HCPP, 1908 [Cd. 4202], *Royal Commission on the Care and Control of the Feeble-Minded*, 188.
96. BCL, BBG, GP/B/2/1/73, July 20, 1904; LGB Letters, GP/B/1/2/1/9, Apr. 12, 1906; GP/B/1/2/1/11, May 3, 1909; HCPP, 1908 [Cd. 4202], *Royal Commission on the Care and Control of the Feeble-Minded*, 50–52.
97. Hutchings, *Monyhull*, 20.
98. HCPP, 1908 [Cd. 4202], *Royal Commission on the Care and Control of the Feeble-Minded*, 15, 307.
99. Hutchings, *Monyhull*, 15–16.
100. Siena, *Venereal Disease*, 5l; this group of diseases is now known as sexually transmitted disease.
101. WALS, HC, PU/WOL/E/1, Dec. 31, 1902; WBG, PU/WOL/A/30, Jan. 2, 1903.
102. WALS, MJ, PU/WOL/2, Apr. 23, 1842; Feb. 11 and 18, 1843; Dec. 14, 1844.
103. Dobson, *Disease*, 32.
104. HCPP, 1913 [Cd. 7029], *Local Government Board. Report on Venereal Diseases, by Dr R. W. Johnstone, with an Introduction by the Medical Officer of the Board* (hereafter *Report on Venereal Diseases*), 11–12.
105. WALS, HC, PU/WOL/E/4, Jan. 29, 1914.
106. HCPP, 1916 [Cd. 8189], *Royal Commission on Venereal Diseases. Final Report of the Commissioners* (hereafter *Royal Commission on Venereal Diseases*), 118–20.
107. Parker, *The Modern Treatment of Syphilitic Diseases*, para. 100–101; copaiba was an oil resin obtained by incising the trunks of several species of *Copaifera*.
108. Wyke, "Hospital Facilities for, and Diagnosis and Treatment," 78–79.
109. HCPP, 1913 [Cd. 7029], *Report on Venereal Diseases*, 20.

NOTES TO PP. 117–123 ?» 257

110. Reinarz, *Health Care*, 110.
111. HCPP, 1913 [Cd. 7029], *Report on Venereal Diseases*, 20.
112. Siena, *Venereal Disease*, 150.
113. TNA, MH12/13288, May 15, 1844; BCL, VGPC, GP/B/2/8/1/2, Jan. 18, 1856; HCPP, 1867–68 (4), 46, 153.
114. BCL, HSC, GP/B/2/3/3/3, June 3, 1873.
115. HCPP, 1877 (260), *Workhouse Unions, England and Wales (Diseases). Returns of General Diseases and of Venereal Diseases, from the Workhouse of Each Union in England and Wales, during the First Week in January 1876; and, of Deaths in Each Such Workhouse during the Period of Twelve Months Ending the 31st Day of December 1875* (hereafter *Returns of General Diseases and of Venereal Diseases*), 10–11, 17.
116. WALS, WBG, PU/WOL/A/5, Aug. 23, 1844; WJ, LS/LO7/79, liv.
117. HCPP, 1916 [Cd. 8189], *Royal Commission on Venereal Diseases*, 118–19.
118. HCPP, 1870 (468–I), *Poor Relief*, 3, 53, 83, 87, 233, 237; HCPP, 1877 (260), *Returns of General Diseases and of Venereal Diseases*, 10–11, 17.
119. TNA, MH12/11675, June 2, 1841.
120. BCL, BBG, GP/B/2/1/18, July 2 and 9, 1856.
121. BCL, VGPC, GP/B/2/8/1/8, Dec. 22, 1880; Jan. 7, 1881.
122. BCL, BBG, GP/B/2/1/57, June 29, 1888.
123. BCL, Western Road House Sub-committee (hereafter WRHSC), GP/B/2/3/15/2, Sept. 4, 1914; HCPP, 1916 [Cd. 8189], *Royal Commission on Venereal Diseases*, 120.
124. HCPP, 1913 [Cd. 7029], *Report on Venereal Diseases*, 21–22.
125. BCL, VGPC, GP/B/2/8/1/7, Nov. 17, 1876; Apr. 20, 1877.
126. Wyke, "Hospital Facilities," 81; Parker, *The Modern Treatment*, para. 1–15.
127. Parker, *The Modern Treatment*, para. 29 and 208.
128. Wyke, "Hospital Facilities," 81–82.
129. Oriel, *The Scars of Venus*, 88–89.
130. HCPP, 1913 [Cd. 7029], *Report on Venereal Diseases*, 16–18.
131. TNA, MH12/11682, Feb. 2, 1855; Jan. 23, 1856.
132. BCL, VGPC, GP/B/2/8/1/2, July 31 and Aug. 7, 1857.
133. BCL, BBG GP/2/1/20, Dec. 2, 1857. Condylomata are wart-like excrescences near the anus or vulva, which occur in the secondary stage of syphilis.
134. WALS, WBG, PU/WOL/A/13, Nov. 15, 1867.
135. HCPP, 1913 [Cd. 7029], *Report on Venereal Diseases*, 22.
136. BCL, HSC, GP/B/2/3/3/14, June 21 and Oct. 11, 1892; Reinarz, *Health Care*, 110.
137. BCL, WRHSC, GP/B/2/3/15/1, July 19, Sept. 20, Nov. 8 and 22, and Dec. 6, 1912.
138. HCPP, 1913 [Cd. 7029], *Report on Venereal Diseases*, 21–22.
139. Smith, "Behind Closed Doors," 321–22.
140. Crowther, "Paupers or Patients?," 47–49.
141. Price, "A Regional Quantitative and Qualitative Study," 315.

142. TNA, MH12/11690, Mar. 8, 1873.
143. WALS, HC, WOL/PU/E/1, Dec. 31, 1902.
144. Blistering was a common method of producing a sore on the skin that would supposedly remove harmful substances responsible for disease. It was carried out by applying an adhesive dressing covered with irritating substances to the skin.
145. BCL, VGPC, GP/B/2/8/1/8, Dec. 9, 1881; HCPP, 1886 (19–Sess.2), *Copies "of Evidence Taken by Inspectors of the Local Government Board at Sworn Inquiry, Held on the 16th and 17th Day of February 1886, to Inquire into Charges Made by the Birmingham Board of Guardians against Dr. A. B. Simpson, Medical Officer of Birmingham Workhouse; and, Report of Inspectors Founded Thereon"*; TNA, MH12/13338, Dec. 17, 1881; Anonymous, "Charge against the Medical Staff," 993; Rogers, "The Alleged Punishment," 33.
146. Scull, *The Most Solitary of Afflictions*, 120–21, 161–62.
147. The Mental Health Taskforce to the NHS in England, *The Five Year Forward View for Mental Health*, 2016, 3, 9–10.

Chapter Four

1. Thomas, "The Old Poor Law," 7; Crowther, "Health Care," 209.
2. BCL, HSC, GP/B/2/3/3/20, July 24, 1900.
3. Hodgkinson, "Poor Law Medical Officers," 301, 306.
4. Hodgkinson, "Poor Law Medical Officers," 302; Brand, "The Parish Doctor," 100.
5. Price, "A Regional, Quantitative and Qualitative Study," 335.
6. Crowther, "Paupers or Patients?," 47–49.
7. Price, "A Regional Quantitative and Qualitative Study," 21, 154; Crowther, *The Workhouse System*, 163.
8. Brand, "The Parish Doctor," 105.
9. Rogers, *Joseph Rogers*, xviii–xix, 60–61.
10. Hodgkinson, *The Origins of the National Health Service*, 399–401.
11. Brand, "The Parish Doctor," 110.
12. Hodgkinson, "Poor Law Medical Officers," 319–20; BCL, LGB Returns, GP/B/18/2/1, Oct. 15, 1856.
13. BCL, BBG, GP/B/2/1/1, Mar. 11, 1823; Bosworth, "Public Healthcare," 206.
14. Loudon, *Medical Care*, 238; the unions were Derby, Lincoln, Bridgewater, Aylesbury, Eton, Shipston, and Newbury.
15. BCL, BBG, GP/B/2/1/3, June 3, 1827; July 8, 1834.
16. Bosworth, "Public Healthcare," 210–11.
17. BCL, BBG, GP/B/2/1/4, July 2, Oct. 8, and Dec. 18, 1844; Mar. 15, 1847.
18. BCL, BBG, GP/B/2/1/4, Feb. 21, 1848.

19. BCL, BBG, GP/B/2/1/6, June 27 and Dec. 11, 1849.
20. BCL, BBG, GP/B/2/1/7, Mar. 15, 1850.
21. BCL, BBG, GP/B/2/1/66–8, Jan. 1850 to Dec. 1899.
22. BCL, General Hospital, Birmingham, Annual Reports, 1857–75.
23. BCL, VGPC, GP/B/2/8/1/8, Mar. 21, 1882.
24. BCL, HSC, GP/B/2/3/3/8, July 4, 1882.
25. Peterson, *The Medical Profession*, 211, 214.
26. Hearn, *Dudley Road Hospital*, 23.
27. BCL, BBG, GP/B/2/1/55, Jan. 5, 1887.
28. In the 1860s, the starting salary of the medical officer at the Battle work-house was £120, Railton and Barr, *Battle Workhouse*, 16.
29. BCL, BBG, GP/B/2/1/15, Apr. 4, 1855.
30. Sydenham College was the rival medical school to Queen's College in Birmingham.
31. BCL, BBG, GP/B/2/1/39, Aug. 10, 1870; Anonymous, "Obituary. Edmund Bancks Whitcombe," 1353.
32. BCL, BBG, GP/B/2/1/39, Aug. 10, 1870; General Purposes and Advisory Sub Committee, GP/B/2/8/2/1, Sept. 23, 1914.
33. Railton and Barr, *Battle Workhouse*, 90.
34. BCL, BBG, GP/B/2/1/11, Oct. 6, 1852. The Asylum for the Infant Poor had been in use since 1797 for pauper children.
35. BCL, VGPC, GP/2/8/1/1, Dec. 31, 1852.
36. BCL, BBG, GP/B/2/1/12, Jan. 5 to Feb. 5, 1853.
37. BCL, BBG, GP/B/2/1/15, Apr. 4, 1855.
38. BCL, Returns, GP/B/18/2/1, Oct. 15, 1856.
39. BCL, BBG, GP/B/2/1/19, Apr. 8 and 15, May 6, 1857.
40. BCL, LGB Returns, GP/B/18/2/1, Oct. 15, 1856.
41. BCL, LGB Returns, GP/B/18/2/1, Oct. 15, 1856.
42. HCPP, 1867–68 (4), *Poor Relief*, 43.
43. Anonymous, "Dr. Edward Smith's Report," 166.
44. Heslop, "The Medical Aspects of Birmingham," 701–2.
45. Anonymous, "The Medical Aspects of Birmingham," 109.
46. BCL, VGPC, GP/B/2/8/1/6, Mar. 13, 1874; July 2, 1875.
47. Ritch, "'Sick, Aged and Infirm,'" 47–49.
48. BCL, Workhouse Inquiry Sub Committee (hereafter WISC), GP/B/2/3/11/1, Jan. 24 and Mar. 22, 1878.
49. BCL, VGPC, GP/B/2/8/1/7, May 3, 1878.
50. Anonymous, "Editorial," 1308.
51. Anonymous, "Birmingham Workhouse Infirmary" (1889), 47.
52. BCL, WIMC, GP/B/2/4/4/2, Jan. 28, 1893; Jan. 25, 1894.
53. BCL, WIMC, GP/B/2/4/4/4, May 8, 1903.
54. Hearn, *Dudley Road Hospital*, 23.
55. BCL, BUB, GP/B/2/1/81, Mar. 19, 1913.
56. BCL, WMC, GP/B/2/3/2/2, Apr. 27, 1894; Mar. 11, 1898.
57. BCL, WMC, GP/B/2/3/2/1, Apr. 11, 1890.

58. BCL, HSC, GP/B/2/3/3/7, June 22, 1880.
59. BCL, WIMC, GP/B/2/4/4/3, July 30, 1900.
60. BCL, WMC, GP/B/2/3/2/3, Feb. 27, 1903.
61. BCL, Infirmary House Sub-committee (hereafter IHSC), GP/B/2/4/5/3, Dec. 21, 1903.
62. BCL, HSC, GP/B/2/3/3/21, Jan. 26, 1904.
63. BCL, HSC, GP/B/2/3/3/19, Apr. 11 and July 11, 1899; GP/B/2/3/3/22, Jan. 8, 1907.
64. BCL, HSC, GP/B/2/3/3/20, Sept. 10, 1901.
65. BCL, LGB Returns, GP/B/5/1/3, Oct. 2, 1901.
66. WALS, WBG, PU/WOL/A/2, Mar. 19, 1839.
67. WALS, WBG, PU/WOL/A/3, Mar. 19, 1841.
68. WALS, WBG, PU/WOL/A/10, Oct. 28 and Nov. 18, 1859.
69. WALS, WBG, PU/WOL/A/6, July 9, 1847; WC, July 7, 1847.
70. WALS, WBG, PU/WOL/A/8, June 24, 1853.
71. WALS, WBG, PU/WOL/A/13, Oct. 5, 1866; WC, Oct. 30, 1866.
72. WALS, WBG, PU/WOL/A/16, Dec. 11, 1874.
73. WALS, General Purposes Committee (hereafter GPC), PU/WOL/D/1, Feb. 28, 1901.
74. WALS, WBG, PU/WOL/A/29, May 10, 1901; PU/WOL/A/30, Aug. 10 and 28, 1903.
75. WALS, WBG, PU/WOL/A/30, Dec. 2 and 18, 1903.
76. Crowther, *The Workhouse System*, 163; Fowler, *Workhouse*, 156; Loudon, *Medical Care*, 50, 63; Digby, *Pauper Palaces*, 171.
77. Brand, "The Parish Doctor," 122; Hodgkinson, "Poor Law Medical Officers," 311.
78. WALS, Resolutions re. Duties of Officers, PU/WOL/L, Oct. 27, 1890; WVC, PU/WOL/H/1, Mar. 16, 1894.
79. WALS, MJ, PU/WOL/U/2, Nov. 4, 1843; June 7, 1845.
80. WALS, WBG, PU/WOL/A/8, Oct. 17, 1851.
81. WALS, WC, Sept. 24, 1851.
82. TNA, MH12/11680, Dec. 30, 1851.
83. WALS, WBG, PU/WOL/A/8, Nov. 7 and 21, Dec. 12, 1851.
84. Price, "A Regional Quantitative and Qualitative Study," 262–64; Klein has demonstrated that failure to visit was the second most common cause of dissatisfaction with general practitioner services in the 1970s, with the manners of practitioners being the first; Klein, *Complaints against Doctors*, 105, 116.
85. Price, "A Regional Quantitative and Qualitative Study," 141, 230, 342; Price, *Medical Negligence*, 96.
86. Price, *Medical Negligence*, 99.
87. Price, "'The Shape of the Iceberg,'" 138.
88. Price, "'The Shape of the Iceberg,'" 136.
89. WALS, WBG, PU/WOL/A/8, Dec. 19, 1851; WC, Feb. 11, 1852; TNA, MH12/11680, Dec. 30, 1851.

90. WALS, *WC*, Feb. 11, 1852.
91. WALS, WBG, PU/WOL/A/8, Feb. 20, June 25, and July 16, 1852; *WC*, 29, Sept. 1852.
92. WALS, *WC*, Dec. 10, 1851.
93. Price, "A Regional Quantitative and Qualitative Study," 231.
94. WALS, WBG, PU/WOL/A/9, 9, Feb. 16 and 23, Mar. 16, 1855; *WC*, Feb. 14, 1855.
95. WALS, WBG, PU/WOL/A/9, Mar. 30, Apr. 13, and May 18, 1855; *WC*, May 23, 1855.
96. WALS, WBG, PU/WOL/A/9, July 27, 1855; *WC*, Aug. 1, 1855.
97. WALS, WBG, PU/WOL/A/10, Feb. 23, 1858; *WC*, Aug. 11, 1858; Sept. 28, 1859.
98. HCPP, 1867–68 (4), *Poor Relief*, 125; Bosworth, "Public Healthcare," 236–37.
99. WALS, WBG, PU/WOL/A/14, Dec. 2, 1870.
100. WALS, WBG, PU/WOL/A/17, Apr. 27, 1877.
101. WALS, WBG, PU/WOL/A/18, Sept. 5, 1879; PU/WOL/A/19, Apr. 14, 1882; *WC*, Aug. 13, 1879.
102. WALS, WBG, PU/WOL/A/18, Aug. 12, 1881.
103. WALS, WBG, PU/WOL/A/23, Apr. 28, 1882; May 16, 1890.
104. WALS, WBG, PU/WOL/A/23, May 15, July 17, Aug. 21, and Dec. 4, 1891.
105. WALS, WVC, PU/WOL/H/1, June 15, 1894.
106. Price, "A Regional Quantitative and Qualitative Study," 209–11.
107. WALS, WVC, PU/WOL/H/2, Feb. 7 and 14, 1896; Apr. 7, 1898.
108. WALS, WBG, PU/WOL/A/30, Jan. 30, 1903; HC, PU/WOL/E/1, Jan. 29 and Feb. 26, 1903.
109. Railton and Barr, *Battle Workhouse*.
110. Bosworth, "Public Healthcare," 235–43.
111. Negrine, "Medicine and Poverty," 57, 63, 66.
112. BCL, BBG, GP/B/2/1/23, Feb. 22, June 8 and 22, 1859.
113. BCL, BBG, GP/B/2/1/26, Aug. 21, 1861.
114. BCL, VGPC, GP/B/2/8/1/3, Aug. 16, 1861.
115. BCL, BBG, GP/B/2/1/26, Sept. 25 and Oct. 9, 1861.
116. In his will, he left a bequest to the National University of Ireland in Dublin on condition that Irish would be a compulsory subject in the university's matriculation examination. It became available to the university in 1923 and was used to fund a journal of Irish studies, *Éigse*, until 1999 and afterward a postdoctoral fellowship; BCL, Register of Wills, 1913, 1469–72. "Journal History," *Éigse: A Journal of Irish Studies*, accessed June 27, 2019, http://www.nui.ie/eigse/journalhistory.html.
117. BCL, BBG, GP/B/2/1/40, Dec. 27, 1871; VGPC, GP/B/2/8/16, Aug. 30, 1872; Jan. 2, 1874; Apr. 16, 1875.
118. BCL, BBG, GP/B/2/1/44, Nov. 10, 1875.
119. TNA, MH12/13326, Mar. 26, 1877.

120. BCL, HSC, GP/B/2/3/3/6, May 1, 1877; VGPC, GP/B/2/8/1/7, Sept. 21, 1877; BBG, GP/B/2/1/45, Sept. 26 and Oct. 24, 1877.
121. BCL, VGPC, GP/B/2/8/1/8, Dec. 9, 1881; BBG, GP/B/2/1/49, Dec. 14, 1881; HCPP, 1886 (19–Sess. 2), *Evidence Taken by Inspectors of the Local Government Board at Sworn Inquiry*, 11, 22; Anonymous, "Charge against the Medical Staff," 993.
122. BCL, VGPC, GP/B/2/8/1/9, Dec. 5, 1884.
123. HCPP, 1886 (19–Sess. 2), *Evidence Taken by Inspectors of the Local Government Board at Sworn Inquiry*, 3–11, 24, 27, 29, 31; Wood's initial temperature was 37.8°C as opposed to the normal upper limit of 36.8°C, and increased to 39.4°C and then to 39.8°C.
124. The raised temperature at the start of the illness was not in keeping with a diagnosis of puerperal fever, although the increase after a few days would suggest the onset of septicemia.
125. BCL, ISC, GP/B/2/4/1/2, Dec. 1, 1885; HCPP, 1886 (19–Sess. 2), *Evidence Taken by Inspectors of the Local Government Board at Sworn Inquiry*, 24.
126. HCPP, 1886 (19–Sess. 2), *Evidence Taken by Inspectors of the Local Government Board at Sworn Inquiry*, 3–11.
127. BCL, ISC, GP/B/2/4/1/2, Jan. 22, 1886.
128. HCPP, 1886 (19–Sess. 2), *Evidence Taken by Inspectors of the Local Government Board at Sworn Inquiry*, 3–11.
129. *Birmingham Daily Post*, June 16, 1886.
130. BCL, BBG, GP/B/2/1/54, Aug. 4, 1886.
131. BCL, LGB Orders, GP/B/1/1/4, Aug. 2, 1886; Incident Book, GP/B (Acc 2009/109), Box 15.
132. BCL, WISC, GP/B/2/3/11/1, Nov. 15, 1877.
133. Price, "A Regional Quantitative and Qualitative Study," 300, 315–17.
134. BCL, WISC, GP/B/2/3/11/1, Jan. 24, 1878.
135. BCL, WISC, GP/B/2/3/11/1, Jan. 24 and Mar. 22, 1878.
136. Price, "A Regional Quantitative and Qualitative Study," 224, has calculated that only 0.4 percent of poor law medical officers received more than £300 annually throughout the nineteenth century; HCPP, 1867–68 (4), *Provincial Workhouses*, 45.
137. Hodgkinson, *Origins of the National Health Service*, 129; Price, "A Regional Quantitative and Qualitative Study," 237.
138. Stewart and King, "Death in Llantrisant," 81.
139. Mulcahy, *Disputing Doctors*, 45, 68–69.
140. Mulcahy, *Disputing Doctors*, 68–69. The majority of cases of complaints quoted by Klein against general practitioners between 1949 and 1971 concerned children and older adults. Klein, *Complaints against Doctors*, 37–57.
141. Mulcahy, *Disputing Doctors*, 68–69.
142. Price, "A Regional, Quantitative and Qualitative Study," 189, 224.
143. Crowther, "Paupers or Patients?," 40.

Chapter Five

1. King, "Poverty, Medicine," 229, 234–35.
2. Rogers, *Joseph Rogers*, 111–12.
3. Warner, *The Therapeutic Perspective*, 1; Rosenberg, "The Therapeutic Revolution," 485.
4. Keele, "Clinical Medicine," 9.
5. Rosenberg, "The Therapeutic Revolution," 485–86.
6. Risse, "Brunonian Therapeutics," 48.
7. Hamilton, *The Healers*, 138.
8. Risse, *Hospital Life in Enlightenment Scotland*, 181.
9. Rosen, *A History of Public Health*, 288.
10. Morrison, *The Workhouse*, 20, 105.
11. BCL, VGPC, GP/B/2/8/1/4, June 17, 1864.
12. BCL, VGPC, June 17, 1864.
13. BCL, HC, GP/B/2/3/1/1, Feb. 7, 1843.
14. Condrau, "Beyond the Total Institution," 80–81.
15. Reinarz, *Health Care*, 151.
16. Price, "Hydropathy in England," 270; Jackson, "Waters and Spas in the Classical World," 1.
17. Price, "Hydropathy in England," 271.
18. Marland and Adams, "Hydropathy at Home," 500–501.
19. Risse, *Hospital Life*, 203, 211.
20. Reinarz, *Health Care*, 110.
21. WALS, WBG, PU/WOL/A/10, Aug. 13, 1858.
22. WALS, *WC*, June 14, 1893.
23. BCL, VGPC, GP/B/2/8/1/1, Aug. 24, 1855.
24. Cantor, "The Contradictions of Specialization," 127.
25. BCL, ISC, GP/B/2/4/1/1, Apr. 20, 1883.
26. Marland and Adams, "Hydropathy at Home," 506.
27. Risse, *Hospital Life*, 203.
28. Ackerknecht, *Medicine at the Paris Hospital*, 61.
29. Ackerknecht, *Medicine at the Paris Hospital*, 61–71; Warner, *Therapeutic Perspective*, 48–50.
30. Warner, "Therapeutic Explanation and the Edinburgh Bloodletting Controversy," 241–42, 254.
31. Warner, *The Therapeutic Perspective*, 117.
32. Kirk and Pemberton, *Leech*, 49–51, 62, 160–63.
33. Kirk and Pemberton, *Leech*, 55, 59; Ackerknecht, *Medicine at the Paris Hospital*, 70.
34. BCL, BBG, GP/B/2/1/5, Jan. 4 and May 25, 1848; GP/B/2/1/6, Apr. 24 and May 22, 1849.
35. BCL, BBG, GP/B/2/1/5, Mar. 13, 1846; BCL, HC, GP/B/2/3/1/1, Aug. 9, 1842.
36. BCL, BBG, GP/B/2/1/4, Dec. 1, 1841.
37. BCL, VGPC, GP/B/2/8/1/5, July 24, 1868.

38. Elliot, "'More Subtle than the Electric Aura,'" 198.
39. Risse, *Hospital Life*, 203, 216–17.
40. Reinarz, *The Birth of a Provincial Hospital*, 28.
41. Rosner, "The Professional Context of Electrotherapeutics," 67, 78; Morus, *Shocking Bodies*, 81–83.
42. Rosner, "The Professional Context of Electrotherapeutics," 64, 70.
43. Morus, *Shocking Bodies*, 84, 126.
44. Rosner, "The Professional Context of Electrotherapeutics," 72–73.
45. BCL, BBG, GP/B/2/1/7, June 19, 1850; GP/B/2/1/8, Oct. 30, 1850; the term *galvanic* derived from Luigi Galvani, an Italian physician, who carried out experiments in which he stimulated frogs' legs with electricity.
46. BCL, ISC, GP/B/2/4/1/1, Feb. 9, 1883.
47. Risse, *Hospital Life*, 221.
48. Pennell and Rich, "Food: 'The Forgotten Medicine,'" *Social History of Medicine* (2016): 5–9, https://academic.oup.com/DocumentLibrary/SOCHIS/food-the-forgotten-medicine-vi.pdf.
49. Brock, "Liebigiana," 201; Lipman, "Vitalism and Reductionism," 185.
50. Warner, "Physiological Theory and Therapeutic Explanation," 241–42.
51. Lipman, "Vitalism and Reductionism," 179–80.
52. Risse, *Hospital Life*, 220–24; Warner, *The Therapeutic Perspective*, 145–46.
53. Warner, *The Therapeutic Perspective*, 117.
54. Risse, *Hospital Life*, 222.
55. HCPP, 1866 [3660], *Dietaries for the Inmates of Workhouses. Report to the President of the Poor Law Board of Dr. Edward Smith, F.R.S., Medical Officer of the Poor Law Board, and Poor Law Inspector*, 20, 54–55.
56. Sheen, *The Workhouse*, 17–18, 61.
57. BCL, BBG, GP/B/2/1/4, Oct. 17 and Dec. 9, 1838; HC, GP/B/2/3/1/1, Nov. 14, 1844.
58. TNA, MH12/13353, May 17, 1886.
59. BCL, WMC, GP/B/2/3/2/3, Dec. 7, 1900; WALS, House Committee (hereafter HC), PU/WOL/E/1, Jan. 25, 1901.
60. WALS, HC, PU/WOL/E/3, Jan. 9, 1908; scurvy results from a dietary deficiency of vitamin C.
61. Lucia, *A History of Wine*, 110, 114, 150; Paul, *Bacchic Medicine*, i, 60.
62. Lucia, *A History of Wine*, 8, 155–56; Paul, *Bacchic Medicine*, iii.
63. Bynum, *Science and Practice*, 17.
64. Risse, "Brunonian Therapeutics," 50, 61.
65. Risse, *Hospital Life*, 225.
66. Warner, "Physiological Theory," 236.
67. Wilks, "Clinical Lecture," 505.
68. Paul, *Bacchic Medicine*, 66; Warner, "Physiological Theory," 240–42, 244.
69. Williams, "The Use of Beverage Alcohol as Medicine," 551.
70. Gairdner, 'Facts and Conclusions," 291–94.
71. Paul, *Bacchic Medicine*, 92, 134; Warner, "Physiological Theory," 256.
72. Paul, *Bacchic Medicine*, 167, 171, 308; Sournia, *A History of Alcoholism*, 70.

73. Sournia, *A History of Alcoholism*, 298–99; Reinarz and Wynter, "The Spirit of Medicine," 138.
74. Lucia, *A History of Wine*, 161–62; Harrison, *Drink and the Victorians*, 38.
75. BCL, BBG, GP/B/2/1/4, Oct. 17, 1838; HC, GP/B/2/3/1/1, Nov. 14, 1844.
76. Hodgkinson, *The Origins of the National Health Service*, 154.
77. Risse, *Hospital Life*, 224.
78. HCPP, 1866 (372), *Metropolitan Workhouse Infirmaries*, 25.
79. Reinarz and Wynter, "The Spirit of Medicine," 136–37.
80. Risse, "Brunonian Therapeutics," 52.
81. HCPP, 1867–68 (4), *Provincial Workhouses*, 16.
82. WALS, WBG, PU/WOL/A/16, Nov. 20 and Dec. 24, 1874.
83. WALS, *WC*, July 3 and Aug, 14, 1867.
84. BCL, BBG, GP/B/2/1/3, Apr. 2, 1833; GP/B/2/1/6, Apr. 24, 1849; HCPP, 1872 (391), 24–25; HCPP, 1870 (468–I), *Poor Relief*, 21; TNA, MH12/13286, MH12/13288.
85. BCL, HSC, GP/B/2/3/3/5, July 25, 1876.
86. HCPP, 1872 (391), *Paupers (Consumption of Liquors). Return Relating to the Consumption of Liquors in Workhouses* (hereafter *Paupers [Consumption of Liquors]*), 22–25, 36.
87. WALS, *WC*, July 11, 1883.
88. WALS, WBG, PU/WOL/A/22, Apr. 6, 1888; HCPP, 1886 (206), *Workhouses (Consumption of Spirits, &c.). Return Showing the Quantity of Spirits, Wine, and Malt Liquors Consumed in Each Workhouse in England and Wales in the Year Ending 31 December 1885, Together with the Expenditure in Each Workhouse for Each Such Kind of Intoxicating Liquor for the Same Period, and Stating the Daily Average Number of Inmates in Each Workhouse during the Same Term; and, Similar Return for Scotland and Ireland*, 5.
89. BCL, VGPC, GP/B/2/8/1/8, June 23, 1882.
90. HCPP, 1895 (44), *Workhouses (Consumption of Spirits). Return Showing the Quantity of Spirits, Wine, and Malt Liquors Consumed in Each Workhouse in England and Wales in 1892 and 1893, with the Expenditure in Each Workhouse for Each Kind of Intoxicating Liquor, Stating the Daily Average Numbers of Inmates in Each Workhouse; and, Similar Returns for Scotland and Ireland (in Continuation of Parliamentary Paper, no. 292, of Session 1892*, 25; BCL, BBG, GP/B/2/1/6, Apr. 9 and 24, 1849.
91. Nicholls, *The Politics of Alcohol*, 138.
92. Harrison, *Drink and the Victorians*, 329.
93. BCL, IHSC, BP/B/2/4/5/2, May 9, 1901.
94. The return in question was HCPP, 1892 (292), *Workhouses (Consumption of Spirits, &c.). Return Showing the Quantity of Spirits, Wine, and Malt Liquors Consumed in Each Workhouse in England and Wales, in the Year Ending 31 December 1891, Together with the Expenditure in Each Workhouse for Each Such Kind of Intoxicating Liquor for the Same Period; and Stating the Daily Average Number of Inmates in Each Workhouse during the Same Term; and, Similar Return for Scotland and Ireland*.

95. WALS, WBG, PU/WOL/A/24, Nov. 25 and Dec. 9, 1892.
96. WALS, WBG, PU/WOL/A/24, Mar. 17, 1893.
97. WALS, HC, PU/WOL/E/2, Mar. 27, 1906.
98. WALS, WBG, PU/WOL/A/28, Sept. 29, Oct. 18 and 27, 1899.
99. WALS, WBG, PU/WOL/A/29, Apr. 11, 1902.
100. WALS, WBG, PU/WOL/A/32, Oct. 18, 1907; Williams, "The Use of Beverage Alcohol," 551.
101. HCPP, 1876 (202), *Wrexham Union (Use of Stimulants)*. *Copy of the Correspondence between the Guardians of the Saint George's Union, Middlesex, and the Guardians of the Wrexham Union, Relating to the Discontinuance of the Use of Stimulants in the Latter Union*, 3–4.
102. Sheen, *The Workhouse*, 20–22.
103. HCPP, 1872 (391), *Paupers (Consumption of Liquors)*, 32–33; 1883 (108), 19; 1895 (44), 36.
104. Warner, *The Therapeutic Perspective*, 62–63.
105. Risse, *Hospital Life*, 192, 198–200; Warner, *The Therapeutic Perspective*, 141.
106. Whorton, *The Arsenical Century*, 236.
107. TNA, MH12/11682, Jan. 23, 1856; Graham, *Modern Domestic Medicine*, 6, 56.
108. WALS, WC, Feb. 14, 1855; WBG, PU/WOL/A/9, Mar. 9, 1855.
109. WALS, WC, Oct. 3, 1866.
110. WALS, WBG, PU/WOL/A/16, Nov. 20 and 27, Dec. 11, 1874.
111. WALS, WBG, PU/WOL/A/20, June 5, 1885.
112. BCL, BBG, GP/B/2/1/3, Nov. 16, 1831.
113. BCL, BBG, GP/B/2/1/6, Dec. 11, 1849; GP/B/2/1/3, July 8, 1834; Jan. 4, 1835; GP/B/2/1/5, Oct. 12, 1847.
114. BCL, BBG, GP/B/2/1/15, Feb. 28, 1855.
115. BCL, ISC, GP/B/2/4/1/4, Nov. 25, 1887.
116. BCL, WMC, GP/B/2/3/2/1, Apr. 11, 1890.
117. BCL, WIMC, GP/B/2/4/4/2, May 15, 1896.
118. Siena, "The Moral Biology," 71, 77, 234.
119. Parish, "History of Scabies," 4–8; Siena, "The Moral Biology," 72–73.
120. HCPP, 1867–68 (4), *Provincial Workhouses*, 8, 26–157.
121. BCL, HC, GP/B/2/3/1/1, Aug. 2, 1842.
122. WALS, MJ, PU/WOL/U/2, Nov. 5, 1842.
123. WALS, WBG, PU/WOL/A/5, Aug. 23, 1844.
124. Anonymous, "Wolverhampton Workhouse," 555, 623.
125. HCPP, 1870 (468–I), *Poor Relief*, 63, 233.
126. BCL, LGB Returns, GP/B/5/1/1–8, 1877–1911.
127. WALS, WC, Sept. 22 and 29, Oct. 13, 1858; Feb. 9, 1859.
128. WALKS, WC, Sept. 1, 1880.
129. WALS, WBG, PU/WOL/A/24, Mar. 3, 1893.
130. Sulfur continues to be recommended as the treatment of choice for children and second option for adults.

131. BCL, BBG, GP/B/2/1/19, June 24, 1857; HCPP, 1867–68 (4), *Provincial Workhouses*, 8.
132. Bynum, *Science and the Practice*, 37–38.
133. Risse, *Hospital Life*, 146.
134. Woodward, "Medicine and the City," 67.
135. HCPP, 1870 (468–I), *Poor Relief*, 56, 57, 63, 327, 329.
136. Woods, "Mortality and Sanitary Conditions," 190.
137. Suckling, "Lobar Pneumonia," 407.
138. BCL, IMC, GP/B/2/4/4/5, Dec. 14, 1908.
139. Senega was the dried root of *Polygala senega*, a plant of the milkwort family. It was in common use as an infusion to treat pneumonia, probably for its perceived action as an expectorant.
140. Terebene is a mixture of dipentene and other hydrocarbons, distilled from oil of turpentine.
141. Suckling, "Pure Terebene in the Treatment of Winter-Cough," 541.
142. See Wilson, "The Historical Decline of Tuberculosis," 366–96; Worboys, "Before McKeown," 148–70; Cronjé, "Tuberculosis and Mortality Decline," 79–101.
143. HCPP, 1907 [Cd.3657], *Thirty-Fifth Annual Report of the Local Government Board, 1905–06. Supplement in Continuation of the Report of the Medical Officer for 1905–06, on Sanatoria for Consumption and Certain Other Aspects of the Tuberculosis Question* (hereafter *Thirty-Fifth Annual Report of the Local Government Board*), 240–47.
144. Wilson, "The Historical Decline of Tuberculosis," 383, 388; this view is supported by Cronjé, "Tuberculosis and Mortality Decline," 82.
145. Cronjé, "Tuberculosis and Mortality Decline," 84–85.
146. HCPP, 1907 [Cd.3657], *Thirty-Fifth Annual Report of the Local Government Board*, 32–36.
147. Cronjé, "Tuberculosis and Mortality Decline," 83, 78.
148. HCPP, 1907 [Cd.3657], *Thirty-Fifth Annual Report of the Local Government Board*, 43, facing page 44.
149. Cronjé, "Tuberculosis and Mortality Decline," 79, 97; Woods, "Mortality and Sanitary Conditions," 180.
150. Wohl, *Endangered Lives*, 130.
151. Dormandy, *The White Death*, 1–2; Bynum, *Spitting Blood*, 2, 5.
152. Bynum, *Spitting Blood*, 91.
153. Worboys, *Spreading Germs*, 194; Mooney, *Intrusive Interventions*, 119.
154. Koch initially labeled the bacillus he identified in the tubercles as *Tubercle bacillus*, but it is now known as *Mycobacterium tuberculosis*. Infection in humans can also occur from the bacillus that infects cows, namely *Mycobacterium bovis*.
155. Dobson, *Disease*, 64.
156. Dormandy, *The White Death*, 22.
157. Worboys, *Spreading Germs*, 225.
158. BCL, WIMC, GP/B/2/3/3/2, Nov. 28, 1890.

159. Worboys, *Spreading Germs*, 218.
160. Worboys, "The Sanatorium Treatment," 50, 52.
161. Burton-Fanning, *The Open-Air Treatment*, 83.
162. Worboys, "The Sanatorium Treatment," 47, 52; Bynum, *Spitting Blood*, 134; Condrau, "Beyond the Total Institution," 80–81.
163. Smith, *The Retreat of Tuberculosis*, 238–39.
164. Cronjé, "Tuberculosis and Mortality Decline," 82; Worboys, "The Sanatorium Treatment," 48.
165. Worboys, "The Sanatorium Treatment," 52, 55–56, 216.
166. Railton and Barr, *Battle Workhouse*, 143.
167. TNA, MH12/13297–99, 13300.
168. HCPP, 1867–68 (4), *Provincial Workhouses*, 46.
169. HCPP, 1870 (468-I), *Poor Relief*, 11, 143, 147.
170. BCL, WIMC, GP/B/2/4/4/3, July 29, 1901; BBG, GP/B/2/1/71, Sept. 3, 1902.
171. BCL, WIMC, GP/B/2/4/4/4, Feb. 17 and Dec. 15, 1902; IHSC, GP/B/2/4/5/3, Dec. 23, 1902; Dormandy, *The White Death*, 166.
172. BCL, WIMC, GP/B/2/4/4/4, Aug. 31 and Oct. 6, 1903.
173. BCL, IHSC, GP/B/2/4/5/3, Sept. 26, 1904; Mar. 6, 1905.
174. BCL, WIMC, GP/B/2/4/4/5, Feb. 25, 1907.
175. BCL, WIMC, GP/B/2/4/4/4, May 21, 1906.
176. BCL, WIMC, GP/B/2/4/4/5, Jan. 27 and Mar. 9, 1908.
177. Condrau, "Beyond the Total Institution," 80–81; Worboys, "The Sanatorium Treatment," 52.
178. BCL, WIMC, GP/B/2/4/4/5, Mar. 9, 1908.
179. Condrau, "Beyond the Total Institution," 80.
180. BCL, WIMC, GP/B/2/4/4/5, Mar. 9, 1908.
181. WALS, New Workhouse Committee, PU/WOL/S/1, Nov. 27, 1901.
182. WALS, Block Plan, Wolverhampton Union Workhouse, DX/120/10/10, 1902.
183. WALS, HC, PU/WOL/E/2, Dec. 15, 1904; Sept. 20, 1906; Oct. 31, 1907; PU/WOL/E/3, June 9, 1910.
184. WALS, HC, PU/WOL/E/1, Feb. 11, 1904.
185. WALS, WBG, PU/WOL/A/33, Apr. 8, 1909.
186. WALS, Special Committees, PU/WOL/P/1, Jan. 25, 1906.
187. BCL, WIMC, GP/B/2/4/4/5, Jan. 10, 1910.
188. BCL, WIMC, GP/B/2/4/4/5, Jan. 11, 1909.
189. BCL, WIMC, GP/B/2/4/4/2, July 29, 1901; GP/B/2/4/4/4, May 21, 1906.
190. Dormandy, *The White Death*, 83–84.
191. Gray, *The Edinburgh City Hospital*, 171.
192. BCL, WIMC, GP/B/2/4/4/5, Dec. 14, 1908; July 11, 1910.
193. Smith, *The Retreat of Tuberculosis*, 105.
194. Bynum, *Spitting Blood*, 142; Condrau, "Beyond the Total Institution," 74–75.

195. WALS, BBG, PU/WOL/A/33, Apr. 8, 1909; HC, PU/WOL/E/4, July 31, Aug. 22 and 27, 1913; PU/WOL/E/5, Apr. 17, 1914.
196. Railton and Barr, *Battle Hospital*, 143–44; BCL, IHSC, GP/B/2/4/5/3, Dec. 23, 1902.
197. HCPP, 1909 [Cd. 4573], *Royal Commission on the Poor Laws and Relief of Distress. Appendix vol. XIV. Report to the Royal Commission on the Poor Laws and Relief of Distress on Poor Law Medical Relief in Certain Unions in England and Wales* (hereafter *Royal Commission on the Poor Laws*), 92.
198. Dormandy, *The White Death*, 148.
199. Dormandy, *The White Death*, 166–67; Smith, *The Retreat of Tuberculosis*, 104–5.
200. Dormandy, *The White Death*, 167.
201. *White swelling* was the term used to denote tubercular infection of the joint.
202. WALS, *WC*, Apr. 4, 1855; TNA, MH12/11682, Apr. 5 and Oct. 27, 1855.
203. WALS, WVC, PU/WOL/H/1, June 15, 1894.
204. TNA, MH12/11682, Feb. 2, 1855; Jan. 23, 1856.
205. BCL, VGPC, GP/B/2/8/1/2, Sept. 4, 1857.
206. BCL, IHSC, GP/B/2/4/5/1, Dec. 19, 1898.
207. BCL, ISC, GP/B/2/4/1/4, Nov. 25, 1887.
208. Kamper and Williams, "The Placebo Effect," 6–9.
209. Warner, *The Therapeutic Perspective*, 4.
210. Negrine, "Medicine and Poverty," 80–81.

Chapter Six

1. Wildman, "Changes in Hospital Nursing," 102.
2. Maggs, "Nurse Recruitment," 23.
3. Borsay and Hunter, *Nursing and Midwifery*.
4. Dingwall, Rafferty, and Webster, *An Introduction to the Social History of Nursing*, 157, 160.
5. White, *Social Change*, 3.
6. Versluysen, "Old Wives' Tales?," 181.
7. Lorentzon, "'Lower than a Scullery Maid,'" 4–15, 11.
8. Abel-Smith, *The Hospitals*, 210; Digby, *Pauper Palaces*, 172; White, *Social Change*, 198.
9. For example, Hawkins, *Nursing and Women's Labour*; Borsay and Hunter, *Nursing and Midwifery*.
10. Helmstadter and Godden, *Nursing before Nightingale*, 72–73, 123.
11. Baly, *Florence Nightingale*, 38, 219.
12. Crowther, *The Workhouse System*, 165.
13. Abel-Smith, *A History of the Nursing Profession*, 9.

14. HCPP, 1866 (469), *Workhouses (Metropolis). Copy of a Circular Issued by the Poor Law Board to the Metropolitan Guardians, Calling upon Them to Appoint Trained Nurses to Attend the Sick in the Workhouses of the Metropolis, Dated May 1865*, 1–2.
15. Anonymous, "The Lancet Sanitary Commission," 19.
16. White, *Social Change*, 78–81.
17. HCPP, 1849 (306), *Poor Law. Return of the Number of Officers Employed in 591 Unions, with the Amount of Salaries, for the Year 1844–5; and Expense of Poor Law Commission for the Year Ended 31 March 1849, &c*, 1.
18. Hodgkinson, *The Origins of the National Health Service*, 570.
19. HCPP, 1896 (371), *The Number of Sick Persons Occupying the Wards for the Sick*, 2–5, 4–5, 28–29; Abel-Smith, *The Hospitals*, 51.
20. HCPP, 1909 [Cd. 4573], *Royal Commission on the Poor Laws*, 48–49.
21. Baly, *Florence Nightingale*, 100.
22. White, *Social Change*, 75.
23. Helmstadter and Godden, *Nursing before Nightingale*, 8, 10, 52.
24. BCL, VGPC, GP/B/2/8/1/1, Dec. 10 and 17, 1852; BBG, GP/B/2/1/12, Dec. 1, 1852; TNA, MH12/13298, Feb. 11, 1852; MH12/13299, July 7, 1853.
25. BCL, HC, GP/B/2/3/1/1, Apr. 4, 1842.
26. Wildman, "The Development of Nursing," 21, 24; Hawkins, *Nursing*, 67–68.
27. WALS, HC, PU/WOL/E/1, June 15 and Oct. 5, 1904.
28. Brown and Stones, *The Male Nurse*, 15; Mackintosh, "A Historical Study of Men in Nursing," 232.
29. TNA, MH12/13326, Mar. 3 and Apr. 13, 1877.
30. TNA, MH12/13290, July 1846.
31. TNA, MH12/13298, Dec. 31, 1851.
32. Smith, "Behind Closed Doors," 307.
33. Maggs, "Nurse Recruitment," 27–28.
34. BCL, HC, GP/B/2/3/1/1, May 28, 1844; CEB, 1841.
35. Abel-Smith, *A History of the Nursing Profession*, 4.
36. Borsay, "Nursing, 1700–1830," 39.
37. Helmstadter and Godden, *Nursing before Nightingale*, 11, 27.
38. White, *Social Change*, 8, 24; Helmstadter and Godden, *Nursing before Nightingale*, 35–37.
39. Helmstadter and Godden, *Nursing before Nightingale*, 25–26.
40. Wildman, "'Docile Bodies,'" 13–17; Helmstadter and Godden, *Nursing before Nightingale*, 59.
41. BCL, BBG, GP/B/2/1/2, June 2, 1818.
42. WALS, Resolutions passed by the Guardians as to the Duties of Officers, PU/WOL/L, Oct. 27, 1890.
43. BCL, HSC, GP/B/2/3/3/22, Apr. 9, 1907.
44. Wildman, "The Development of Nursing," 21.

45. WALS, WBG, PU/WOL/A/14, Mar. 18, 1870.
46. WALS, WBG, PU/WOL/A/30, Oct. 10, 1902.
47. BCL, IMC, GP/B/2/4/4/6, Feb. 27, 1911.
48. BCL, IC(H), GP/B/2/4/8/1, Sept. 10, 1913.
49. Negrine, "Medicine and Poverty," 106, 111.
50. Railton and Barr, *Battle Workhouse*, 37–38.
51. WALS, WBG, PU/WOL/A/2, Dec. 3 and 27, 1839.
52. WALS, WBG, PU/WOL/A/2, Feb. 21 and May 15, 1840; Jan. 1, 1841; CEB, 1841.
53. WALS, WBG, PU/WOL/A/3, June 24, 1842; May 26, 1843; MJ, PU/WOL/U/2, May 27, 1843.
54. WALS, WBG, PU/WOL/A/4, July 7 and 14, 1843; MJ, PU/WOL/U/2, July 8, 1843.
55. WALS, MJ, PU/WOL/U/2, May 3, 1845.
56. WALS, PU/ WOL/A/12, Mar. 31, 1865; BCL, VGPC, GP/B/2/8/1/5, Mar. 23, 1866.
57. WALS, PU/WOL/A/11, May 11 and 18, June 1, 1860; *WC*, May 23, 1860; CEB, 1861.
58. WALS, WBG, PU/WOL/A/5, June 11, 1847; TNA, MH12/11677, July 16 and Aug. 16, 1845.
59. WALS, *WC*, June 23, 1847.
60. WALS, WBG, PU/WOL/A/6, July 16 and Aug. 13, 1847; CEB, 1851.
61. TNA, MH12/13298, Jan. 22 and Feb. 11, 1852.
62. WALS, WBG, PU/WOL/A/11, July 4, 1862.
63. Higgs, *Life*, 131.
64. WALS, WBG, PU/WOL/A/8, Oct. 29, 1852; Mar. 30, 1855; *WC*, Apr. 4, 1855.
65. WALS, WBG, PU/WOL/A/9, Oct. 3, 1856.
66. WALS, WBG, PU/WOL/A/13, Jan. 18 and Feb. 1, 1867; Jan 3, 1868.
67. WALS, WBG, PU/WOL/A/19, Nov. 11, 1881.
68. WALS, WBG, PU/WOL/A/16, Aug. 13, Oct. 1 and 22, 1875.
69. WALS, WBG, PU/WOL/A/18, 19, Mar. 25, Apr. 23, and Sept. 24, 1880.
70. WALS, WBG, PU/WOL/A/11, Jan. 11 and 18, 1861; May 9 and 23, 1862.
71. WALS, WBG, PU/WOL/A/12, Jan. 25 and Feb. 8, 1867.
72. WALS, WBG, PU/WOL/A/18, Apr. 2, 1880; PU/WOL/A/24, Jan. 12, 1893.
73. WALS, WBG, PU/WOL/A/15, June 13, 1873; *WC*, June 18 and July 30, 1873.
74. WALS, WBG, PU/WOL/A/9, Sept. 12 and 19, 1856.
75. WALS, WBG, PU/WOL/A/12, Aug. 4, 1865; *WC*, Apr. 19, 1865.
76. WALS, WBG, PU/WOL/A/13, Apr. 24 and July 17, 1868.
77. WALS, *WC*, July 6, 1870.
78. WALS, *WC*, Aug. 25 and Sept. 8, 1871.
79. WALS, WBG, PU/WOL/A/15, Dec. 29, 1871; Jan. 5, 1872.
80. WALS, WBG, PU/WOL/A/16, Feb. 11, 1876.

81. White, *Social Change*, 74; Wildman, "The Development of Nursing," 22.
82. WALS, WBG, PU/WOL/A/18, June 18, 1880.
83. WALS, WBG, PU/WOL/A/18, Feb. 2, 1882.
84. WALS, MJ, PU/WOL/U/2, Apr. 16, 1842; WBG, PU/WOL/A/22, Apr. 6, 1888.
85. WALS, WBG, PU/WOL/A/16, July 31 and Aug. 21, 1874; *WC*, Feb. 17, 1875.
86. HCPP, 1867–68 (4), *Provincial Workhouses*, 153; WALS, *WC*, July 11, 1866, and Apr. 4, 1888; WBG, PU/WOL/A/22, Apr. 6, 1888. The figures are not directly comparable, as the first excludes those "of unsound mind" from the patient total, and the second excludes "idiots and imbeciles," but they give a fair estimate of the increase in the nurses' workload.
87. White, *Social Change*, 26, 74.
88. Maggs, "Nurse Recruitment," 33; he found that 16 percent of probationers in the early twentieth century left their training early for this reason.
89. Helmstadter and Godden, *Nursing before Nightingale*, 53, 188, 191.
90. BCL, BBG, GP/B/2/1/2, Feb. 11, 1818; July 1, 1823.
91. Wildman, "The Development of Nursing," 22.
92. BCL, HC, GP/B/2/3/1/1, Mar. 29 and Apr. 5, 1842.
93. BCL, HC, GP/B/2/3/1/1, June 7 and 14, July 5 and 19, 1842.
94. BCL, BBG, GP/B/2/1/5, July 8, 1845.
95. BCL, HC, GP/B/2/3/1/1, July 11, 1843; Apr. 16 and May 28, 1844.
96. BCL, BBG, GP/B/2/1/4, Oct. 11, 1842.
97. BCL, BBG, GP/B/2/1/4, July 31 and Aug. 14, 1845.
98. BCL, BBG, GP/B/2/1/6, June 26, 1849.
99. BCL, BBG, Apr. 24, Apr. 9 to Dec. 24, 1849.
100. Wildman, "The Development of Nursing," 24.
101. BCL, HC, GP/B/2/3/1/1, Jan. 2, 1844.
102. BCL, HC, GP/B/2/3/1/1, June 13, 1843; Mar. 26 and Nov. 5, 1844; Feb. 26, 1845; BBG, GP/B/2/1/5, Feb. 3, 1846; GP/B/2/1/6, May 29, 1849.
103. BCL, BBG, GP/B/2/1/7, Mar. 19, 1850; CEB, 1851.
104. BCL, BBG, GP/B/2/1/11, June 16 and Sept. 22, 1852.
105. BCL, BBG, GP/B/2/1/18, May 7, July 16 and 23, 1856.
106. BCL, *Returns Relating to the Numbers of Officers and Servants*, GP/B/16/2/1, Oct. 15, 1856.
107. BCL, VGPC, 2/8/1/5, Mar. 25, 1866.
108. HCPP, 1866 (372), *Metropolitan Workhouse Infirmaries*; 1867–68 (4), *Provincial Workhouses*.
109. HCPP, 1866 (372), *Metropolitan Workhouse Infirmaries*, 23–24, 31–32; HCPP, 1867–68 (4), *Provincial Workhouses*, 26–157.
110. HCPP, 186–768 (4), *Provincial Workhouses*, 26–157; Smith noted the nursing experiment using trained nurses was taking place at the time of his visit and gave it a favorable mention.
111. HCPP, 1867–68 (4), *Provincial Workhouses*, 152–53.
112. BCL, HSC, GP/B/2/3/3/4, Nov. 17, 1874; Feb. 9 and 23, 1875.

113. Wildman, "The Development of Nursing," 22.
114. BCL, HSC, GP/B/2/3/3/5, Apr. 18, 1876; the amount was based on her salary, plus a notional amount for board and lodgings.
115. BCL, WISC, GP/B/2/3/11/1, Mar. 23, 1878; VGPC, GP/B/2/8/1//7, May 3, 1878; BBG, GP/B/2/1/46, July 31, 1878; CEB, 1881.
116. TNA, MH12/13336, Jan. 31, 1881.
117. TNA, MH12/13338, Dec. 15, 1881.
118. TNA, MH12/13298, Dec. 31, 1851.
119. BCL, VGPC, GP/B/2/8/1/8, Oct. 28, 1881; CEB, 1881.
120. Hawkins, *Nursing*, 148.
121. BCL, VGPC, GP/B/2/8/1/8, Nov. 25, 1881.
122. BCL, ISC, GP/B/2/4/1/1, July 28, 1882; GP/B/2/4/1/2, Nov. 2, 1883; GP/B/2/4/1/4, Jan. 6, 1888.
123. WALS, WBG, PU/WOL/A/28, Mar. 9, 1900.
124. BCL, BBG, GP/B/2/1/51, Dec. 12, 1883.
125. BCL, ISC, GP/B/2/4/1/1, Mar. 9, 1883; Oct. 3, 1884.
126. TNA, MH12/13349, Dec. 3, 1885.
127. BCL, GP/B/(ACC 2009/109), Box 15.
128. Pickstone, *Medicine and Industrial Society*, 217.
129. BCL, HSC, GP/B/2//3/2/12, June 23, 1891; WMC, GP/B/2/3/2/1, July 10, 1891.
130. BCL, HSC, GP/B/2/3/3/13, Sept. 8, 1891.
131. BCL, WMC, GP/B/2/3/2/4, May 4 and June 29, 1906; HSC, GP/B/2/3/3/22, June 26, 1906.
132. BCL, WMC, GP/B/2/3/2/5, Jan. 10 and Feb. 5, 1908.
133. BCL, WMC, GP/B/2/3/2/6, June 16, 1911.
134. For example, Crowther, *The Workhouse System*, 188; Digby, *Pauper Palaces*, 172.
135. White, *Social Change*, 198–99.
136. HCPP, 1902 [Cd. 1367], *Report of the Departmental Committee Appointed by the President of the Local Government Board to Enquire into the Nursing of the Sick Poor in Workhouses. Part II* (hereafter *Report of the Departmental Committee*), 56.
137. Abel-Smith, *A History of the Nursing Profession*, 40.
138. White, *Social Change*, 33–34; HCPP, 1867–68 (4), *Provincial Workhouse*, 112.
139. Baly, *Florence Nightingale*, 90–100.
140. BCL, ISC, GP/B/2/4/1/2, Nov. 2 and Dec. 6, 1883; GP/B/2/4/1/4, Nov. 4, 1887; May 18, 1888.
141. BCL, IMC, GP/B/2/4/4/1, Dec. 21, 1888.
142. BCL, IMC, GP/B/2/4/4/1, Aug. 17, 1888; BBG, GP/B/2/1/57, June 29 and Sept. 19, 1888.
143. White, *Social Change*, 96, 100.
144. BCL, IMC, GP/B/2/4/4/1, June 20, 1889; GP/B/2/4/4/2, Jan. 26, 1894.
145. TNA, MH12/13365, Feb. 26, 1892.

146. Abel-Smith, *A History of the Nursing Profession*, 23–24.
147. HCPP, 1896 (371), *The Number of Sick Persons Occupying the Wards for the Sick*, 26–29; Wildman, "The Development of Nursing," 23.
148. Anonymous, "On Nursing in Workhouse Infirmaries," 857–59; Maggs, *The Origins of General Nursing*, 90.
149. BCL, IHSC, GP/B/2/4/5/1, Oct. 23, 1899.
150. Wildman, "The Development of Nursing," 23.
151. HCPP, 1902 [Cd. 1367], *Report of the Departmental Committee*, 158.
152. BCL, IHSC, GP/B/2/4/5/4, Mar. 26, 1906.
153. WALS, WBG, PU/WOL/A/24, June 9 and July 21, 1893; WVC, PU/WOL/H/1, May 19 and June 9, 1893.
154. WALS, *WC*, July 26, 1893.
155. WALS, WBG, PU/WOL/A/24, Feb. 2 and 16, July 6, 1894; *WC*, June 20, 1893.
156. Lorentzen, "'Lower than a Scullery Maid," 9.
157. HCPP, 1902 [Cd. 1366], 9.
158. WALS, WBG, PU/WOL/A/25, Oct. 9, 1896; WVC, PU/WOL/H/2, Oct. 1, 1897.
159. BCL, IHSC, GP/B/2/4/5/3, Feb. 9, 1903.
160. WALS, WVC, PU/WOL/11/2, Mar. 24 and July 24, 1896; Jan. 28 and Feb. 11, 1898.
161. WALS, WBG, PU/WOL/A/27, May 13 and 20, June 3, 1898.
162. HCPP, 1902 [Cd. 1366], *Report of the Departmental Committee Appointed by the President of the Local Government Board to Enquire into the Nursing of the Sick Poor in Workhouses. Part I*, 155.
163. WALS, WBG, PU/WOL/A/28, June 8, 1900.
164. WALS, GPC, PU/WOL/E/1, Dec. 2, 1903.
165. WALS, HC, PU/WOL/E/2, Nov. 12, 1907.
166. WALS, WBG, PU/WOL/A/31, July 29, 1904; PU/WOL/A/34, Apr. 1, 1910.
167. WALS, WBG, PU/WOL/A/31, July 28, 1905; HC, PU/WOL/E/2, Mar. 9, 1905.
168. WALS, HC, PU/WOL/E/1, June 4, 1903; Feb. 23, 1905.
169. WALS, SC, PU/WOL/P/1, Nov. 30, 1906.
170. WALS, SC, PU/WOL/P/1, Nov. 30, 1906.
171. WALS, HC, PU/WOL/E/2, July 25, 1907.
172. WALS, HC, PU/WOL/E/2, Mar. 5, 1908.
173. BCL, HC, GP/B/2/3/1/1, June 13, 1843.
174. BCL, HSC, GP/B/2/3/3/8, July 4, 1882; ISC, GP/B/2/4/1/1, Nov. 10, 1882.
175. BCL, ISC, 2/4/1/2, Sept. 4, 1855.
176. WALS, WBG, PU/WOL/A/15, June 13, 1873.
177. WALS WBG, PU/WOL/A/33, Jan. 3, 1908.
178. WALS, HC, PU/WOL/E/4, Jan. 4, 1912.
179. Borsay and Hunter, *Nursing and Midwifery*, 21.

180. WALS, WBG, PU/WOL/A/13, Sept. 25, 1868; Jan. 19, 1869.
181. BCL, HC, GP/B/2/3/1/1, Jan. 16, 1844.
182. Helmstadter and Godden, *Nursing before Nightingale*, 12, 18, 39.
183. BCL, VGPC, GP/B/2/2/1/1, May 12, 1854.
184. BCL, WMC, GP/B/2/3/2/1, June 15, 1888.
185. WALS, MJ, PU/WOL/U/2, Sept. 9, 1843.
186. WALS, WBG, PU/WOL/A/16, May 14, 1875.
187. WALS, WVC, PU/WOL/H/2, Dec. 1, 1899.
188. WALS, WBG, PU/WOL/A/33, Dec. 20, 1907.
189. Crowther, *The Workhouse System*, 166; Hodgkinson, *The Origins of the National Health Service*, 169.
190. Price, *Medical Negligence*, 127.
191. King, "Nursing under the Old Poor Law," 588–622.
192. Helmstadter and Godden, *Nursing before Nightingale*.
193. King, "Nursing under the Old Poor Law," 12–13.
194. Maggs, "Nurse Recruitment," 23.
195. Gamarnikow, "Nurse or Woman," 110.
196. Gamarnikow, "Sexual Division of Labour," 114; Mackintosh, "A Historical Study of Men in Nursing," 233.
197. Hart, *Nurses and Politics*, 102.
198. Dingwall, "The Place of Men in Nursing," 199, 202.
199. BCL, BBG, GP/B/2/1/51, Dec. 12, 1883.
200. Hawkins, *Nursing*, 77.

Chapter Seven

1. Hitchcock, "Review of 'Jonathan Reinarz and Leonard Schwarz,'" 821–23.
2. King, *Sickness, Medical Welfare*, 114, 253–54, 332.
3. HCPP, 1870 (468-I), *Poor Relief*, 12–14, 19–21, 29.
4. Pickstone, *Medicine and Industrial Society*, 178.
5. Stewart and King, "Death in Llantrisant," 81.
6. Price, "'The Shape of the Iceberg,'" 129–46.
7. Price, "A Regional, Quantitative and Qualitative Study," 109–10, 339.
8. Price, *Medical Negligence*, 13, 126–27.
9. Ritch, "History of Geriatric Medicine," 372–73.
10. BCL, BBG, GP/B/2/1/61, Feb. 1, 1893.
11. BCL, VGPC, GP/B/2/8/1/9, Sept. 26, 1884.
12. BCL, WIMC, GP/B/2/4/4/4, Dec. 15, 1902; Bright's disease is a group of diseases characterized by inflammation of the kidneys and edema of the lower body.
13. WALS, *WC*, May 22, 1895.

Bibliography

Archival Sources

Birmingham Central Library, Archives and Heritage Service, Birmingham
House of Commons Parliamentary Papers
Royal College of Physicians of London
The National Archives, London
Wolverhampton Archives and Local Studies, Wolverhampton

Published Sources

Abel-Smith, Brian. *A History of the Nursing Profession*. London: Heinemann, 1960.
———. *The Hospitals 1800–1948: A Study in Social Administration in England and Wales*. London: Heinemann, 1964.
Ackerknecht, Erwin H. *Medicine at the Paris Hospital 1794–1848*. Baltimore, MD: Johns Hopkins University Press, 1967.
Aitken, W. C. "Brass and Brass Manufactures." In *Birmingham and the Midland Hardware District*, edited by Samuel Timmins, 225–380. London: Frank Cass & Co. Ltd., 1967.
Anderson, Julia, and Ana Carden-Coyne. "Enabling the Past: New Perspectives in the History of Disability." *European Review of History* 14, no. 4 (2007): 447–57.
Anonymous. "Birmingham." *The Lancet* 1 (1874): 109.
———. "Birmingham Workhouse Infirmary." *The Lancet* 1 (1889): 47.
———. "Birmingham Workhouse Infirmary. A Case of Peritonitis Following Parturition." *The Lancet* 2 (1891): 1276–77.
———. "Charge against the Medical Staff of the Birmingham Workhouse." *British Medical Journal* 2 (1881): 993.
———. "Dr. Edward Smith's Reports on the Treatment of the Sick in Selected Provincial Workhouses." *The Lancet* 1 (1868): 166–68.
———. "Editorial." *The Lancet* 2 (1888): 1244–45.
———. "The Lancet Sanitary Commission for Investigating the State of the Infirmaries of Workhouses." *The Lancet* 2 (1865): 14–22.

———. "The Lancet Sanitary Commission for Investigating the State of the Infirmaries of Workhouses. Country Workhouse Infirmaries. No. IV. Wolverhampton Workhouse, Staffordshire." *The Lancet* 2 (1867): 555–56.

———. "Obituary. Edmund Bancks Whitcombe." *British Medical Journal* 1 (1911): 1353.

———. "On Nursing in Workhouse Infirmaries." *British Medical Journal* 2 (1896): 857–62.

———. "Reports of Medical Officers of Health." *The Lancet* 2 (1902): 178.

———. "Reports of the Old Cholera Haunts and Modern Fever Nests of London." *The Lancet* 2 (1865): 656–58.

Ashforth, David. "The Urban Poor Law." In *The New Poor Law in the Nineteenth Century*, edited by Derek Fraser, 128–48. London: Macmillan Press, 1976.

Ayers, Gwendoline M. *England's First State Hospitals and the Metropolitan Asylums Board 1867–1930*. London: Wellcome Institute of the History of Medicine, 1971.

Baly, Monica E. *Florence Nightingale and the Nursing Legacy*. London: Croom Helm, 1986.

Barling, S. G. *The History of the Birmingham Medical School 1825–1925*. Birmingham, UK: Cornish Brothers Ltd., 1925.

Barnsby, G. J. *Social Conditions in the Black Country 1800–1900*. Wolverhampton, UK: Integrated Publishing Services, 1980.

Bentley, A. O. *A Text-book of Pharmaceutics*. London: Bailliere, Tindall, and Cox, 1933.

Bergen, Amanda N. "The Blind, the Deaf and the Halt." PhD diss., University of Leeds, 2004.

Booth, Charles. *The Aged Poor in England and Wales*. London: Macmillan and Co., 1894.

Borsay, Anne. *Disability and Social Policy in Britain Since 1750: A History of Exclusion*. Basingstoke, UK: Palgrave Macmillan, 2005.

———. "History, Power and Identity." In *Disability Studies Today*, edited by Colin Barnes, Mike Oliver, and Len Barton, 98–119. Cambridge: Polity Press, 2002.

———. "Nursing, 1700–1830: Families, Communities, Institutions." In *Nursing and Midwifery in Britain Since 1700*, edited by Anne Borsay and Billlie Hunter. Basingstoke, UK: Palgrave Macmillan, 2012.

Borsay, Anne, and Billie Hunter, eds. *Nursing and Midwifery in Britain Since 1700*. Basingstoke, UK: Palgrave Macmillan, 2012.

Bosworth, Ennis C. "Public Healthcare in Nottingham 1750–1911." PhD diss., University of Nottingham, 1998.

Boulton, Jeremy, Romola Davenport, and Leonard Schwarz. "'These ANTE-CHAMBERS OF THE GRAVE?' Mortality, Medicine and the Workhouse in Georgian London, 1725–1824." In *Medicine and the Workhouse*, edited by Jonathan Reinarz and Leonard Schwarz. Rochester: University of Rochester Press, 2013.

Boulton, Jeremy, and Leonard Schwarz. "The Medicalisation of a Parish Workhouse in Georgian Westminster: St. Martin in the Fields, 1725–1824." *Family & Community History* 17, no. 2 (2014): 122–40.

Bradley, Sarah, Pam Jones, and Jane Somerwell. "Who Cared? Death, Dirt and Disease in the Bromsgrove Poor Law Union." In *Pauper Prisons, Pauper Palaces: The Victorian Poor Law in the East and West Midlands 1834–1871*, edited by Paul Carter and Kate Thompson, 75–101. Beauchamp, UK: Matador, 2018.

Brand, Jeanne L. *Doctors and the State: The British Medical Profession and Government Action in Public Health, 1870–1912*. Baltimore, MD: Johns Hopkins University Press, 1965.

———. "The Parish Doctor: England's Poor Law Medical Officers and Medical Reform, 1870–1900." *Bulletin of the History of Medicine* 35, no. 2 (1961): 97–122.

Briggs, Asa. *History of Birmingham*. Vol. 2, *Borough and City, 1865–1938*. London: Oxford University Press, 1952.

Brock, W. H. "Liebigiana: Old and New Perspectives." *History of Science* 19, no. 3 (1981): 201–18.

Brown, R. G. S., and R. W. H. Stones. *The Male Nurse*. London: G. Bell & Sons, 1973.

Buchan, W. *Domestic Medicine*. 6th ed. London: Strachan, T. Cadell, and J. Balfour, 1799.

Bunce, J. T. "The Social and Economical Aspects of Birmingham." In *Birmingham and the Midland Hardware District*, edited by Samuel Timmins, 683–88. London: Frank Cass & Co. Ltd., 1967.

Burch, Susan, and Ian Sutherland. "Who's Not Yet Here? American Disability History." *Radical History Review* 94 (Winter 2006): 127–47.

Burton-Fanning, F. W. *The Open-Air Treatment of Tuberculosis*. London: Cassell, 1909.

Butler, Graham A. "Disease, Medicine and the Urban Poor in Newcastle-upon-Tyne, c. 1750–1850." PhD diss., Newcastle University, 2012.

Bynum, Helen. *Spitting Blood: The History of Tuberculosis*. Oxford: Oxford University Press, 2012.

Bynum, W. F. "Cullen and the Study of Fevers in Britain, 1760–1820." *Medical History*, Supplement, no. 1 (1981): 135–47.

———. *Science and the Practice of Medicine in the Nineteenth Century*. Cambridge: Cambridge University Press, 1994.

Cantor, D. "The Contradictions of Specialization: Rheumatism and the Decline of the Spa in Inter-war Britain." In "The Medical History of Waters and Spas," edited by Roy Porter. *Medical History* Supplement 10 (1990): 127–44.

Clark, Michael J. "The Rejection of Psychological Approaches to Mental Disorder in Late Nineteenth-Century British Psychiatry." In *Madhouses, Mad-Doctors, and Madmen: The Social History of Psychiatry in the Victorian Era*, edited by Andrew Scull, 272–39. London: Athlone Press, 1981.

Clouston, Thomas S. *Unsoundness of Mind*. New York: E. P. Dutton and Company, 1911.

Cockin, Tim. *The Staffordshire Encyclopaedia*. Stoke-on-Trent, UK: Malthouse Press, 2006.

Condrau, Flurin. "Beyond the Total Institution: Towards a Reinterpretation of the Tuberculosis Sanatorium." In *Tuberculosis Then and Now*, edited by Flurin Condrau and Michael Worboys, 72–99. Montreal, QC: McGill-Queen's University Press, 2010.

Creighton, Charles. *A History of Epidemics*. Vol. 2, 2nd ed. London: F. Cass, 1965.

Crompton, Frank. *Workhouse Children*. Stroud, UK: Sutton, 1997.

Cronjé, Gillian. "Tuberculosis and Mortality Decline in England and Wales, 1851–1910." In *Urban Disease and Mortality in Nineteenth-Century England*, edited by Robert Woods and John Woodward, 79–101. London: Batsford Academic and Educational, 1984.

Crowther, Anne. "Health Care and Poor Relief in Provincial England." In *Health Care and Poor Relief in 18th and 19th Century Northern Europe*, edited by Ole P. Grell, Andrew Cunningham, and Robert Jütte, 203–19. Aldershot, UK: Ashgate, 2002.

Crowther, M. A. "Paupers or Patients? Obstacles to Professionalisation in the Poor Law Medical Service before 1914." *Journal of the History of Medicine* 39, no. 1 (1984): 33–54.

———. *The Workhouse System 1834–1929*. London: Methuen, 1981.

Currie, Margaret R. *Fever Hospital and Fever Nurses: A British Social History of Fever Nurses: A National Service*. London: Routledge, 2004.

Davies, J. Redfern. "Birmingham Workhouse Infirmary." *British Medical Journal* 1 (1858): 677.

———. "On the Radical Cure of Varicocele." *The Lancet* 2 (1861): 60.

Davies, Redfern. "Birmingham Workhouse Infirmary." *British Medical Journal* 1 (1859): 284.

———. "Remarks on the Operative and Mechanical Treatment of Prolapsus Uteri." *The Lancet* 1 (1864): 407–8.

Denham, Michael J. "The History of Geriatric Medicine and Hospital Care of the Elderly in England between 1929 and the 1970s." PhD diss., University of London, 2004.

———. "The Surveys of the Birmingham Chronic Sick Hospitals, 1948–1960s." *Social History Medicine* 19, no. 2 (2006): 279–93.

Dick, Malcolm. "The City of a Thousand Trades, 1700–1945." In *Birmingham: The Workshop of the World*, edited by Carl Chinn and Malcolm Dick, 125–57. Liverpool, UK: Liverpool University Press, 2016.

Digby, Anne. *Making a Medical Living: Doctors and Patients in the English Market for Medicine, 1720–1911*. Cambridge: Cambridge University Press, 1994.

———. *Pauper Palaces*. London: Routledge and Kegan Paul, 1978.

———. *The Poor Law in Nineteenth-Century England and Wales*. London: Historical Association, 1982.

Dingwall, Robert, Anne Marie Rafferty, and Charles Webster, eds. *An Introduction to the Social History of Nursing*. London: Routledge, 1988.
———. "The Place of Men in Nursing." In *Readings in Nursing*, edited by Malcolm M. Colledge and Dan Jones, 199–209. Edinburgh: Churchill Livingstone, 1979.
Dobson, Mary. *Disease, the Extraordinary Stories behind History's Deadliest Killers*. London: Quercus, 2007.
Dormandy, Thomas. *The White Death*. London: Hambledon Press, 1999.
Driver, Felix. *Power and Pauperism: The Workhouse System 1834–1884*. Cambridge: Cambridge University Press, 2004.
Eadie, Mervyn J., and Peter F. Bladin. *A Disease Once Sacred: A History of the Medical Understanding of Epilepsy*. Eastleigh, UK: John Libbey and Company Ltd., 2001.
Eden, Sir Frederick Morton. *The State of the Poor*. Vol. 3. London: B. & J. White, 1797.
Edwards, Claudia. "Age-Based Rationing of Medical Care in Nineteenth-Century England." *Community and Change* 14, no. 2 (1999): 227–65.
Elliot, Paul. "'More Subtle than the Electric Aura': Georgian Medical Electricity, the Spirit of Animation and the Development of Erasmus Darwin's Psychophysiology." *Medical History* 52, no. 2 (2008): 195–220.
Finer, S. E. *The Life and Times of Sir Edwin Chadwick*. London: Routledge, 1997.
Fissell, Mary E. *Patients, Power, and the Poor in Eighteenth-Century Bristol*. Cambridge: Cambridge University Press, 1991.
Flinn, M. W. "Medical Services under the New Poor Law." In *The New Poor Law in the Nineteenth Century*, edited by Derek Fraser, 45–56. London: Macmillan Press, 1976.
Fowler, Simon. *Workhouse: The People, the Places, the Life behind Doors*. Richmond, UK: National Archives, 2007.
Fraser, Derek. *The Evolution of the British Welfare State*. Basingstoke, UK: Palgrave Macmillan, 2003.
Friedlander, Walter J. *The History of Modern Epilepsy: The Beginning, 1865–1914*. London: Greenwood Press, 2001.
Gairdner, W. T. "Facts and Conclusions as to the Use of Alcoholic Stimulants in Typhus Fever." *The Lancet* 1 (1864): 291–94.
Gamarnikow, E. "Nurse or Woman: Gender and Professionalism in Reformed Nursing 1860–1923." In *Anthropology and Nursing*, edited by Pat Holden and Jenny Littlewood, 110–29. London: Routledge, 1991.
———. "Sexual Division of Labour; The Case for Nursing." In *Feminism and Materialism*, edited by Annette Kuhn and AnnMarie Wolpe, 1–10. London: Routledge and Kegan Paul, 1978.
Gehrke, Jules P. "A Radical Endeavor: Joseph Chamberlain and the Emergence of Municipal Socialism in Birmingham." *American Journal of Economics and Sociology* 75, no. 1 (2016): 23–51.
General Council of Medical Education and Registration of the United Kingdom. *The British Pharmacopoeia 1932*. London: The General Medical Council, 1932.

Gestrich, Andres, Elizabeth Hurren, and Steven King. "Narratives of Poverty and Sickness in Europe 1780–1938: Sources, Methods and Experiences." In *Poverty and Sickness in Modern Europe*, edited by Andreas Gestrich, Elizabeth Hurren, and Steven King, 1–34. London: Continuum, 2012.

———, eds. *Poverty and Sickness in Modern Europe*. London: Continuum, 2012.

Gorsky, Martin. "Creating the Poor Law Legacy: Institutional Care for Older People before the Welfare State." *Contemporary British History* 29, no. 4 (2012): 441–65.

Gorsky, Martin, John Mohan, and Tim Willis. "A 'Splendid Spirit of Co-operation': Hospital Contributory Schemes in Birmingham before the National Health Service." In *Medicine and Society in the Midlands 1750–1950*, edited by Jonathan Reinarz, 167–91. Birmingham, UK: Midland History, 2007.

Graham, Thomas J. *Modern Domestic Medicine*. 10th ed. London: Simpkin and Marshall, 1848.

Gray, James A. *The Edinburgh City Hospital*. East Linton, UK: Tuckwell Press, 1999.

Green, David R. "Icons of the New System: Workhouse Construction and Relief Practices in London under the Old and New Poor Law." *The London Journal* 34, no. 3 (2009): 264–84.

———. "Pauper Protests: Power and Resistance in Early Nineteenth-Century London Workhouses." *Social History* 31, no. 2 (2006): 137–59.

Griffith, George. *History of the Free-Schools, Colleges, Hospitals and Asylums of Birmingham*. London: William Tweedie, 1861.

Hamilton, David. *The Healers: A History of Medicine in Scotland*. Edinburgh: Canongate, 1981.

Hamlin, Christopher. *Public Health and Social Justice in the Age of Chadwick: Britain, 1800–1854*. Cambridge: Cambridge University Press, 1998.

Hardy, Anne. *The Epidemic Streets, Infectious Disease and the Rise of Preventive Medicine, 1856–1900*. Oxford: Clarendon Press, 1993.

———. *Health and Medicine in Britain since 1860*. Basingstoke, UK: Palgrave, 2001.

Harrison, Brian H. *Drink and the Victorians: The Temperance Question in England, 1815–72*. Staffordshire, UK: Keele University Press, 1994.

Hart, Chris. *Nurses and Politics: The Impact of Power and Practice*. Basingstoke, UK: Palgrave Macmillan, 2004.

Hawkins, Sue. *Nursing and Women's Labour in the Nineteenth Century*. Abingdon, UK: Routledge, 2010.

Hearn, George W. *Dudley Road Hospital, 1887–1987*. Birmingham, UK: Postgraduate Centre, Dudley Road Hospital, 1987.

Helmstadter, Carol, and Judith Godden. *Nursing before Nightingale, 1815–1899*. Farnham, UK: Ashgate, 2011.

Hennock, E. P. *Fit and Proper Persons: Ideal and Reality in Nineteenth-Century Urban Government*. London: Edward Arnold, 1973.

———. *The Origins of the Welfare State in England and Germany, 1850–1914: Social Policies Compared*. Cambridge: Cambridge University Press, 2007.

Heslop, T. P. "The Medical Aspects of Birmingham." In *Birmingham and the Midland Hardware District*, edited by Samuel Timmins, 689–703. London: Frank Cass & Co. Ltd., 1967.

Higgs, Michelle. *Life in the Victorian and Edwardian Workhouse*. Stroud, UK: Tempus, 2007.

Hill, Alfred. "The Epidemic of Small-Pox in Birmingham." *Public Health* 8 (1895–96): 5–6.

———. "Remarks on the Incidence of Diphtheria in Birmingham." *Public Health* 8 (1895–96): 342–44.

———. "Reports of Medical Officers of Health." *The Lancet* 2 (1902): 178.

Hitchcock, Tim. "Review of 'Jonathan Reinarz and Leonard Schwarz (eds.), *Medicine and the Workhouse*.'" *Social History of Medicine* 27, no. 4 (2014): 821–23.

Hodgkinson, Ruth G. *The Origins of the National Health Service: The Medical Services of the New Poor Law 1834–71*. London: Wellcome Historical Medical Library, 1967.

———. "Poor Law Medical Officers of England, 1834–1871." *Journal of History of Medicine and Allied Sciences* 11, no. 2 (1956): 299–338.

———. "Provision for Pauper Lunatics 1834–1871." *Medical History* 10, no. 2 (1966): 142.

Hopkins, Donald R. *Princes and Peasants. Smallpox in History*. Chicago: University of Chicago Press, 1983.

Hopkins, Eric. *Birmingham, the Making of the Second City 1850–1939*. Stroud, UK: Tempus, 2001.

Hughes, Bill. "The Constitution of Impairment: Modernity and the Aesthetic of Oppression." *Disability Society* 14, no. 2 (2002): 155–72.

———. "Disability and the Body." In *Disability Studies Today*, edited by Colin Barnes, Mike Oliver, and Len Barton, 58–76. Cambridge: Polity Press, 2002.

Humphreys, Robert. "The Poor Law and Charity: The Charity Organisation Society in the Provinces." PhD diss., University of London, 1991.

Hurren, Elizabeth T. "Poor Law versus Public Health: Diphtheria, Sanitary Reform, and the 'Crusade' against Outdoor Relief, 1870–1900." *Social History of Medicine* 18, no. 3 (2005): 399–418.

Hutchings, Deborah. *Monyhull 1908–1998: A History of Caring*. Studley, UK: Brewin Books, 1998.

Hutton, William. *An History of Birmingham*. 6th ed. Birmingham, UK: James Guest, 1835.

Jackson, David G. "The Medway Union Workhouse, 1876–1881: A Study Based on the Admission and Discharge Registers and the Census Enumerators' Books." *Local Population Studies* 75 (2005): 11–32.

Jackson, R. "Waters and Spas in the Classical World." In "The Medical History of Waters and Spas," edited by Roy Porter. *Medical History* Supplement 10 (1990): 1–13.

Jones, Christine. "Disability in Herefordshire, 1851–1911." *Local Population Studies* 87 (2011): 29–44.

Kamper, S. J., and C. M. Williams, "The Placebo Effect: Powerful, Powerless or Redundant?" *British Journal of Sports Medicine* 47, no. 1 (2013): 6–9.

Keele, Kenneth D. "Clinical Medicine in the 1860s." In *Medicine and Science in the 1860s*, edited by F. N. L. Poynter, 1–11. London: Wellcome Institute of the History of Medicine, 1968.

Kenwood, Henry. "Notes on the Origin of Diphtheria." *Public Health* 8 (1895–96): 344–45.

Kerr, Matthew N. "Sites of Complaint and Complaining; Fever and Smallpox Hospitals in Late-Victorian London." In *Complaints, Controversies and Grievances in Medicine*, edited by Jonathan Reinarz and Rebecca Wynter, 205–22. London: Routledge, 2014.

Kidd, Alan. *State, Society, and the Poor in Nineteenth-Century England.* Basingstoke, UK: Macmillan, 1999.

King, Steven. "Nursing under the Old Poor Law in Midland and Eastern England 1780–1834." *Journal of the History of Medicine and Allied Science* 70, no. 4 (2015): 588–622.

———. *Poverty and Welfare in England 1700–1850.* Manchester, UK: Manchester University Press, 2000.

———. "Poverty, Medicine and the Workhouse in the Eighteenth and Nineteenth Centuries." In *Medicine and the Workhouse*, edited by Jonathan Reinarz and Leonard Schwarz, 228–51. Rochester, NY: University of Rochester Press, 2013.

———. "Regional Patterns in the Treatment of the Sick Poor, 1800–40: Rights, Obligations and Duties in the Rhetoric of Paupers." *Family and Community History* 10, no. 1 (2007): 61–75.

———. *Sickness, Medical Welfare and the English Poor, 1750–1834.* Manchester, UK: Manchester University Press, 2018.

———. "Thinking and Rethinking the New Poor Law." *Local Population Studies* 99 (2017): 5–19.

King, Steven, and Alannah Tomkins. "Introduction." In *The Poor in England, 1700–1850: An Economy of Makeshifts*, edited by Steven King and Alannah Tomkins, 1–35. Manchester, UK: Manchester University Press, 2003.

Kirk, Robert G. W., and Neil Pemberton. *Leech.* London: Reaktion Books, 2013.

Klein, Rudolph. *Complaints against Doctors: A Study in Professional Accountability.* London: C. Knight, 1973.

Lane, Joan. *Social History of Medicine: Health, Healing and Disease in England, 1750–1950.* London: Routledge, 2001.

Langford, John A. *Modern Birmingham and Its Institutions.* Birmingham, UK: William Downing, 1871.

Lawrence, Christopher. *Medicine in the Making of Modern Britain, 1700–1920.* London: Routledge, 1994.

Lees, Lynn Hollen. *The Solidarities of Strangers: The English Poor Laws and the People, 1700–1948.* Cambridge: Cambridge University Press, 1998.

Levene, Alysa. "Between Less Eligibility and the NHS: The Changing Place of Poor Law Hospitals in England and Wales, 1929–39." *Twentieth Century British History* 20, no. 3 (2009): 322–45.

Lipman, Timothy O. "Vitalism and Reductionism in Liebig's Thought." *Isis* 58, no. 2 (1967): 167–85.

Lloyd, Jordan. "On Acute Intestinal Obstruction and Its Treatment by Abdominal Section, with Illustrative Cases." *The Lancet* 1 (1890): 794–96, 844–46.

———. "Reports on Medical and Surgical Practice in the Hospitals and Asylums of Great Britain, Ireland, and the Colonies: Birmingham Workhouse Infirmary." *British Medical Journal* 1 (1892): 16.

Logan, W. P. D. "Mortality in England and Wales from 1848 to 1947." *Population Studies* 4, no. 2 (1950): 132–78.

Lorentzon, Maria. "'Lower than a Scullery Maid.'" *International History of Nursing Journal* 7, no. 3 (2003): 4–15.

Loudon, Irvine. *Medical Care and the General Practitioner 1750–1850*. Oxford: Clarendon Press, 1986.

———. "The Nature of Provincial Medical Practice in Eighteenth-Century England." *Medical History* 29, no. 1 (1985): 1–32.

———. *The Tragedy of Childbed Fever*. Oxford: Oxford University Press, 2000.

Loudon, I. S. L. "Leg Ulcers in the Eighteenth and Early Nineteenth Centuries." *Journal of the Royal College of General Practitioners* 31, no. 226 (1981): 263–73.

Loveridge, Henry. "Wolverhampton Trades." In *Birmingham and the Midland Hardware District*, edited by Samuel Timmins, 117–21. London: Frank Cass & Co. Ltd., 1967.

Lucia, Salvatore P. *A History of Wine as Therapy*. Philadelphia, PA: J. B. Lippincott Company, 1963.

Luckin, Bill. "Evaluating the Sanitary Revolution: Typhus and Typhoid in London, 1851–1900." In *Urban Disease and Mortality in Nineteenth-Century England* edited by Robert Woods and John Woodward, 102–19. London: Batsford Academic and Educational, 1984.

MacKinnon, Mary. "The Use and Misuse of Poor Law Statistics 1857 to 1912." *Historical Methods* 21, no. 1 (1988): 5–19.

Mackintosh, Carolyn. "A Historical Study of Men in Nursing." *Journal of Advanced Nursing* 26, no. 2 (1997): 232–36.

Maggs, Christopher. "Nurse Recruitment to Four Provincial Hospitals 1881–1921." In *Rewriting Nursing History*, edited by Celia Davies, 18–40. London: Croom Helm, 1980.

———. *The Origins of General Nursing*. London: Croom Helm, 1983.

Marland, Hilary. *Medicine and Society in Wakefield and Huddersfield 1780–1870*. Cambridge: Cambridge University Press, 1987.

Marland, Hilary, and Jane Adams. "Hydropathy at Home: The Water Cure and Domestic Healing in Mid-Nineteenth-Century Britain." *Bulletin of the History of Medicine* 83, no. 3 (2009): 499–529.

Mayne, Alan. *The Imagined Slum: Newspaper Representation in Three Cities, 1870–1914*. Leicester, UK: Leicester University Press, 1993.

McKeown, Thomas, and R. G. Record. "Reasons for the Decline of Mortality in England and Wales during the Nineteenth Century." *Population Studies* 16, no. 2 (1962): 94–122.

Mercer, Alexander. *Infections, Chronic Disease, and the Epidemiological Transition: A New Perspective.* Rochester, NY: University of Rochester Press, 2014.

Mooney, Graham. "Infectious Diseases and Epidemiologic Transition in Victorian Britain? Definitely." *Social History of Medicine* 20, no. 3 (2007): 600.

———. *Intrusive Interventions: Public Health, Domestic Space, and Infectious Disease Surveillance in England, 1840–1914.* Rochester, NY: University of Rochester Press, 2015.

———. "'A Tissue of the Most Flagrant Anomalies': Smallpox Vaccination and the Centralization of Sanitary Administration in Nineteenth-Century London." *Medical History* 41, no. 3 (1991): 261–90.

Mooney, Graham, Bill Luckin, and Andrea Tanner. "Patient Pathways: Solving the Problem of Institutional Mortality in London during the Later Nineteenth Century." *Social History of Medicine* 12, no. 2 (1999): 227–69.

Morris, R. J. *Cholera 1832: The Social Response to an Epidemic.* London: Croom Helm, 1976.

Morrison, Kathryn. *The Workhouse: A Study of Poor-Law Buildings in England.* Swindon, UK: English Heritage, 1999.

Morus, Iwan Rhys. *Shocking Bodies: Life, Death and Electricity in Victorian England.* Stroud, UK: History Press, 2011.

Mulcahy, Linda. *Disputing Doctors: The Socio-Legal Dynamics of Complaints about Medical Care.* Maidenhead, UK: Open University Press, 2003.

Negrine, Angela. "Medicine and Poverty: A Study of the Poor Law Medical Services of the Leicester Union 1876–1914." PhD diss., University of Leicester, 2008.

———. "Practitioners and Paupers." In *Medicine and the Workhouse*, edited by J. Reinarz and L. Schwarz, 192–211. Rochester, NY: University of Rochester Press, 2013.

Nicholls, James. *The Politics of Alcohol: A History of the Drink Question in England.* Manchester, UK: Manchester University Press, 2009.

Omran, Abdel R. "The Epidemiological Transition." *Milbank Memorial Fund Quarterly* 49, no. 4 (1971): 509–38.

Oriel, J. David. *The Scars of Venus: A History of Venereology.* London: Springer-Verlag, 1994.

Parish, Lawrence C. "History of Scabies." In *Cutaneous Infestations and Insect Bites*, edited by Milton Orkin and Howard Maibach, 3–8. New York: Dekker, 1985.

Parker, Langston. *The Modern Treatment of Syphilitic Diseases.* Philadelphia, PA: A. Waldie, 1840.

Paul, Harry W. *Bacchic Medicine: Wine and Alcohol Therapies from Napoleon to the French Paradox.* Amsterdam: Rodopi, 2001.

Pelling, Margaret. *Cholera, Fever and English Medicine, 1825–1865.* Oxford: Oxford University Press, 1978.

Pennell, S., and R. Rich. "Food: 'The Forgotten Medicine,'" *Social History of Medicine* (2016). https://academic.oup.com/DocumentLibrary/SOCHIS/food-the-forgotten-medicine-vi.pdf.

Peyton, Edward. "Manufacture of Iron and Brass Bedsteads." In *Birmingham and the Midland Hardware District*, edited by Samuel Timmins, 624–27. London: Frank Cass & Co. Ltd., 1967.

Pickstone, John V. *Medicine and Industrial Society: A History of Hospital Development in Manchester and Its Regions 1752–1946.* Manchester, UK: Manchester University Press, 1985.

Pinches, Sylvia M. "Charities in Warwickshire in the Eighteenth and Nineteenth Centuries." PhD diss., University of Leicester, 2000.

Pinker, Robert. *English Hospital Statistics, 1861–1938.* London: Heinemann, 1966.

Peterson, M. Jeanne. *The Medical Profession in Mid-Victorian London.* Berkeley: University of California Press, 1978.

Price, Kim P. *Medical Negligence in Victorian Britain: The Crisis of Care under English Poor Law, c. 1834–1900.* London: Bloomsbury, 2015.

———. "A Regional, Quantitative and Qualitative Study of the Employment, Disciplining and Discharging of Workhouse Medical Officers of the New Poor Law throughout Nineteenth-Century England and Wales." PhD diss., Oxford Brookes University, 2008.

———. "'The Shape of the Iceberg': Doctors and Neglect under the New Poor Law, c.1871–1900." In *Complaints, Controversies and Grievances in Medicine*, edited by J. Reinarz and R. Wynter, 128–53. London: Routledge, 2014.

Price, Robin. "Hydropathy in England 1840–1870." *Medical History* 25, no. 3 (1981): 269–80.

Railton, Margaret, and Marshall Barr. *Battle Workhouse and Hospital 1867–2005.* Reading, UK: Berkshire Medical Heritage Centre, 2005.

Razell, Peter. *The Conquest of Smallpox.* Firle, UK: Caliban Books, 1977.

Reinarz, Jonathan. *The Birth of a Provincial Hospital: The Early Years of the General Hospital, Birmingham, 1765–1790.* Stratford-upon-Avon, UK: Dugdale Society, 2003.

———. *Health Care in Birmingham: The Birmingham Teaching Hospitals 1779–1939.* Woodbridge, UK: Boydell Press, 2009.

———. "Investigating the 'Deserving' Poor: Charity and the Voluntary Hospitals in Nineteenth-Century Birmingham." In *Medicine, Charity and Mutual Aid: The Consumption of Health and Welfare in Britain, c. 1550–1950*, edited by Anne Borsay and Peter Shapely, 111–33. Aldershot, UK: Ashgate, 2007.

Reinarz, Jonathan, and Alistair Ritch. "Exploring Medical Care in the Nineteenth-Century Provincial Workhouse: A View from Birmingham." In *Medicine and the Workhouse*, edited by Jonathan Reinarz and Leonard Schwarz, 140–63. Rochester, NY: University of Rochester Press, 2013.

Reinarz, Jonathan, and Leonard Schwarz, eds. *Medicine and the Workhouse.* Rochester, NY: University of Rochester Press, 2013.

Reinarz, Jonathan, and Rebecca Wynter. "The Spirit of Medicine: The Use of Alcohol in Nineteenth-Century Medical Practice." In *Drink in the Eighteenth and Nineteenth Centuries*, edited by Susanne Schmid and Barbara Schmidt-Haberkamp, 121–41. London: Pickering & Chatto, 2014.

Richardson, Harriet. *English Hospitals 1660–1948*. Swindon, UK: Royal Commission on the Historical Monuments of England, 1998.

Riley, James C. *Sick, Not Dead: The Health of British Workingmen during the Mortality Decline*. Baltimore, MD: Johns Hopkins University Press, 1997.

Riley, J. W. "Operation for Strangulated Femoral Hernia in a Man Ninety Years of Age; Recovery." *The Lancet* 2 (1879): 110.

Risse, Guenter B. "Brunonian Therapeutics: New Wine in Old Bottles?" *Medical History* Supplement, no. 8 (1988): 46–62.

———. *Hospital Life in Enlightenment Scotland: Care and Teaching at the Royal Infirmary of Edinburgh*. Cambridge: Cambridge University Press, 1986.

Ritch, Alistair E. S. "English Poor Law Institutional Care for Older People: Identifying the 'Aged and Infirm' and the 'Sick' in Birmingham Workhouse, 1852–1912." *Social History of Medicine* 27, no. 1 (2014): 64–85.

———. "History of Geriatric Medicine: From Hippocrates to Marjory Warren." *Journal of the Royal College of Physicians of Edinburgh* 42, no. 4 (2012): 368–74.

———. "Medical Care in the Workhouses in Birmingham and Wolverhampton, 1834–1914." PhD diss., University of Birmingham, 2015.

———. "New Poor Law Medical Care in the Local Health Economy." *Local Population Studies* 99 (2017): 42–55.

———. "'Sick, Aged and Infirm' Adults in the New Birmingham Workhouse, 1852–1912." MPhil diss., University of Birmingham, 2010.

Rogers, Joseph. "The Alleged Punishment of Sick Paupers." *British Medical Journal* 1 (1882): 33.

Rogers, Thorold, ed. *Joseph Rogers, M.D. Reminiscences of a Workhouse Medical Officer*. London: T. Fisher Unwin, 1889.

Rosen, George. *A History of Public Health*. New York: MD Publications, 1958.

Rosenberg, Charles E. "The Therapeutic Revolution: Medicine, Meaning, and Social Change in Nineteenth-Century America." *Perspectives in Biology and Medicine* 26 (Summer 1977): 485–506.

Rosner, Lisa. "The Professional Context of Electrotherapeutics." *Journal of the History of Medicine and Allied Sciences* 43, no. 1 (1988): 64–82.

Rothery, Karen. "'Who Do They Think They Are?' An Analysis of the Boards of Guardians in Hertfordshire." *Local Population Studies* 99 (2017): 20–30.

Scott, D. F. *The History of Epileptic Therapy*. Carnforth, UK: Parthenon Publishing Group, 1993.

Scull, Andrew. *The Most Solitary of Afflictions: Madness and Society in Britain 1700–1900*. London: Yale University Press, 1993.

———. "The Social History of Psychiatry in the Victorian Era." In *Madhouses, Mad-Doctors, and Madmen: The Social History of Psychiatry in the Victorian Era*, edited by Andrew Scull, 1–4. London: Athlone Press, 1981.

Shave, Samantha. "'Immediate Death or a Life of Torture Are the Consequences of the System': The Bridgewater Union Scandal and Policy Change." In *Medicine and the Workhouse*, edited by Jonathan Reinarz and Leonard Schwarz, 164–91. Rochester, NY: University of Rochester Press, 2013.

————. *Pauper Policies: Poor Law Practice in England, 1780–1850*. Manchester, UK: Manchester University Press, 2017.

Sheard, Sally. "Reluctant Providers? The Politics and Ideology of Municipal Hospital Finance 1870–1914." In *Financing Medicine: The British Experience Since 1750*, edited by Martin Gorsky and Sally Sheard, 112–29. London: Routledge, 2006.

Sheen, Alfred. *The Workhouse and Its Medical Officer*. Bristol, UK: John Wright & Co., 1890.

Siena, Kevin. "Contagion, Exclusion and the Unique Medical World of the Eighteenth-Century Workhouse." In *Medicine and the Workhouse*, edited by Jonathan Reinarz and Leonard Schwarz, 19–39. Rochester, NY: University of Rochester Press, 2013.

————. "The Moral Biology of 'The Itch' in Eighteenth-Century Britain." In *A Medical History of Skin: Scratching the Surface*, edited by Jonathan Reinarz and Kevin Siena, 71–84. London: Pickering & Chatto, 2013.

Siena, Kevin P. *Venereal Disease, Hospitals and the Urban Poor: London's "Foul Wards," 1600–1800*. Rochester, NY: University of Rochester Press, 2004.

Smith, F. B. *The People's Health 1830–1910*. London: Croom Helm, 1979.

————. *The Retreat of Tuberculosis*. London: Croom Helm, 1998.

Smith, John B. "The Governance of Wolverhampton, 1848–1888." PhD diss., University of Leicester, 2001.

Smith, Leonard. "Behind Closed Doors: Lunatic Asylum Keepers, 1800–60." *Social History of Medicine* 1, no. 3 (1988): 302–27.

————. *"Cure, Comfort and Safe Custody": Public Lunatic Asylums in Early Nineteenth Century England*. London: Leicester University Press, 1999.

————. "The Pauper Lunatic Problem in the West Midlands, 1815–1850." *Midland History* 21, no. 2 (1996): 106.

————. "'A Sad Spectacle of Hopeless Mental Degradation': The Management of the Insane in West Midlands Workhouses, 1815." In *Medicine and the Workhouse*, edited by Jonathan Reinarz and Leonard Schwarz, 103–20. Rochester, NY: University of Rochester Press, 2013.

Sneyder, Sharon, and David Mitchell. "Afterword–Regulated Bodies: Disabled Studies and the Controlling Profession." In *Social Histories of Disability and Deformity*, edited by David M. Turner and Kevin Stagg, 179–85. London: Routledge, 2006.

Sournia, Jean-Charles. *A History of Alcoholism*. Oxford: Basil Blackwell, 1990.

Stanley, Peter. *For Fear of Pain: British Surgery, 1790–1850*. Amsterdam: Rodopi, 2003.

Stewart, John, and Steven King. "Death in Llantrisant: Henry Williams and the New Poor Law in Wales." *Rural History* 15, no. 1 (2004): 69–87.

Stone, Deborah A. *The Disabled State*. Philadelphia, PA: Temple University Press, 1984.

Suckling, C. W. "Lobar Pneumonia." *The Lancet* 2 (1884): 407.

———. "Pure Terebene in the Treatment of Winter-Cough." *British Medical Journal* 1 (1886): 541.

Szreter, Simon. "The Importance of Social Intervention in Britain's Mortality Decline c.1850–1914." *Social History of Medicine* 1, no. 1 (1988): 1–37.

Thomas, Eric G. "The Old Poor Law and Medicine." *Medical History* 24, no. 1 (1980): 1–19.

Tildesley, J. E. "Wolverhampton Trades: Addenda." In *Birmingham and the Midland Hardware District*, edited by Samuel Timmins, 121–24. London: Frank Cass & Co. Ltd., 1967.

Tildesley Norman A. *A History of Willenhall*. Willenhall, UK: Willenhall Urban District Council, 1952.

Timmerman, Carsten. "Chronic Illness and Disease History." In *Oxford Handbook of the History of Medicine*, edited by Mark Jackson, 393–410. Oxford: Oxford University Press, 2011.

Timmins, Samuel. "The Industrial History of Birmingham." In *Birmingham and the Midland Hardware District*, edited by Samuel Timmins, 207–24. London: Frank Cass & Co. Ltd., 1967.

Tolley, Paul L. "The Birmingham, Aston and Kings Norton Boards of Guardians, and the Politics and Administration of the Poor Law, circa 1836–1912." PhD diss., De Montfort University, 1994.

Tomkins, Alannah. "The Excellent Example of the Working Class: Medical Welfare, Contributory Funding and the North Staffordshire Infirmary from 1815." *Social History of Medicine* 21, no. 1 (2008): 13–30.

———. "'Labouring on a Bed of Sickness': The Material and Rhetorical Deployment of Ill-health in Male Pauper Letters." In *Poverty and Sickness in Modern Europe*, edited by Andreas Gestrich, Elizabeth Hurren, and Steven King, 51–68. London: Ashgate, 2012.

Tröhler, Ulrich. "Surgery (Modern)." In *Companion Encyclopaedia of the History of Medicine*, edited by W. F. Bynum and Roy Porter, 984–1028. London: Routledge, 1993.

Turner, David M. "Introduction." In *Social Histories of Disability and Deformity*, edited by David M. Turner and Kevin Stagg, 1–9. London: Routledge, 2006.

Upton, Chris. *The Birmingham Parish Workhouse, 1730–1840*. Hatfield, UK: University of Hertfordshire Press, 2019.

———. *A History of Birmingham*. Chichester, UK: Phillimore, 1984.

———. *A History of Wolverhampton*. Chichester, UK: Phillimore, 1998.

Vernon, James. *Distant Strangers: How Britain Became Modern*. Berkeley: University of California Press, 2014.

Versluysen, M. C. "Old Wives' Tales? Women Healers in English History." In *Rewriting Nursing History*, edited by Celia Davies, 175–99. London: Croom Helm, 1980.

Walton, John. "The Treatment of Pauper Lunatics in Victorian England." In *Madhouses, Mad-Doctors, and Madmen: The Social History of Psychiatry in the Victorian Era*, edited by Andrew Scull, 166–90. London: Athlone Press, 1981.

Ward, Roger. "Birmingham: A Political Profile, 1700–1940." In *Birmingham: The Workshop of the World*, edited by Carl Chinn and Malcolm Dick, 159–91. Liverpool, UK: Liverpool University Press, 2016.

Warner, John H. "Physiological Theory and Therapeutic Explanation in the 1860s: The British Debate on the Medical Use of Alcohol." *Bulletin of the History of Medicine* 54, no. 2 (1980): 235–57.

———. "Therapeutic Explanation and the Edinburgh Bloodletting Controversy: Two Perspectives on the Medical Meaning of Science in the Mid-Nineteenth Century." *Medical History* 24, no. 3 (1980): 241–58.

———. *The Therapeutic Perspective: Medical Practice, Knowledge, and Identity in America, 1820–1885.* Cambridge, MA: Harvard University Press, 1986.

Webb, Sidney and Beatrice. *The State and the Doctor.* London: Longmans, Green and Co., 1910.

Weisz, George. *Chronic Disease in the Twentieth Century: A History.* Baltimore, MD: Johns Hopkins Press, 2014.

White, Rosemary. *Social Change and the Development of the Nursing Profession: A Study of the Poor Law Nursing Service 1848–1948.* London: Henry Kimpton Publishers, 1978.

Whorton, James C. *The Arsenical Century.* Oxford: Oxford University Press, 2010.

Wildman, Stuart. "Changes in Hospital Nursing in the West Midlands, 1841–1901." In *Medicine and Society in the Midlands 1750–1950*, edited by Jonathan Reinarz, 98–114. Birmingham, UK: Midland History, 2007.

———. "The Development of Nursing at the General Hospital, Birmingham, 1779–1919." *International History of Nursing Journal* 4, no. 3 (1999): 20–28.

———. "'Docile Bodies' or 'Impudent' Women: Conflicts between Nurses and Their Employers, in England, 1880–1914." In *Medizin, Gesellschaft und Geschichte*, edited by Robert Jutte, 9–20. Stuttgart, Germany: Franz Steiner Verlag, 2014.

———. "*He's Only a Pauper Whom Nobody Owns": Caring for the Sick in the Warwickshire Poor Law Unions, 1934–1914.* Stratford-upon-Avon, UK: Dugdale Society, 2016,

Wilks, Samuel. "Clinical Lecture on the Indiscriminate Use of Alcoholic Stimulants in Disease." *The Lancet* 1 (1867): 505–7.

Williams, Karel. *From Pauperism to Poverty.* London: Routledge and Kegan Paul, 1981.

Williams, Sarah E. "The Use of Beverage Alcohol as Medicine, 1790–1860." *Journal of Studies in Alcohol* 41, no. 5 (1980): 543–66.

Wilson, Leonard G. "The Historical Decline of Tuberculosis in Europe and America: Its Causes and Significance." *Journal of the History of Medicine and Allied Sciences* 45, no. 3 (1990): 366–96.

Wohl, Anthony S. *Endangered Lives, Public Health in Victorian Britain.* London: J. M. Dent & Sons Ltd., 1983.

Woods, Robert. "Mortality and Sanitary Conditions in Late Nineteenth-Century Birmingham." In *Urban Disease and Mortality in Nineteenth-Century England,* edited by Robert Woods and John Woodward, 176–202. London: Batsford Academic and Educational, 1984.

Woods, Robert, and John Woodward. "Mortality, Poverty and the Environment." In *Urban Disease and Mortality in Nineteenth-Century England,* edited by Robert Woods and John Woodward, 19–36. London: Batsford Academic and Educational, 1984.

Woodward, John. *To Do the Sick No Harm: A Study of the British Voluntary Hospital System to 1875.* London: Routledge and Kegan Paul, 1974.

———. "Medicine and the City: The Nineteenth Century Experience." In *Urban Disease and Mortality in Nineteenth-Century England,* edited by Robert Woods and John Woodward, 65–78. London: Routledge and Kegan Paul, 1984.

Worboys, Michael. "Before McKeown: Explaining the Decline of Tuberculosis in Britain, 1880–1930." In *Tuberculosis Then and Now,* edited by Flurin Condrau and Michael Worboys, 148–70. Montreal, QC: McGill-Queen's University Press, 2010.

———. "The Sanatorium Treatment for Consumption in Britain, 1890–1914." In *Medical Innovations in Historical Perspective,* edited by John V. Pickstone, 47–71. New York: Palgrave MacMillan, 1991.

———. *Spreading Germs, Disease Theories and Medical Practice in Britain, 1865–1900.* Cambridge: Cambridge University Press, 2000.

Wright, J. S. "The Jewellery and Gilt Toy Trades." In *Birmingham and the Midland Hardware District,* edited by Samuel Timmins, 452–62. London: Frank Cass & Co. Ltd., 1967.

Wyke, T. J. "Hospital Facilities for, and Diagnosis and Treatment of, Venereal Disease in England, 1800–1870." *British Journal of Venereal Diseases* 49, no. 1 (1973): 78–85.

Youngson, A. J. *The Scientific Revolution in Victorian Medicine.* London: Croom Helm, 1979.

Index

Printed in the United States
By Bookmasters